# Antimicrobial Chemotherapy

# Antimicrobial Chemotherapy

## SEVENTH EDITION

### Professor Peter Davey
Lead for Clinical Quality Improvement
Medical Education Institute
University of Dundee

### Professor Mark Wilcox
Consultant / Head of Microbiology
Leeds Teaching Hospitals NHS Trust
Professor of Medical Microbiology & Sir Edward Brotherton Chair of Bacteriology
University of Leeds
Lead on *C. difficile* infection
Public Health England

### Professor William Irving
Professor and Honorary Consultant in Virology
University of Nottingham and Nottingham University Hospitals NHS Trust

### Professor Guy Thwaites
Director of the Oxford University Clinical Research Unit
and the Wellcome Trust Major Overseas Research Programme, Viet Nam
Senior Research Fellow
Nuffield Department of Medicine
University of Oxford
Honorary Consultant in Infectious Diseases and Clinical Microbiology
Guy's and St Thomas' NHS Foundation, London

## OXFORD
### UNIVERSITY PRESS

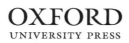
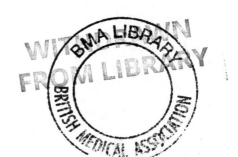

# OXFORD
UNIVERSITY PRESS

Great Clarendon Street, Oxford, OX2 6DP,
United Kingdom

Oxford University Press is a department of the University of Oxford.
It furthers the University's objective of excellence in research, scholarship,
and education by publishing worldwide. Oxford is a registered trade mark of
Oxford University Press in the UK and in certain other countries

First Edition published by Ballière Tindall in 1983
Second Edition published in 1989
Third Edition published in 1995
Fourth Edition published in 2000
Reprinted in 2001, 2003 (twice), 2004, 2005
Fifth Edition published in 2007
Sixth Edition published in 2012
Seventh Edition published in 2015

Impression: 1

Published in the United States of America by Oxford University Press
198 Madison Avenue, New York, NY 10016, United States of America

British Library Cataloguing in Publication Data
Data available

Library of Congress Control Number: 2014958214

ISBN 978–0–19–968977–4

Printed in Great Britain by
Clays Ltd, St Ives plc

# Preface

Almost everyone in the developed world will receive several antibiotic courses during their lifetime. It is therefore not surprising that most clinicians and dentists will prescribe these drugs on a regular basis throughout their professional career. Indeed, several antibiotics figure among the most frequent of all prescribed drugs.

Antibiotics are not only life-saving with regard to severe infections, such as pneumonia, meningitis, and endocarditis, but are also responsible for controlling much of the morbidity associated with non-life-threatening infectious disease; illness is abbreviated, return to normal activities is hastened, risk of infection transmission may be reduced and there is often economic benefit to the individual, as well as society, by reducing the number of working days lost. In addition, infectious complications of many commonly conducted surgical procedures are now preventable by the use of peri-operative antibiotic prophylaxis. Likewise procedures such as bone marrow and organ transplantation are also possible because of the effective control of complicating infections. These benefits are well known to healthcare professionals and to the public who no longer fear infection in the way earlier generations did. The very success of antimicrobial chemotherapy has led to a perception that such agents are generally safe and that industry will continue to generate new agents to ensure the effective control of most infectious problems.

Antibiotics have largely been derived from natural sources, mainly from environmental bacteria and fungi. Their use in clinical medicine has been one of the major successes of the past century. The term 'antibiotic' was coined by Selman A Waksman, who recognized that these 'naturally derived substances were antagonistic to the growth of other micro-organisms in high dilution.' Over the years, other agents have been developed by chemical synthesis. More recently much effort has been applied to identifying genomic research based products. The term 'antimicrobial agents' captures all such compounds which in turn have been subdivided into antibacterial, antifungal, antiparasitic (anthelminthic and antiprotozoal) and antiviral agents according to the target pathogen. However, this purist approach is often ignored in practice and the term antibiotic is somewhat loosely applied to all these agents. The reader will find all such terms in use in this book.

Antibiotics are unique among therapeutic agents in that they target invading micro-organisms rather than any pathological process arising from host cells or tissues. Furthermore, unlike other classes of drug, micro-organisms have the inherent or acquired ability to evade or inactivate antimicrobial activity of these drugs. Such resistance presents a major threat to sustaining effective treatment and prevention of infectious disease. In addition, there is increasing recognition of the importance of the normal bacterial flora of the human body and of the consequences of collateral damage from the use of antibacterials, such as the risk of *Clostridium difficile* infection.

Indeed, controlling antibiotic resistance is one of the greatest challenges facing healthcare professionals and the public and is likely to remain so. While new drugs, vaccines and better diagnostic methods are still a requirement, the fundamental issue is to ensure that existing agents are used effectively. This can only be achieved by ensuring those doctors, dentists, and, increasingly, other healthcare professionals who use these agents in the care of their patients, pursue good prescribing practice.

Good prescribing practice is the product of sound education, with particular emphasis on the acquisition of appropriate knowledge, skills, and professional behaviour. Good science informs good practice and since the knowledge base for prescribing practice is continuously expanding, the need for life-long learning is self-evident.

Patient safety remains paramount in medicine. This is of particular importance since antibiotics are often used in the management of mild to moderate community infections and the prophylaxis of infections. The safety of antibiotics is monitored closely during drug development, at licensing and in clinical use. Since no drug is free from side effects, it is essential that the balance of risks and benefits of prescribing is understood by the prescribing practitioner. With more than 100 antimicrobial compounds currently available in the UK, this remains a particular challenge.

Setting forth the principles of rational antimicrobial chemotherapy is the whole purpose of this book. In revisiting the contents, we welcome Dr Guy Thwaites among the editors. All chapters have been revised, several rewritten and a new chapter introduced on Antimicrobial Stewardship, Surveillance of Antimicrobial Consumption and Its Consequences to reflect the changes that have taken place in guiding prescribing practices.

However, the basic plan of the book remains unchanged and much of the material provided by former authors has been retained attesting to its durability. As such, it reflects the vision of Professor David Greenwood, who was the inspiration for this book and Professor Roger Finch, who guided the first six editions so successfully.

We sincerely hope that this 7th edition of *Antimicrobial Chemotherapy* will continue to furnish students and all healthcare professionals throughout the world with the necessary framework for understanding what antimicrobial agents will and will not do, and provide a firm basis for their informed use in the treatment and control of infection.

March 2015
P.D.
M.W.
W.I.
G.T.

# Contents

# List of abbreviations

| | | | | |
|---|---|---|---|---|
| 5FC | flucytosine | EMA | European Medicines Agency |
| AASLD | American Association for the Study of Liver Disease | EoT | end of treatment |
| | | EoTR | end of treatment response |
| ACT | artemisinin combination treatment | ESAC | European Surveillance of Antibiotic Consumption |
| ADR | adverse drug reaction | | |
| AIDS | acquired immune deficiency syndrome | ESBL | extended spectrum β-lactamases |
| ALT, | alanine aminotransferase | EVR | early virological response |
| ASA | American Society of Anesthesiologists | FDA | Food and Drug Administration |
| ATC | anatomical therapeutic chemical | G6PD | glucose-6-phosphate dehydrogenase |
| AZT | azidothymidine (Zidovudine) | | |
| BAN | British Approved Name | GABA | gamma-amino butyric acid |
| BARDA | Biomedical Advanced Research and Development Authority | GAIN | Generating Antibiotic Incentives Now |
| BNF | *British National Formulary* | GRE | glycopeptide-resistant enterococci |
| BNFC | children's version of the *British National Formulary* | HAART | highly active antiretroviral therapy |
| cART | combination antiretroviral therapy | HBsAg | hepatitis B surface antigen |
| CDC | Centers for Disease Control | HBV | hepatitis B virus |
| CDI | *Clostridium difficile* infection | HCV | hepatitis C virus |
| cEVR | complete early virological response | HHV-6 | human herpesvirus 6 |
| CMV | cytomegalovirus | HIV | human immunodeficiency virus |
| COPD | chronic obstructive pulmonary disease | HLA | human leukocyte antigen |
| CRB | carbapenem-resistant bacteria | HPV | human papillomavirus |
| CRP | C-reactive protein | HSE | herpes simplex virus encephalitis |
| CSF | cerebrospinal fluid | IDU | idoxuridine |
| CSM | Committee on Safety of Medicines | IE | infective endocarditis |
| DAA | directly acting antivirals | IFN | interferon |
| DDD | defined daily dose | IGRA | interferon-γ release assay |
| DEET | diethyltoluamide | IL | interleukin |
| DHPG | dihydroxypropoxymethylguanine | IL-28B | interleukin-28B |
| DNA | pol DNA polymerase | IMI | Innovative Medicines Initiative |
| DRM | drug resistance mutation | INN | International Non-Proprietary Name (specified)IRES internal ribosomal entry site |
| EASL | European Association for the Study of the Liver | | |
| EBV | Epstein–Barr virus | IRIS | immune reconstitution inflammatory syndrome |
| ECDC | European Centre for Disease Prevention and Control | | |
| | | IV | intravenous |
| EDTA | ethylenediaminetetraacetic acid | IVOST | intravenous to oral switch therapy |
| eGFR | estimated glomerular filtration rate | LRTI | lower respiratory tract infections |
| EIA | enzyme immunoassay | LVM | lamivudine |

| | | | |
|---|---|---|---|
| MALDI-TOF | matrix-assisted laser desorption/ionization time of flight | pEVR | partial early virological response |
| MDR-TB | multidrug-resistant tuberculosis | PJI | prosthetic joint infection |
| MERS-CoV | Middle East respiratory syndrome coronavirus | PI | protease inhibitor |
| | | PICC | peripherally inserted central catheters |
| MIC | minimum inhibitory concentration | PPD | purified protein derivative |
| MHRA | Medicines and Healthcare Products Regulatory Agency | PVL | Panton–Vallentine leukocidin (toxin) |
| MIR | magnetic resonance imaging | QIDP | qualified infectious disease product |
| miR-122 | microRNA-122 | rINN | recommended International Non-Proprietary Name |
| MMR | measles, mumps, and rubella (vaccination) | RR | relapser-responder |
| mRNA | messenger RNA | rRNA | ribosomal RNA |
| MRSA | methicillin-resistant *Staphylococcus aureus* | RSV | respiratory syncytial virus |
| | | RT | reverse transcriptase |
| MSM | men who have sex with men | RTI | reverse transcriptase inhibitors |
| MSQ | mental state questionnaire | RV | ribavirin |
| NA | neuraminidase | RVR | rapid virological response |
| NANBH | non-A non-B hepatitis | SAB | *Staphylococcus aureus* bacteraemia |
| NCR | non-coding region | SARS-CoV | severe acute respiratory syndrome |
| NICE | National Institute for Health and Clinical Excellence | ScRAP | Scottish Reduction in Antimicrobial Prescribing |
| NNIS | National Nosocomial Infections Surveillance | SIRS | systemic inflammatory response syndrome |
| NNRTI | non-nucleoside analogue reverse transcriptase inhibitor | SNP | single nucleotide polymorphism |
| | | SVR | sustained virological response |
| NR | non-response | SVR12 | sustained virological response determined at 12 weeks after the end of treatment |
| NRTI | nucleos(t)ide analogue reverse transcriptase inhibitor | | |
| NSAID | non-steroidal anti-inflammatory drug | SVR24 | sustained virological response determined at 24 weeks after the end of treatment |
| OPAT | outpatient parenteral antimicrobial therapy | | |
| | | TB | tuberculosis |
| ORF | open reading frame | TESSy | The European Surveillance System |
| ORION | *Outbreak Reports and Intervention studies Of Nosocomial* (infection) | TK | thymidine kinase |
| | | USAN | United States Adopted NameVRE vancomycin-resistant enterococcal |
| PAS | *para*-aminosalicylic acid | | |
| PBP | penicillin-binding protein | VZV | varicella-zoster virus |
| PCR | polymerase chain reaction | WHO | World Health Organization |
| PEG | pegylated interferon | XDR | extensively drug resistant |
| PEP | post-exposure prophylaxis | XDR-TB | extensively drug-resistant tuberculosis |

# 1

# General properties of antimicrobial agents

# Chapter 1

# Mechanisms of action and resistance to modern antibacterials, with a history of their development

## Introduction to mechanisms

The 'antibiotic revolution' began in the early 1940s when Howard Florey and his colleagues in Oxford developed Alexander Fleming's penicillin into a major therapeutic compound and Selman Waksman in the United States began his systematic pursuit of antibiotics from soil microorganisms. In the twenty-first century we have a huge range of antimicrobial drugs in our therapeutic armoury. At the same time we face increasing problems with antimicrobial resistance and emergence of bacteria that are resistant to all available antibacterial drugs. Antibacterial drugs have a wide range of mechanisms of action, inhibiting a number of key functions within those organisms (Table 1.1). However, through a variety of mechanisms, bacteria have also evolved an equally impressive array of mechanisms for resistance to antibacterial drugs (Fig. 1.1). In subsequent chapters of this book, the mechanisms of action and development of resistance to antimicrobial drugs will be discussed in detail. However, for those who are interested, here is a brief history of antimicrobial development.

## Mechanisms of selective action on bacterial versus mammalian cells

Unlike mammalian cells bacteria have a cell wall, and disruption of cell wall synthesis is the target site for the β-lactam antibiotics (penicillins, cephalosporins, carbapenems, monobactams) and for glycopeptides (vancomycin, teicoplanin).

Most other antibacterials are metabolic inhibitors of targets that are present in mammalian cells but the drugs are either selective for bacterial enzymes or are not transported into mammalian cells (Table 1.1).

## Mechanisms of resistance

The effectiveness of antibacterials is dependent on two main factors: first, the amount that reaches the target site and, second, the affinity of the antibacterial for the target site.

Most resistance to antibacterials occurs either because the drug is prevented from reaching the target site in sufficient quantity to inhibit growth, or the drug is prevented from working at the target site. Resistance is either intrinsic (preceded the use of antibacterials in animals or humans) or has been acquired through mutation or transfer of resistance determinants (see Chapter 11; Fig. 1.1).

**Table 1.1** Bacterial targets for common antibacterial drugs and the mechanism for their selective action on bacterial versus mammalian cells.

| Bacterial target | Antibacterial class | Representatives | Selective action |
|---|---|---|---|
| Cell wall synthesis | β-Lactams | Penicillins | Mammalian cells do not have a cell wall. In bacteria, disruption of their rigid cell wall is lethal. |
| | | Cephalosporins | |
| | | Carbapenems | |
| | | Monobactams | |
| | Glycopeptides | Vancomycin | |
| | | Teicoplanin | |
| Tetrahydrofolate synthesis | Sulphonamides | Sulphamethoxazole | Sulphonamides act on dihydrofolate synthetase, which is not present in mammalian cells. |
| | Diaminopyrimidines | Trimethoprim | Trimethoprim is a selective inhibitor of bacterial dihydrofolate reductase and does not significantly inhibit the bacterial enzyme. |
| DNA synthesis | Quinolones | Ciprofloxacin | Selective inhibition of bacterial DNA gyrase, which prevents DNA supercoiling, and bacterial topoisomerase, which prevents the separation of DNA strands. |
| | | Levofloxacin | |
| | Nitroimidazoles | Metronidazole | Metronidazole does interact with mammalian DNA but can only be transported into anaerobic bacteria; therefore, its activity is restricted to these bacteria. |
| RNA synthesis | Rifamycins | Rifampicin | Selective inhibition of bacterial DNA-dependent RNA polymerase. |
| Protein synthesis | Aminoglycosides | Gentamicin | Selective interaction with bacterial ribosomes, do not interact with mammalian ribosomes. |
| | | Amikacin | |
| | Macrolides and related compounds | Erythromycin | |
| | | Clarithromycin | |
| | | Clindamycin (a lincosamide) | |
| | Tetracyclines and related compounds | Doxycycline | These drugs do inhibit mammalian ribosomes but are poorly transported into mammalian cells. However, some glycines that have been synthesized are too toxic for clinical use. |
| | | Tigecycline (a glycine) | |
| | Oxazolidinones | Linezolid | Selective interaction with bacterial ribosomes; however, linezolid is only relatively selective, and long-term use is associated with bone marrow dyscrasia. |
| Permeability | Lipopeptides | Daptomycin | Selective depolarization of bacterial cell membranes, causing potassium efflux and prevention of synthesis of essential macromolecules. |

Source: data from Sebastian G. B. Ames, *Antimicrobial Chemotherapy*, Oxford Infections Disease Library, Oxford University Press, Oxford, UK, Copyright © Oxford University Press 2010.

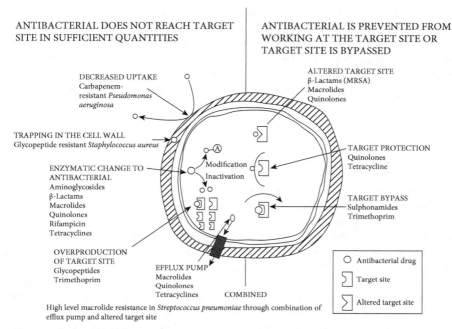

ANTIBACTERIAL DOES NOT REACH TARGET
SITE IN SUFFICIENT QUANTITIES

ANTIBACTERIAL IS PREVENTED FROM
WORKING AT THE TARGET SITE OR
TARGET SITE IS BYPASSED

DECREASED UPTAKE
Carbapenem-
resistant *Pseudomonas
aeruginosa*

ALTERED TARGET SITE
β-Lactams (MRSA)
Macrolides
Quinolones

TRAPPING IN THE CELL WALL
Glycopeptide resistant *Staphylococcus aureus*

ENZYMATIC CHANGE TO
ANTIBACTERIAL
Aminoglycosides
β-Lactams
Macrolides
Quinolones
Rifampicin
Tetracyclines

Modification
Inactivation

TARGET PROTECTION
Quinolones
Tetracycline

TARGET BYPASS
Sulphonamides
Trimethoprim

OVERPRODUCTION
OF TARGET SITE
Glycopeptides
Trimethoprim

EFFLUX PUMP
Macrolides
Quinolones
Tetracyclines     COMBINED

○  Antibacterial drug

⊃  Target site

⊃  Altered target site

High level macrolide resistance in *Streptococcus pneumoniae* through combination of
efflux pump and altered target site

**Fig. 1.1** Mechanisms of resistance to common antibacterials.

## The foundations of modern chemotherapy

Oddly, in view of later developments, the foundations of twentieth-century chemotherapy were built on a search for antiprotozoal agents, as it was to the newly discovered parasites of malaria and African sleeping sickness (trypanosomiasis) that Paul Ehrlich first turned his attention. He reasoned that, since these parasites could be differentiated from the tissues of infected patients by various dyes in the laboratory, such substances might display a preferential affinity for the parasites in the body as well. In a phrase, such dyes might exhibit *selective toxicity*.

Progress with development of antimicrobials from dyes was slow until the discovery of the first broad-spectrum antibacterial agents, the sulphonamides. This discovery came about by another of those happy accidents with which the history of chemotherapy is littered. In 1932 Gerhard Domagk, an experimental pathologist working in the laboratories of the Bayer wing of the IG Farbenindustrie consortium, tested a number of dyes synthesized by his colleagues, Fritz Mietzsch and Josef Klarer. In one such compound, Prontosil red, a sulphonamide group had been linked to a red dye in the hope of improving the binding to bacterial cells, as it was known that this modification improved binding of the dye to fibres. Remarkably, mice treated with Prontosil red survived an otherwise fatal infection with haemolytic streptococci; however, when the compound was tested against streptococci in vitro, it was found to have no antibacterial activity whatsoever. This paradox was explained by the Tréfouëls and their colleagues in France when they showed that, in the experimental animal, sulphanilamide was liberated from the dye. It was this colourless compound—hitherto unsuspected of possessing any antimicrobial activity—that was responsible for the astonishing properties of Prontosil.

As a chemical, sulphanilamide had been synthesized and described as early as 1908, and Bayer were unable to protect the discovery by patent. Naturally, many other firms seized the opportunity to market the drug; thus, by 1940, sulphanilamide itself was available under many different trade names, and a start had been made on producing the numerous sulphonamide derivatives that subsequently appeared. One proprietary version marketed in the United States, 'Elixir Sulfanilamide', was formulated in diethylene glycol and killed over 100 people. This event led to a law giving the Food and Drug Administration power to regulate the licensing of new drugs in the United States. Such was the situation when penicillin appeared on the scene as a potential therapeutic agent in 1940.

## Antibiotics

### Penicillin

When Howard Florey and his team at the Sir William Dunn School of Pathology in Oxford first took an interest in penicillin in the mid-1930s, the concept of antibiosis and its therapeutic potential was not new. In fact, moulds had been used empirically in folk remedies for infected wounds for centuries, and the observation that organisms, including fungi, sometimes produced substances capable of preventing the growth of others was as old as bacteriology itself. One antibiotic substance, pyocyanase, produced by the bacterium *Pseudomonas aeruginosa*, had actually been used therapeutically at the turn of the twentieth century by instillation into wounds.

Thus, when Alexander Fleming interrupted a holiday to visit his laboratory in St Mary's Hospital in early September 1928 to make his famous observation on a contaminated culture plate of staphylococci, he was merely one in a long line of workers who had noticed similar phenomena. However, it was Fleming's observation that sparked off the events that led to the development of penicillin as the first antibiotic in the strict sense of the term.

The actual circumstances of Fleming's discovery have become interwoven with myth and legend. Attempts to reproduce the phenomenon have led to the conclusion that the lysis of staphylococci in the area surrounding a contaminant *Penicillium* colony on Fleming's original plate could have arisen only by an extraordinary concatenation of accidental events, including the vagaries of temperature of an English summer.

Early attempts to exploit penicillin foundered, partly through a failure to purify and concentrate the substance. Fleming made some attempts to use crude filtrates in superficial infections and there is documentary evidence that, in Sheffield, Cecil George Paine, a former student of Fleming, successfully treated gonococcal ophthalmia with filtrates of *Penicillium* cultures as early as 1930. However, it was left to Ernst Chain, a German refugee who had been recommended to Florey as a biochemist, to obtain a stable extract of penicillin. Chain had been set the task of investigating naturally occurring antibacterial substances (including lysozyme, another of Fleming's discoveries) as a biochemical exercise. It was with his crude extracts that the first experiments were performed in mice and men. Since these extracts contained less than 1 per cent pure penicillin, it is fortunate that problems of serious toxicity were not encountered.

Further development of penicillin was beyond the means of wartime Britain, and Florey visited the United States in 1941 with his assistant, Norman Heatley, to enlist the support of the American authorities and drug firms. Once Florey had convinced them of the potential of penicillin, progress was rapid and, by the end of the Second World War, bulk production of penicillin was in progress, and the drug was beginning to become readily available.

### Cephalosporins

The discovery of the cephalosporins (which are structurally related to the penicillins) is equally extraordinary. Between 1945 and 1948, Giuseppe Brotzu, former rector of the University of

Cagliari, Sardinia, investigated the microbial flora of a sewage outflow in the hope of discovering naturally occurring antibiotic substances. One of the organisms recovered from the sewage was a *Cephalosporium* mould that displayed striking inhibitory activity against several bacterial species—including *Salmonella typhi*, the cause of typhoid and now considered a serotype of *Sal. enterica*—that were beyond the reach of penicillin at that time. Brotzu carried out some preliminary bacteriological and clinical studies and published some encouraging results in a local house journal. However, he lacked the facilities to develop the compound further, and nothing more might have been heard of the work if he had not sent a reprint of his paper to a British acquaintance, Dr Blyth Brooke, who drew it to the attention of the Medical Research Council in London. They advised contacting Howard Florey, and Brotzu sent the mould to the Sir William Dunn School in 1948.

The first thing to be discovered by the Oxford scientists was that the mould produced two antibiotics, which they called cephalosporin P and cephalosporin N, because the former inhibited Gram-positive organisms (e.g. staphylococci and streptococci) whereas the latter was active against Gram-negative organisms (e.g. *Escherichia coli* and *Sal. typhi*). Neither of these substances is a cephalosporin in the sense that the term is used today: cephalosporin P proved to be an antibiotic with a steroid-like structure, and cephalosporin N turned out to be a penicillin (adicillin). The forerunner of the cephalosporins now in use, cephalosporin C, was detected later as a minor component on fractionation of cephalosporin N. Such a substance could easily have been dismissed but it was pursued because it exhibited some attractive properties, notably, stability to the enzymes produced by some staphylococcal strains that were by then threatening the effectiveness of penicillin.

## Antibiotics from soil

The development of penicillin, cephalosporin C, and, subsequently, their numerous derivatives represents only one branch of the antibiotic story. The other main route came through an investigation into antimicrobial substances produced by microorganisms in soil. The chief moving spirit was Selman A. Waksman, an émigré from the Ukraine, who had taken up the study of soil microbiology in the United States as a young man. In 1940 Waksman initiated a systematic search for non-toxic antibiotics produced by soil microorganisms, notably actinomycetes, a group that includes the *Streptomyces* species that were to yield many therapeutically useful compounds. Waksman was probably influenced in his decision to undertake this study by the first reports of penicillin and by the discovery by an ex-pupil, René Dubos, of the antibiotic complex tyrothricin in culture filtrates of *Bacillus brevis*.

Waksman's first discoveries were, like Dubos's tyrothricin, too toxic for systemic use, although they included actinomycin, a compound later used in cancer chemotherapy. The real breakthrough came in 1943 with the discovery by Waksman's research student, Albert Schatz, of streptomycin, the first aminoglycoside antibiotic, which was found to have a spectrum of activity that neatly complemented penicillin by inhibiting many Gram-negative bacilli and—very importantly at that time—*Mycobacterium tuberculosis*. It remained the staple treatment for tuberculosis (together with some synthetic compounds; see 'Non-antibiotic antibacterial compounds') until the antibiotic rifampicin—named after the 1955 French gangster film *Rififi*—was introduced in 1968.

The success of streptomycin stimulated the pharmaceutical houses to join the chase in the years following the end of the Second World War. Soil samples by the hundreds of thousands from all over the world were screened for antibiotic-producing microorganisms. Thousands of antibiotic substances were discovered and rediscovered and, although most failed preliminary toxicity tests, by the mid-1950s representatives of most of the major families of antibiotics, including aminoglycosides, chloramphenicol, tetracyclines, and macrolides, had been found.

Since 1960 few truly novel antibiotics have been discovered, although a surprising number of naturally occurring molecular variations on the penicillin structure have emerged. A more fruitful approach, especially with penicillins and cephalosporins, has been to modify existing agents chemically in order to derive semi-synthetic compounds with improved properties.

## Non-antibiotic antibacterial compounds

Alongside developments in naturally occurring antibiotics, chemists and microbiologists have also been successful in seeking synthetic chemicals with antibacterial activity. Most of these agents have emerged through an indefinable mixture of biochemical know-how and luck rather than the rational targeting of vulnerable processes within the microbial cell.

The first important advance came with the discovery of *para*-aminosalicylic acid and isoniazid as effective antituberculosis drugs in the early 1950s, ushering in the era of reliable triple therapy (with streptomycin) for tuberculosis. Among the rest, the nitrofurans have a long history stretching back to before the Second World War but attracted little attention until the development of nitrofurantoin in the early 1950s. The diaminopyrimidine, trimethoprim, was first synthesized in America by George Hitchings and his colleagues in 1956.

Commercially, the most successful synthetic antibacterial agents have been the quinolones. The original compound, nalidixic acid, discovered in the 1960s as a by-product of the synthesis of the antimalarial agent chloroquine, was of minor importance but, after an unpromising start, quinolones began to assume a more significant role in the 1980s, when derivatives such as norfloxacin and ciprofloxacin emerged that exhibited much better activity against a broader spectrum of bacteria.

## Antifungal, antiparasitic, and antiviral agents

The revolution in therapy brought about by the numerous antibacterial 'wonder drugs' was not mirrored in infections caused by other microbes, but considerable progress in the treatment of non-bacterial infection was nevertheless made in the second half of the twentieth century.

Treatment of fungal infections was the first to benefit. In 1949, at the height of the search for naturally occurring antibacterial compounds, Elizabeth Hazen and Rachel Brown discovered an antibiotic with surprisingly good antifungal activity. They named it nystatin after the New York State Department of Health in whose laboratories they worked. The related polyene, amphotericin, was developed by scientists at Squibb in the 1950s. Another antifungal antibiotic, griseofulvin, had been described as early as 1939 but not used in human medicine until 1958, following the work by James Gentles in Glasgow on dermatophyte infections in experimental animals. A major step forward occurred in the 1970s with the discovery in Germany and Belgium of the unexpectedly broad-spectrum antifungal activity of certain nitroimidazole derivatives such as clotrimazole and ketoconazole (which offered the added advantage that it could be given orally), leading to the later development of the triazoles fluconazole and itraconazole. The most recent class of antifungals, the echinocandins, are the result of screening fermentation products for novel antibiotics. These act by inhibiting fungal wall glucan synthesis and include caspofungin, which is used in the treatment of systemic candidiasis and aspergillosis.

Among antiprotozoal agents, most progress was made among antimalarial agents, starting with the development in America after the Second World War of a pre-war German discovery, chloroquine, and culminating in the successful testing of artemisinin, the active ingredient of the ancient Chinese herbal remedy qinghaosu, in the late 1970s. Many other protozoal diseases fared less well but patients suffering from amoebic dysentery, giardiasis, and trichomonal vaginitis (and those with infections caused by anaerobic bacteria) benefited from the development in France around 1960 of metronidazole, a synthetic compound based on the structure of a naturally occurring antibiotic, azomycin.

Even helminthic disease treatment was to profit from the intense research activity, albeit through investigations into drugs for worm infections of farm animals. Remarkably, by the early 1980s, three anthelminthic compounds—praziquantel, albendazole, and ivermectin—were available, which between them offered safe and effective treatment for a diverse range of human worm infections.

For many years, antimicrobial agents played a very minor part in the treatment of viral infections, although the prevention of a number of viral diseases through the use of vaccines was outstandingly effective. Antiviral chemotherapy became a clinical reality in 1962 with the testing of idoxuridine (IDU) for herpes simplex, and methisazone for smallpox. However, IDU was teratogenic and had a narrow therapeutic index, and methisazone was rendered redundant by the success of smallpox vaccination. The first real breakthrough came with the development of the nucleoside analogue aciclovir by Gertrude Ellion's team at Burroughs Wellcome in 1978. This agent has excellent selective toxicity because it has to be activated by a viral enzyme (thymidine kinase) that is produced only in cells infected with herpesviruses. It is 10 times more active than IDU and has minimal toxicity even with high dose intravenous administration. The identification of HIV as the cause of AIDS in 1981 stimulated the pharmaceutical industry to produce an array of drugs targeted at a variety of viral gene products that have transformed the prognosis of HIV infection. Although eradication is still not possible, the introduction of highly active, combination antiretroviral chemotherapy (HAART) in the mid-1990s resulted in sustained control of viral replication for many patients. The first agents to be discovered were the nucleoside reverse transcriptase inhibitors (e.g. zidovudine), which are analogues of the naturally occurring deoxynucleotides and compete with them for incorporation in the growing viral DNA chain. The non-nucleoside reverse transcriptase inhibitors (e.g. efavirenz) bind to a different site of the enzyme and block its activity through allosteric inhibition. Subsequent developments targeted HIV protein synthesis (protease inhibitors), entry inhibitors, and inhibitors of viral integrase, an enzyme which is key to viral DNA incorporation into the host chromosome. The most recent— and still emerging—success story in antivirals is the development of directly acting antiviral agents that target specific gene products of hepatitis C virus, such as the NS3/4a protease and the NS5b polymerase.

In 1967 William Stewart, the Surgeon General of the United States of America, said 'The time has come to close the book on infectious diseases. We have basically wiped out infection in the United States'. Fifty years on, the limitations of antimicrobial therapy are all too apparent. Microbes have shown amazing versatility in avoiding, withstanding, or repelling the antibiotic onslaught, while parallel medical advances have provided a large and increasing group of vulnerable patients for them to attack. Antimicrobial agents are essential tools of modern medicine but the battle against infection is far from won. The challenge now is to preserve the remarkable achievements of the twentieth century by learning to use these powerful drugs more judiciously as well as finding new ways to develop new compounds.

## Further Reading

Greenwood, D. (2008) *Antimicrobial Drugs: Chronicle of a Twentieth Century Medical Triumph*. Oxford: Oxford University Press.

## Chapter 2

# Inhibitors of bacterial cell wall synthesis

## Introduction to inhibitors

The essence of antimicrobial chemotherapy is selective toxicity—to kill or inhibit the microbe without harming the host (patient). In bacteria, a prime target for attack is the cell wall, since practically all bacteria (with the exception of mycoplasmas) have a cell wall, whereas mammalian cells lack this feature. Several types of antibiotics, notably β-lactam agents (penicillins, cephalosporins, and their relatives) and glycopeptides (vancomycin and teicoplanin) take advantage of this difference. Some compounds used in the treatment of tuberculosis and leprosy act on the specialized mycobacterial cell wall (see 'Antimycobacterial agents' in Chapter 4).

In general, bacterial cell walls conform to two basic patterns, which are distinguished by the Gram stain. Gram-positive (staphylococci, streptococci, etc.) and Gram-negative (escherichia, pseudomonas, klebsiella, etc.) bacteria respond differently to agents that target the cell wall, and it is helpful to understand the basis for this difference.

## Cell wall construction

In both Gram-positive and Gram-negative bacteria, the cell wall is formed from a cross-linked chain of alternating units of N-acetylglucosamine and N-acetylmuramic acid, known as peptidoglycan or mucopeptide. The process of synthesis is illustrated in outline in Fig. 2.1, together with the main sites where cell wall active antimicrobial agents act.

In Gram-positive organisms, the cell wall structure is thick (about 30 nm), tightly cross-linked, and interspersed with polysugarphosphates (teichoic acids), some of which have a lipophilic tail buried in the cell membrane (lipoteichoic acids). Gram-negative bacteria, in contrast, have a relatively thin (2–3 nm), loosely cross-linked peptidoglycan layer and no teichoic acid.

External to the Gram-negative peptidoglycan is a membrane-like structure, composed chiefly of lipopolysaccharide and lipoprotein and which prevents large molecules such as glycopeptides from entering the cell. Small hydrophilic molecules enter Gram-negative bacilli through aqueous channels (porins) within the outer membrane. Differential activity among some groups of antibiotics, notably the penicillins and cephalosporins, is influenced by their ability to negotiate these porins, and this, in turn, reflects the size and ionic charge of substituents in individual agents.

## β-Lactam antibiotics

Penicillins, cephalosporins, and certain other antibiotics belong to a family of compounds collectively known as β-lactam antibiotics, which all possess a β-lactam ring. In penicillins the β-lactam ring is fused to a thiazolidine ring, whereas cephalosporins have a fused β-lactam/dihydrothiazine ring structure. The β-lactam ring is the Achilles' heel of these antibiotics, because many bacteria possess enzymes (β-lactamases; see Chapter 10) that can break open this part of the molecule, rendering it antibacterially inactive.

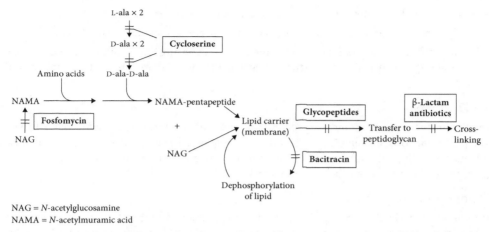

NAG = N-acetylglucosamine
NAMA = N-acetylmuramic acid

**Fig. 2.1** Simplified scheme of bacterial cell wall synthesis showing the sites of action of cell wall–active antibiotics.

## Penicillins

The original preparations of penicillin were found on analysis to be mixtures of four closely related compounds (penicillin F, G, K, and X). Benzylpenicillin (penicillin G), often simply called 'penicillin', was chosen for further development because it exhibited the most attractive properties; a manufacturing process was developed in which *Penicillium chrysogenum* was used to produced benzylpenicillin almost exclusively.

Early attempts to modify this structure relied on presenting the *Penicillium* mould that produced penicillin with different side-chain precursors during the manufacturing process. Later a method was discovered of removing the side-chain of benzylpenicillin and instead adding other chemical groupings, thus creating 'semi-synthetic penicillins'.

Benzylpenicillin revolutionized the treatment of many potentially lethal bacterial infections, such as scarlet fever, puerperal sepsis, bacterial endocarditis, pneumococcal pneumonia, staphylococcal sepsis, meningococcal meningitis, gonorrhoea, syphilis (and other spirochaetal diseases), anthrax, and many anaerobic infections. The overwhelming importance of benzylpenicillin as a major breakthrough in therapy may be gauged from the fact that it remains today the treatment of choice for many of these diseases.

However, resistance has eroded the value of benzylpenicillin. Nearly all staphylococci and many strains of gonococci are now resistant. Pneumococci exhibiting reduced susceptibility to benzylpenicillin became increasingly prevalent in some parts of the world. Such strains are of two types: those for which the minimum inhibitory concentration (MIC) of benzylpenicillin is increased from the usual value of about 0.02 mg/l to 0.1–1 mg/l, and those for which the MIC exceeds 1 mg/l. The former are sufficiently sensitive to enable the antibiotic to be used successfully in high dosage, except in pneumococcal meningitis. However, penicillin is not clinically reliable in infections with strains exhibiting the higher level of resistance.

Despite its attractive properties, benzylpenicillin is not the perfect antimicrobial agent:

◆ it exhibits a restricted antibacterial spectrum;

◆ it causes hypersensitivity reactions in a small proportion of recipients;

◆ it is broken down by gastric acidity when administered orally;

- it is eliminated from the body at a spectacular rate by the kidneys; and
- it is hydrolysed by β-lactamases produced by many bacteria, including staphylococci.

Subsequent developments have been aimed at overcoming these inherent weaknesses while retaining the attractive properties of benzylpenicillin: high intrinsic activity and lack of toxicity.

## Acid stability

The first major success in improving the pharmacological properties of penicillin was achieved with phenoxymethylpenicillin (penicillin V). This compound has properties very similar to those of benzylpenicillin but is acid stable and so achieves better and more reliable serum levels when given orally, at the expense of being marginally less active.

## Prolongation of plasma levels

Most β-lactam antibiotics are rapidly excreted, with plasma half-lives of 1–3 h. Benzylpenicillin is even more rapidly eliminated, and several strategies are used in order to maintain effective levels in the body. The blockbuster approach is simply to give very high doses. Alternatively, oral probenecid can be co-administered, as this agent competes for sites of active tubular secretion in the kidney, slowing down the elimination of penicillin. In addition, insoluble derivatives of penicillin can be injected intramuscularly and act as depots from which antibiotic is slowly liberated. Originally, mixtures of penicillin with oily or waxy excipients were used but insoluble salts, such as procaine penicillin, were later developed. In this way, an inhibitory concentration of penicillin can be maintained in the bloodstream for up to 24 hours; extremely insoluble salts, such as benzathine penicillin, release penicillin even more slowly (consequently achieving lower concentrations).

## Extension of spectrum

Broadening the spectrum of benzylpenicillin to encompass Gram-negative bacilli was first achieved by adding an amino group to the side-chain to form ampicillin. Ampicillin is slightly less active than benzylpenicillin against Gram-positive cocci and is equally susceptible to staphylococcal β-lactamase. However, it displays much improved activity against some enterobacteria, including *Escherichia coli*, *Salmonella enterica*, and *Shigella* spp. as well as against *Haemophilus influenzae*. Oral absorption is relatively poor but can be improved by esterifying the molecule to form so-called prodrugs, such as pivampicillin (see 'Absorption' in Chapter 14). Such compounds are split by non-specific tissue esterases in the intestinal mucosa to release ampicillin during absorption. Improved absorption has also been more simply achieved by a minor modification to the molecule to produce amoxicillin.

Another alteration to the penicillin molecule yielded mecillinam (known as amdinocillin in the United States), which is active against ampicillin-sensitive enterobacteria and some of the more resistant Gram-negative bacilli. However, mecillinam displays no useful activity against Gram-positive cocci. It is poorly absorbed when given orally, but a prodrug form, pivmecillinam, can be given by mouth.

Temocillin, a penicillin in which the β-lactam ring carries a methoxy group that renders it stable to most β-lactamases (as in cephamycins; see 'Parenteral compounds with improved β-lactamase stability'), has an unusual spectrum. It is moderately active against many Gram-negative bacilli but has no useful activity against *Pseudomonas aeruginosa*, Gram-positive cocci, or anaerobic organisms. It was largely abandoned but a rise in prevalence of Gram-negative bacilli that produce broad-spectrum β-lactamases has prompted its reintroduction.

## Antipseudomonal penicillins

None of the agents so far mentioned has any activity against *Ps. aeruginosa*, an important opportunist pathogen, especially in burns, cystic fibrosis, and intensive care and immunocompromised patients. A simple carboxyl derivative of benzylpenicillin, carbenicillin, was found to have weak but useful activity and was used for a time in high dosage. It has been superseded by ticarcillin, the thienyl variant of carbenicillin and by a group of ureido derivatives of ampicillin, including azlocillin and piperacillin. These antipseudomonal penicillins must be administered by injection but two esterified carbenicillin prodrugs, carfecillin and carindacillin, are available in some countries.

## Antistaphylococcal penicillins

By the end of the 1950s, 80 per cent of staphylococci isolated in hospitals were resistant to benzylpenicillin because of their ability to produce penicillinase (β-lactamase). The appearance of these resistant organisms, which spread markedly in hospitals, stimulated research into derivatives that were insusceptible to β-lactamase hydrolysis. Success was achieved with methicillin (no longer generally available), nafcillin, and a group called isoxazolylpenicillins: oxacillin, cloxacillin, dicloxacillin, and flucloxacillin. The isoxazolylpenicillins, particularly flucloxacillin, are well absorbed when given orally and are most widely used. They are highly bound to serum protein in the body but this does not adversely affect their therapeutic efficacy.

Resistance to penicillinase-stable penicillins is caused not by inactivating enzymes but by alterations to the penicillin target (see 'Mode of action of β-lactam antibiotics'). Staphylococci of this type were originally characterized by resistance to methicillin and, although this compound is no longer used in treatment, they are still known as methicillin-resistant staphylococci. Resistance extends to all β-lactam agents and often accompanies resistance to gentamicin and other antibiotics (multiresistant staphylococci). Some strains fully display the resistance phenotype only at a reduced growth temperature or in the presence of high salt concentrations. Particularly troublesome are methicillin-resistant *Staphylococcus aureus* strains (MRSA), which are an important cause of health-care- and, in some settings, community-associated infection.

The spectrum of activity of the most important penicillins in clinical use is shown in Table 2.1.

## Cephalosporins

Cephalosporins generally exhibit a somewhat broader spectrum than penicillins, though, idiosyncratically, they lack activity against enterococci. They are mostly stable to staphylococcal β-lactamase and often lack cross-allergenicity with penicillins (see 'Gonorrhoea' in Chapter 24).

The original cephalosporin, cephalosporin C, was never marketed but has given rise to a large family of compounds that continues to expand. There are many more cephalosporins than penicillins (Table 2.2). Alterations at either end of the molecule may profoundly affect antibacterial activity but, as a generalization, substituents at the C-3 position have more influence on pharmacokinetic properties. For example, cefotaxime is only slowly altered by liver enzymes because of such a substitution. The altered cephalosporin is usually less active than the parent antibiotic and may display altered pharmacokinetic behaviour but there is little evidence that the clinical effectiveness is impaired. Several cephalosporins, including cefamandole, cefotetan, cefmenoxime, cefoperazone, and the oxacephem latamoxef possess a complex side-chain at the C-3 position that has been implicated in haematological side effects in some patients (see 'Parenteral compounds with improved β-lactamase stability').

The earliest cephalosporins, cefalotin and cefaloridine, are not absorbed when given orally and are very susceptible to a wide variety of enzymes produced by Gram-negative organisms

**Table 2.1** Summary of the antibacterial properties of selected penicillins.[a]

| Penicillin | Staphylococci | | Streptococci | Neisseria spp. | Haemophilus influenzae | Enterobacteria | | Pseudomonas aeruginosa | Anaerobes |
|---|---|---|---|---|---|---|---|---|---|
| | Activity | Stability[a] | | | | Activity | Stability[b] | | |
| Benzylpenicillin | Very good | Poor | Very good | Very good | Fair | – | – | – | Variable |
| Phenoxymethylpenicillin | Very good | Poor | Very good | Good | Poor | – | – | – | Variable |
| Ampicillin Amoxicillin | Good | Poor | Very good | Very good | Good | Good | Poor | – | Variable |
| Piperacillin Ticarcillin | Good | Poor | Good | Good | Good | Variable | Variable | Good | Fair |
| Cloxacillin Flucloxacillin | Good | Good | Fair | Fair | Poor | – | – | – | Fair |
| Mecillinam | – | – | – | Fair | Poor | Good | Variable | Poor | Poor |
| Temocillin | – | – | – | Good | Good | Good | Very good | – | – |

[a] –, no useful activity.

[b] Stability to β-lactamases of these organisms.

**Table 2.2** Categorization of cephalosporins in clinical use.

| Parenteral compounds | | | Oral compounds | | |
|---|---|---|---|---|---|
| Cefalotin | Cefacetrile | Ceforanide | Cefalexin[a] | Cefaloglycin | Cefroxadine |
| Cefaloridine | Cefapirin | Cefonicid | Cefradine[a] | Cefadroxil[a] | Cefatrizine |
| Cefazolin | Cefazedone | Ceftezole | Cefaclor | Cefprozil[a] | Loracarbef[b] |
| Cefamandole | | | | | |
| **Compounds with improved β-lactamase stability** | | | **Compounds with improved β-lactamase stability** | | |
| Cefuroxime[a] | Cefmetazole | Cefotiam | *Non-esterified* | *Esterified* | |
| Cefoxitin | Cefotetan | Cefminox | Cefixime[a] | Cefuroxime axetil[a] | |
| | | | Ceftibuten | Cefpodoxime proxetil[a] | |
| **Compounds with improved intrinsic activity and β-lactamase stability** | | | Cefdinir | Cefetamet pivoxil | |
| | | | | Cefteram pivoxil | |
| Cefotaxime[a] | Cefmenoxime | Latamoxef[c] | | Cefotiam hexetil | |
| Ceftriaxone[a] | Ceftizoxime | Flomoxef[c] | | Cefditoren pivoxil | |
| Cefodizime | Cefuzonam | | | Cefcapene pivoxil | |
| **Compounds distinguished by activity against *Pseudomonas aeruginosa*** | | | | | |
| *Broad spectrum* | *Medium spectrum* | *Narrow spectrum* | | | |
| Ceftazidime[a] | Cefoperazone | Cefsulodin | | | |
| Cefpirome[a] | Cefpimizole | | | | |
| Cefepime | Cefpiramide | | | | |
| **Compounds distinguished by activity against MRSA** | | | | | |
| Ceftaroline | | | | | |

[a] Compound available in the United Kingdom (as of 2006).

[b] Strictly a carbacephem.

[c] Strictly oxacephems.

(see Chapter 10). As with penicillins, developments within the cephalosporin family were aimed at devising compounds with more attractive properties: oral absorption or other improved pharmacological properties, stability to inactivating enzymes, better intrinsic activity, or a combination of these features.

Cephalosporins display diverse properties that tend to be grouped according to their relative activity against Gram-positive and Gram-negative bacteria, *Ps. aeruginosa*, and most recently MRSA. It is also helpful to distinguish between cephalosporins (the majority) that have to be administered parenterally and those that can be given orally (Table 2.2). Cephalosporins are commonly described as first, second, third, fourth and, most recently, fifth generation compounds. These loose terms refer to

- early compounds such as cefalotin and cefalexin that were available before about 1975 (first generation);
- β-lactamase stable compounds such as cefuroxime and cefoxitin (second generation);

- compounds such as cefotaxime and ceftazidime that combine β-lactamase stability with improved intrinsic activity (third generation); ceftazidime, but not cefotaxime, has good activity against *Ps. aeruginosa*;

- compounds such as cefepime and cefpirome that are similar to ceftazidime, that is, with good activity against enterobacteria and *Ps. aeruginosa* but better Gram-positive activity (fourth generation); and

- recently developed compounds, including ceftaroline and ceftobiprole, which are the first examples of β-lactams/cephalosporin drugs that have useful activity against MRSA and are referred to as anti-MRSA (or fifth generation) cephalosporins. Ceftobiprole has modestly better activity than ceftaroline against Gram-negative bacteria, while the reverse is true for Gram-positives.

## Parenteral compounds susceptible to enterobacterial β-lactamases

Cephalosporins in this group are of limited clinical value and have been largely superseded by other derivatives; all have been abandoned in the United Kingdom. Cefazolin has the unusual property of being excreted in fairly high concentration in bile; cefamandole exhibits a modestly expanded spectrum. Others, including cefapirin, ceforanide, and cefonicid, offer no discernible advantage over earlier congeners such as cefalotin.

## Parenteral compounds with improved β-lactamase stability

An important advance was achieved with the development of cephalosporins that exhibit almost complete stability to the common β-lactamases of enterobacteria such as *E. coli* and *Klebsiella aerogenes*. The first of these were cefuroxime and cefoxitin, the latter being one of a group of cephalosporins collectively called cephamycins. Other cephamycins available in some countries include cefotetan, cefmetazole, and cefminox. The cephamycins are unusual in displaying useful activity against anaerobes of the *Bacteroides fragilis* group.

These compounds have been overshadowed by the appearance of cephalosporins that combine almost complete stability to most β-lactamases with much improved intrinsic activity. Cefotaxime was the forerunner of this group, but several others are available: ceftizoxime and cefmenoxime are similar to cefotaxime; ceftriaxone displays a sufficiently long plasma half-life to warrant once-daily administration; cefodizime is said to possess immunomodulating properties.

Latamoxef (moxalactam), which is strictly an oxacephem, also displays activity analogous to that of cefotaxime and its relatives but differs in possessing useful activity against *Bact. fragilis* and related anaerobes. However, latamoxef has lost favour owing to toxicity problems and is no longer widely available.

## Compounds distinguished by antipseudomonal activity

*Ps. aeruginosa* is not susceptible to most cephalosporins and, as with penicillins, considerable efforts have been made to find derivatives that include this important opportunist pathogen in their spectrum. Ceftazidime, cefpirome, and cefepime add activity against *Ps. aeruginosa* to broad-spectrum activity comparable with that of cefotaxime and its congeners. These compounds have established a useful role in the management of *Ps. aeruginosa* infections in seriously ill patients. However, the antistaphylococcal activity is suspect, and cefpirome may have some advantage in this respect. Cefepime retains activity against some opportunist Gram-negative bacilli that develop resistance to cefotaxime and its relatives.

Among other antipseudomonal cephalosporins, cefoperazone, cefpimizole, and cefpiramide are not distinguished by any unusual activity against other organisms, and cefsulodin is extraordinary in being virtually inactive against bacteria other than *Ps. aeruginosa*.

Ceftolozane is a new antipseudomonal cephalosporin that, in combination with the β-lactamase inhibitor tazobactam, is in the late stage of clinical trials.

Ceftolozane/tazobactam has a spectrum of activity that includes many Gram-negative pathogens, including some *Ps. aeruginosa* strains that are resistant to carbapenems, piperacillin/tazobactam, and other cephalosporins.

## Oral cephalosporins

Early development of the cephalosporins yielded cefalexin, a compound of modest activity, particularly in terms of its bactericidal action against Gram-negative bacilli, but which is virtually completely absorbed when given orally. Many other oral derivatives are structurally minor variations on the cefalexin theme. These include cefradine (properties indistinguishable from those of cefalexin), cefaclor (more active against the important respiratory pathogen *H. influenzae*), cefadroxil (modestly extended plasma half-life), and cefprozil (improved intrinsic activity). Loracarbef is a carbacephem (carbon replacing sulphur in the fused-ring structure), but is otherwise structurally identical to cefaclor. Not surprisingly, its properties closely resemble those of cefaclor.

Cefixime and ceftibuten are structurally unrelated to cefalexin. They display much improved activity against most Gram-negative bacilli but at the expense of antistaphylococcal (and, in the case of ceftibuten, antipneumococcal) activity, which is very poor. Another compound of this type, cefdinir, appears to lack these defects.

The principle of esterification to produce prodrugs with improved oral absorption has also been applied to cephalosporins. Two such compounds, cefuroxime axetil and cefpodoxime proxetil, are available in the United Kingdom; cefteram pivoxil, cefetamet pivoxil, cefotiam hexetil, cefditoren pivoxil, and cefcapene pivoxil are marketed elsewhere. These esters are fairly well absorbed by the oral route and deliver the parent drug into the bloodstream. Cefpodoxime, cefteram, and cefetamet are more active than the others against most organisms within the spectrum, although cefetamet has poor activity against staphylococci.

A summary of the antimicrobial spectrum of the most important cephalosporins is presented in Table 2.3.

## Other β-lactam agents

In addition to penicillins and cephalosporins, various other compounds display a β-lactam ring in their structure (Fig. 2.2). Clavulanic acid, a naturally occurring substance obtained from *Streptomyces clavuligerus*, and two penicillanic acid sulphones, sulbactam and tazobactam, have little useful antibacterial activity but act as β-lactamase inhibitors. They are used in combination with β-lactamase-labile agents with a view to restoring their activity: clavulanic acid is combined with amoxicillin (co-amoxiclav; available both orally and intravenously) or ticarcillin; sulbactam with ampicillin; and tazobactam with piperacillin. These combination agents have become extremely widely used, particularly in hospitals, and there is now evidence of the emergence of resistance notably among Gram-negative bacilli. This is situation is complicated because of uncertainties about how best to measure susceptibility to two drugs as opposed to one, and variations across the world in the threshold concentrations used to define resistant strains.

Structurally novel compounds that exhibit antibacterial activity in their own right include the carbapenems (imipenem, doripenem, meropenem, panipenem, and ertapenem) and aztreonam, one of a group of compounds collectively known as monobactams and which have a β-lactam ring but no associated fused-ring system. Imipenem is readily hydrolysed by a dehydropeptidase located in the mammalian kidney and is administered together with the dehydropeptidase inhibitor

**Table 2.3** Summary of the spectrum of antibacterial activity of cephalosporins.[a]

| Cephalosporin | Staphylococci | Streptococci[b] | Neisseria spp. | Haemophilus influenzae | Enterobacteria | Pseudomonas aeruginosa | Bacteroides spp. |
|---|---|---|---|---|---|---|---|
| Cefuroxime | Good | Very good | Good | Good | Good | – | – |
| Cefotaxime | Good | Very good | Very good | Very good | Very good | Poor | Poor |
| Ceftriaxone | | | | | | | |
| Ceftazidime | Fair | Good | Very good | Very good | Very good | Good | Poor |
| Cefpirome | Good | Very good | Very good | Very good | Very good | Good | – |
| Ceftaroline | Good[c] | Very good | Good | Good | Good | – | Poor |
| Cefalexin | Good | Good | Poor | Poor | Variable | – | – |
| Cefradine | | | | | | | |
| Cefadroxil | | | | | | | |
| Cefaclor | Good | Good | Fair | Good | Variable | – | – |
| Cefixime | Poor | Very good | Good | Good | Very good | – | – |
| Cefprozil | Good | Good | Very good | Very good | Very good | – | – |
| Cefpodoxime | Good | Very good | Very good | Good | Very good | – | – |

[a] –, no useful activity.

[b] Enterococci are resistant to all cephalosporins.

[c] Includes activity against MRSA.

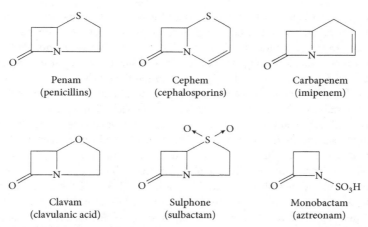

**Fig. 2.2** Basic molecular structures of β-lactam antibiotics currently available (examples in parentheses).

cilastatin. Aztreonam is also β-lactamase stable but, in contrast to carbapenems, the activity is restricted to aerobic Gram-negative bacteria.

The carbapenems are stable to most bacterial β-lactamases and exhibit the broadest spectrum of all β-lactam antibiotics, with high activity against nearly all Gram-positive bacteria (but not MRSA and some enterococci) and all Gram-negative bacteria (with the exception of ertapenem, including *Ps. aeruginosa*), including anaerobes (other than intracellular bacteria such as chlamydiae). Carbapenems are generally considered as the last line of defence in bacterial infection and tend to be reserved for life-threatening infection, especially when empirical therapy is required because the causative pathogen is unknown. Given this place in the therapeutic armamentarium, a most worrying development is the recent rapid emergence of new types of carbapenemases, enzymes produced predominantly by Gram-negative bacteria, which render these valuable agents inactive. There are increasing reports of hospital-based outbreaks of various carbapenem-resistant bacteria (CRB) in some countries, including Greece, the United Kingdom, India, Israel, Italy, and the United States (Chapter 10). Infections caused by CRB are extremely problematic to treat, and these are a major focus for the development of new antibiotics.

## Factors affecting β-lactam agents

Penicillins and other β-lactam antibiotics are categorized as bactericidal agents but this is true only when bacteria are actively dividing. Moreover, the way bacteria respond to β-lactam antibiotics is affected by subtle differences in the mode of action. Several other features of the response that may sometimes have therapeutic implications have also been discovered.

## Mode of action of β-lactam agents

All β-lactam antibiotics interfere with the final cross-linking reaction that gives the cell wall its strength (Fig. 2.1). However, several forms of the enzyme that performs this reaction are needed to maintain the complex molecular architecture of the cell, and these are differentially inhibited by various β-lactam agents. These target enzymes belong to a group of proteins to which penicillin and other β-lactam antibiotics bind (penicillin-binding proteins (PBPs)). *E. coli*, the best-studied species, has seven of these proteins, numbered la, lb, 2, 3, 4, 5, and 6 in order of decreasing molecular weight. PBPs 4–6 are thought to be unconnected with the antibacterial effect of β-lactam agents, since mutants lacking these proteins do not seem to be disabled in any way. Binding to the remainder has been correlated with the various morphological effects of β-lactam antibiotics on Gram-negative bacilli. Thus, cefalexin and its close congeners, as well as aztreonam, bind almost exclusively to PBP 3 and inhibit the division process, causing the bacteria to grow as long filaments. The amidinopenicillin mecillinam binds preferentially to PBP 2 and causes a generalized effect on the cell wall so that the bacteria gradually assume a spherical shape. Most other β-lactam antibiotics bind to PBPs 1–3 and, in sufficient concentration, induce the formation of osmotically fragile, wall-deficient forms (called spheroplasts), which typically emerge at the cell wall growth site as the cell starts to divide. Some morphological events are illustrated in Fig. 2.3 An important consequence of differences in binding is that compounds such as cefalexin, aztreonam, and mecillinam, which bind only to PBP 3 or PBP 2, are much more slowly bactericidal to Gram-negative bacilli that those that bind PBPs 1, 2, and 3. The recently developed anti-MRSA cephalosporins are active by virtue of improved affinity for the PBP that is present in MRSA strains (PBP 2a).

In Gram-negative bacilli, rupture of spheroplasts can be quantitatively prevented by raising the osmolality of the growth medium, so cell death appears to be an osmotic phenomenon. The lethal

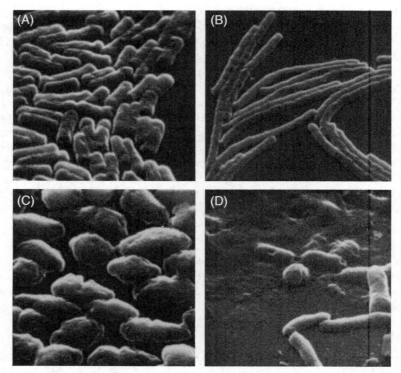

**Fig. 2.3** Morphological effects of penicillins and cephalosporins on Gram-negative bacilli (scanning electron micrographs). (A) Normal *E. coli* cells. (B) *E. coli* exposed to cefalexin, 32 mg/l, for 1 hour. Reproduced from Greenwood D, O'Grady F, The Two Sites of Penicillin Action in Escherichia coli, *Journal of Infectious Diseases*, Volume 128, Number 6, pp. 91–4, Copyright © 1973, by permission of Oxford University Press.

event in Gram-positive organisms, which have much thicker cell walls, appears to be autolysis triggered by the release of lipoteichoic acid following exposure to β-lactam antibiotics.

## Optimal dosage effect

A further complication in Gram-positive organisms is that increasing the concentration of β-lactam antibiotics often results in a reduced bactericidal effect. The mechanism of this effect (known as the Eagle phenomenon after its discoverer) is obscure but may be related to the multiple sites of penicillin action and the fact that cell death occurs only during active growth: saturating a relatively insusceptible PBP may rapidly halt growth and thereby prevent the lethal events that normally follow inhibition of another PBP by lower drug levels.

## Persisters, and penicillin tolerance

In both Gram-positive and Gram-negative bacteria, a proportion of the population, called persisters, survive exposure to β-lactam antibiotics at concentrations that are lethal to the rest of the culture. In addition, some strains of staphylococci and streptococci display 'tolerance' to β-lactam antibiotics, dying much more slowly than usual. The therapeutic significance, if any, of persisters is unknown but penicillin tolerance has been implicated in therapeutic failures in bacterial endocarditis, where bactericidal activity is important for treatment success (see 'Infective endocarditis' in Chapter 26).

## Postantibiotic effect

Much has also been made of laboratory observations that the antimicrobial activity of β-lactam agents may persist for an hour or more after the drug is removed. This effect is not confined to β-lactam agents and is more consistently demonstrated with Gram-positive than with Gram-negative organisms. Theoretically, knowledge of postantibiotic effects might influence the choice of dosages, but in practice they are too erratic to be used in this way, even if the laboratory observations could be convincingly shown to have clinical relevance, which is presently not the case.

# Glycopeptides

The glycopeptides vancomycin and teicoplanin are complex heterocyclic molecules consisting of a multipeptide backbone to which are attached various substituted sugars. These compounds bind to acyl-D-alanyl-D-alanine in peptidoglycan, thereby preventing the addition of new building blocks to the growing cell wall (Fig. 2.1). Glycopeptides are too bulky to penetrate the external membrane of Gram-negative bacteria, so the spectrum of activity is virtually restricted to Gram-positive organisms. Acquired resistance used to be uncommon but resistant strains of enterococci are now widely prevalent and staphylococci exhibiting reduced susceptibility are causing concern. Avoparcin, a glycopeptide formerly used in animal husbandry (now banned in the European Union), has been implicated in generating resistance in enterococci but human use of glycopeptides is equally important. Some Gram-positive genera, including *Lactobacillus*, *Pediococcus*, and *Leuconostoc*, are inherently resistant to glycopeptides but these organisms are seldom implicated in disease.

## Vancomycin

This antibiotic is widely used for the treatment of infections caused by staphylococci that are resistant to methicillin and other β-lactam antibiotics, and for serious infections with Gram-positive organisms in patients who are allergic to penicillin. It is very poorly absorbed when given by mouth and must be given by injection. Oral administration is indicated in the treatment of antibiotic-associated *Clostridium difficile* infection (see 'Antibiotic-associated diarrhoea and CDI' in Chapter 25).

Early preparations of vancomycin contained impurities that gave the drug a reputation for toxicity. The purified formulations now available are much safer but renal and ototoxicity still occur, particularly with high dosage. The drug is given by slow intravenous infusion (typically over 1–2 hours) to avoid 'red man syndrome'.

## Teicoplanin

This is a naturally occurring mixture of several closely related compounds with a spectrum of activity similar to that of vancomycin, although some coagulase-negative staphylococci (*Staph. epidermidis*, *Staph. haemolyticus*, etc.) are less susceptible to teicoplanin. Some strains of enterococci that are resistant to vancomycin (those with the VanB phenotype; see Table 11.4 in Chapter 11) retain susceptibility to teicoplanin. Unlike vancomycin, teicoplanin can be administered by intramuscular injection; it also has a much longer plasma half-life than vancomycin and a reduced propensity to cause adverse reactions.

## Telavancin

Telavancin is a recently launched, once-daily, injectable, lipoglycopeptide that has increased bactericidal properties compared with vancomycin and teicoplanin. This may relate to multimodal activity, that is, a cell membrane depolarizing effect in addition to conventional glycopeptide cell wall action. There are restrictions on its use because of concerns about possible renal toxicity and teratogenicity (meaning it should ideally be avoided in pregnancy).

## Dalbavancin and oitavancin

These lipoglycopeptide antibiotics are in the late stage of clinical development. They notably have very long plasma half-lives, which mean they can be given once or twice in total to treat skin and soft-tissue infections (for which they have been studied most intensively to date). Such infrequent administration offers the potential for outpatient treatment of some infections that otherwise would have necessitated hospital admission/stay.

# Other cell wall active agents

## Fosfomycin

Fosfomycin is a naturally occurring antibiotic originally obtained from a species of *Streptomyces* isolated in Spain. Fosfomycin inhibits the pyruvyl transferase enzyme that brings about the condensation of phosphoenolpyruvate and *N*-acetylglucosamine in the formation of *N*-acetylmuramic acid (Fig. 2.1). Gram-positive cocci are less susceptible than Gram-negative rods. The precise level of activity is a matter of dispute, since the in-vitro activity can be manipulated by altering the test medium. Glucose-6-phosphate potentiates the activity against many Gram-negative bacilli by inducing the active transport of fosfomycin into the bacterial cell.

Fosfomycin is formulated as the sodium salt for parenteral use but is unsuitable for oral administration. It is well tolerated, and the ready emergence of bacterial resistance that is observed in vitro does not appear to have been a major problem in treatment. The trometamol (tromethamine) salt is highly soluble, well absorbed, excreted in high concentration in urine, and can be given orally. Although fosfomycin is used for assorted purposes in some countries, its efficacy in serious infection is in doubt. The oral formulation is increasingly used for uncomplicated urinary tract infections (no fever or flank pain) caused by Gram-negative bacteria producing extended spectrum β-lactamases (ESBLs), for which sometimes few if any other suitable oral antibiotics are available.

## Bacitracin   `Topical use only`

Bacitracin is a cyclic peptide antibiotic, made up of about 10 amino acids joined in a ring. It was first obtained from a strain of *Bacillus subtilis* grown from the infected wound of a 7-year-old girl, Margaret Tracy, in whose honour the antibiotic was named.

The spectrum of activity of bacitracin and related cyclic peptides such as gramicidin and tyrocidine is restricted to Gram-positive organisms. These compounds are too toxic for systemic use but are found in topical preparations. Bacitracin is used in microbiology laboratories to help identify *Streptococcus pyogenes*, which is exquisitely susceptible. Bacitracin acts by preventing regeneration of the lipid carrier in the cell membrane (Fig. 2.1).

## Cycloserine

Cycloserine has broad-spectrum but rather feeble antibacterial activity and is now used only against multiresistant *Mycobacterium tuberculosis* (see 'Tuberculosis' in Chapter 10). Antituberculosis agents that act on special features of the mycobacterial cell wall are discussed in Chapter 3.

## Key points

### Penicillins

◆ Benzylpenicillin (penicillin G) is the original penicillin and still the best against streptococci and spirochaetes.

◆ Amoxicillin (oral)/ampicillin (injection) is used if broader spectrum is needed.

◆ Flucloxacillin is best for staphylococci (except MRSA).

◆ Piperacillin and ticarcillin are usually given with a β-lactamase inhibitor (tazobactam/clavulanic acid) for serious infection, especially if there is a risk of pseudomonas infection.

### Cephalosporins

◆ Cefuroxime is a good broad-spectrum, intravenous workhorse antibiotic.

◆ Cefotaxime and ceftriaxone are more active than cefuroxime and are used for serious infections.

◆ Ceftazidime is reserved for serious infections, especially if there is a risk of pseudomonas infection.

◆ Cefalexin, cefradine, and cefaclor: oral absorption is their chief virtue.

◆ All cephalosporins are associated with a risk of inducing *C. difficile* infection.

## Further reading

Finch, R. G., Greenwood, D., Norrby, S. R., and Whitley, R. J. (2010) *Antibiotic and Chemotherapy* (9th edn). London: Elsevier.

# Chapter 3

# Inhibitors of bacterial protein synthesis

## Introduction to inhibitors

The remarkable process by which proteins are manufactured on the ribosomal conveyor belt according to a blueprint provided by the cell nucleus is of fundamental importance to cell life. Although the general mechanism is thought to be universal, the process as it occurs in bacterial cells is sufficiently different from mammalian protein synthesis to offer scope for the selective toxicity required of therapeutically useful antimicrobial agents. The chief difference involves the actual structure of the protein and RNA components of the ribosomal workshop.

In order to understand how the various inhibitors of protein synthesis work, it is helpful to be aware of the main features of the process (Fig. 3.1). The first step is the formation of an initiation complex, consisting of messenger RNA (mRNA), transcribed from the appropriate area of a DNA strand, two ribosomal subunits, and methionyl transfer RNA (tRNA; N-formylated in bacteria) which occupies the 'peptidyl donor' site (P-site) on the larger ribosomal subunit. Aminoacyl tRNA appropriate to the next codon to be read slots into place in the aminoacyl 'acceptor' site (A-site), and an enzyme called peptidyl transferase attaches the methionine to the new amino acid with the formation of a peptide bond. The mRNA and the ribosome now move with respect to one another so that the dipeptide is translocated from the A-site to the P-site, and the next codon of the mRNA is aligned with the A-site in readiness for the next aminoacyl tRNA. The process continues to accumulate amino acids in the nascent peptide chain according to the order dictated by mRNA until a 'nonsense' codon is encountered, which signals chain termination.

The selective activity of therapeutically useful inhibitors of protein synthesis is far from absolute. Some, such as tetracyclines and clindamycin, have sufficient activity against eukaryotic ribosomes to be of value against certain protozoa. Moreover, the mitochondria of mammalian and other eukaryotic cells (which may have been derived from endosymbiotic bacteria during the course of evolution) carry out protein synthesis that is susceptible to some antibiotics used in therapy. The selectivity of these antibiotics is, therefore, due not only to structural differences in the ribosomal targets but also access to, and affinity for, those targets.

Inhibitors of bacterial protein synthesis with sufficient selectivity to be useful in human therapy include aminoglycosides, chloramphenicol, tetracyclines, fusidic acid, macrolides, lincosamides, streptogramins, oxazolidinones, and mupirocin.

## Aminoglycosides

### Classification

The first aminoglycoside, streptomycin, which was discovered in 1943 (see 'Antibiotics from soil' in Chapter 1), was later found to be just one of a large family of related antibiotics produced by various species of *Streptomyces* and *Micromonospora*. Aminoglycosides derived from the latter genus, such as gentamicin, are distinguished in their spelling by an 'i' rather than a 'y' in the

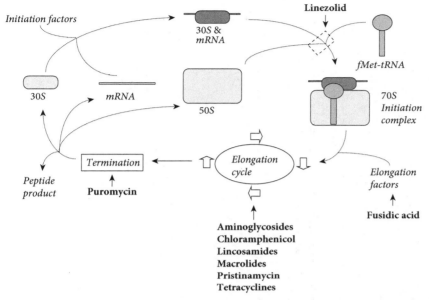

**Fig. 3.1** Schematic to show protein synthesis in bacteria, with examples of key sites at which anti-microbial agents intervene; 30S, 30S ribosomal subunit; 50S, 30S ribosomal subunit; fMet-tRNA, formylmethionyl tRNA.

'-mycin' suffix. Structurally, most aminoglycosides consist of a linked ring system composed of amino sugars and an aminosubstituted cyclic polyalcohol (aminocyclitol). One antibiotic usually included with this group, spectinomycin, contains no aminoglycoside substituent and is properly regarded as a pure aminocyclitol.

The aminoglycosides most commonly used in medicine, including gentamicin and tobramycin, belong to the kanamycin group. The designation 'kanamycin', 'gentamicin', or 'neomycin' indicates a family of closely related compounds, and commercial preparations usually contain a mixture of these. For example, gentamicin, as used therapeutically, is a mixture of several structural variants of the gentamicin C complex.

## General properties

The aminoglycosides are potent, broad-spectrum bactericidal agents that are very poorly absorbed when given orally and are therefore administered by injection for systemic infection or topically. Their spectrum includes most Gram-negative bacilli and staphylococci but not streptococci and anaerobes. Activity against streptococci can often be improved via use in conjunction with penicillins, with which aminoglycosides interact synergically. Aminoglycosides penetrate poorly into mammalian cells and thus are of limited value in infections caused by intracellular bacteria. Some members of the group display important activity against *Mycobacterium tuberculosis* or *Pseudomonas aeruginosa*. All of them display considerable toxicity affecting both the inner ear and the kidney (Table 3.1).

## Aminoglycoside assay

Because of their toxicity, the use of aminoglycosides requires careful laboratory monitoring to make sure that plasma concentrations are adequate but not so high that toxic levels are reached.

**Table 3.1** Summary of the antibacterial spectrum and toxicity of some aminoglycosides.

| Aminoglycoside | Activity against | | | | | Relative degrees of: | |
|---|---|---|---|---|---|---|---|
| | Staphylococci | Streptococci | Enterobacteria | Pseudomonas aeruginosa | Mycobacterium tuberculosis | Ototoxicity | Nephrotoxicity |
| Streptomycin* | Good | Poor | Good | Poor | Good | + + + | + |
| Kanamycin | Good | Poor | Good | Poor | Good | + + | + + |
| Gentamicin | Good | Fair | Good | Good | Poor | + + | + + |
| Tobramycin | Good | Poor | Good | Good | Poor | + + | + + |
| Netilmicin | Good | Poor | Good | Good | Poor | + | + |
| Amikacin | Good | Poor | Good | Good | Good | + + | + |
| Neomycin | Good | Poor | Good | Poor | Fair | + + + | + + + |

* Streptomycin: mainly tuberculosis.

Assays should be performed if treatment is for longer than 48 hours, particularly if there is any renal impairment, and always in older patients. Indeed, it might be considered negligent if a patient developed side effects attributable to aminoglycoside therapy and the drug concentration(s) had not been monitored.

The therapeutic range of concentrations of aminoglycosides such as gentamicin in plasma was originally thought to be 2–10 mg/l but it is far from certain that single high peak concentrations correlate simply with adverse effects. Indeed, it is now common to use once-daily aminoglycoside therapy, which requires a dosage that achieves relatively high peak concentrations and low trough levels (<1 mg/l) before the next dose is administered. Such regimens have been shown to be as safe as conventional multidose therapy.

## Mode of action

Streptomycin binds to a particular ribosomal protein, and a single amino acid change in this protein results in streptomycin resistance (aminoglycosides in the kanamycin and neomycin groups bind at a different site and are generally unaffected by this). Several effects of the binding of streptomycin and other aminoglycosides have been noted, including a tendency to cause misreading of certain codons in mRNA and thus resulting in the production of defective proteins, some of which may affect membrane integrity. Other evidence suggests that the primary site of action is the formation of non-functioning initiation complexes, or the inhibition of the translocation step in polypeptide synthesis. None of these hypotheses fully explains the potent bactericidal activity of aminoglycosides compared with other inhibitors of protein synthesis. Aminoglycosides enter bacteria by an active transport process involving respiratory quinines (which are absent in streptococci and anaerobes).

## Streptomycin

The use of streptomycin has declined with the appearance of other aminoglycosides, although it is still a component of several antituberculosis regimens recommended by the World Health Organization (see Chapter 30). It is also used in the treatment of some rarer conditions, including plague, brucellosis, bartonellosis, and tularaemia, possibly for want of adequate evidence that more modern agents might be effective.

## Neomycin group

Neomycin is the most ototoxic of the aminoglycosides and is now little used, except in topical preparations; even this use is discouraged because of the risk of promoting the emergence of aminoglycoside resistance. It has also been given orally together with other agents to sterilize the gut (e.g. before abdominal surgery or in patients in intensive care units), but the inactivity of aminoglycosides against anaerobes ensures that most of the gut flora escapes, and the procedure is not without risk of systemic toxicity. Framycetin, a common component of topical preparations, is identical to neomycin B.

One aminoglycoside of the neomycin group, paromomycin, is unusual in being active against the protozoa causing amoebic dysentery and leishmaniasis as well as some tapeworms. However, other drugs are preferred in the treatment of these parasitic diseases (see Chapter 35).

## Kanamycin group

Important members of this large group include kanamycin itself, gentamicin, tobramycin, netilmicin, and a semi-synthetic derivative of kanamycin A, amikacin.

The spectrum of activity of kanamycin is similar to that of streptomycin (and includes *Mycob. tuberculosis*) but it retains activity against streptomycin-resistant strains and is less likely to cause vestibular damage. Kanamycin has largely been superseded by gentamicin and tobramycin (deoxykanamycin B), which are more active against many enterobacteria and, more importantly, *Ps. aeruginosa*. This has been a major factor in the popularity of these agents for the 'blind' therapy of serious infection before the results of laboratory tests are known. The relative merits of gentamicin and tobramycin have been the subject of much debate. Tobramycin appears to be marginally less toxic and slightly more active against *Ps. aeruginosa*; against other susceptible bacteria, gentamicin probably has the edge. Netilmicin (*N*-acetyl sisomicin) is said to be somewhat less toxic than its predecessors.

Other members of the kanamycin group, including sisomicin, dibekacin, micronomicin (gentamicin C2b), ribostamycin, and astromicin, are available in some countries. These aminoglycosides offer little advantage over gentamicin or tobramycin, although some have patterns of stability different from those of aminoglycoside-modifying enzymes (see 'Aminoglycosides' under 'Inactivation or modification mechanisms' in Chapter 11).

Amikacin and arbekacin are semi-synthetic aminoglycoside derivatives that were specifically developed to resist most aminoglycoside-modifying enzymes, although they have lower intrinsic activity than gentamicin or tobramycin. Amikacin is most widely used and is popular in units troubled by gentamicin resistance. Strains of bacteria that are resistant to gentamicin by non-enzymic mechanisms are cross-resistant to amikacin and other aminoglycosides.

## Spectinomycin

Spectinomycin is only used occasionally for the treatment of gonorrhoea in patients who are either hypersensitive to penicillin or infected with gonococci that are resistant to penicillin and other options (see 'Gonorrhoea' in Chapter 24).

## Chloramphenicol

Chloramphenicol was one of the first therapeutically useful antibiotics to appear from systematic screening of *Streptomyces* strains in the wake of the discovery of streptomycin in the 1940s. Although it is a naturally occurring compound, it is a relatively simple molecule and can readily be synthesized. Attempts to modify the structure have generally resulted in a marked loss of activity (thiamphenicol is an exception).

Pure chloramphenicol is very insoluble in water and tastes extremely bitter. These problems have been overcome by prodrug forms of the antibiotic: chloramphenicol palmitate and stearate to improve palatability, and chloramphenicol succinate to improve solubility for injection. These prodrugs lack antibacterial activity but serve to release chloramphenicol in the body; they should not be used for laboratory tests of bacterial sensitivity.

Chloramphenicol acts by inhibiting the peptidyl transferase reaction—the step at which the peptide bond is formed—on bacterial ribosomes (Fig. 3.1). The spectrum of activity embraces most Gram-positive and Gram-negative bacteria and also extends to chlamydiae and rickettsiae, strictly intracellular bacteria that cause a variety of infections, including trachoma, psittacosis, and typhus (Table 3.2).

The action of chloramphenicol against enterobacteria is largely bacteriostatic but, against some bacteria, including the Gram-positive cocci, it may display quite potent bactericidal activity. The drug also possesses the important properties of diffusing well into cerebrospinal fluid and of penetrating into cells—a very useful feature in the treatment of diseases such as typhoid, typhus, and other conditions where intracellular bacteria are involved. Resistance to chloramphenicol is generally uncommon, although resistant strains of the typhoid bacillus, *Salmonella enterica* serotype Typhi, cause serious problems in areas of the world where the disease is endemic.

**Table 3.2** Summary of the antibacterial spectrum of inhibitors of protein synthesis in common use.[a]

| Antibiotic | Staphylococci | Streptococci | Neisseria spp. | Haemophilus influenzae | Enterobacteria | Pseudomonas aeruginosa | Anaerobes | Rickettsiae and chlamydiae | Mycoplasmas |
|---|---|---|---|---|---|---|---|---|---|
| Aminoglycosides | Good | Poor | Fair | Fair | Good | Variable | – | – | Fair |
| Chloramphenicol | Good | Good | Good | Good | Good | Poor | Good | Good | Fair |
| Clindamycin | Very good | Good | – | – | – | – | Good | Fair | Variable |
| Fusidic acid | Very good | Fair | Good | – | – | – | Fair | – | – |
| Macrolides | Very good | Very good | Good | Good | – | – | Fair | Good | Variable |
| Mupirocin | Very good | Very good | Good | Good | – | – | – | – | – |
| Linezolid | Very good | Very good | Poor | Poor | – | – | Poor | .... | .... |
| Streptogramins | Very good | Very good | Good | Good | – | – | Fair | .... | .... |
| Tetracyclines | Good | Good | Good | Good | Good[b] | Poor | Fair | Good | Good |
| Tigecycline | Very good | Very good | Good | Good | Good[b,c] | Poor | Good | | |

[a] –, no useful activity; ...., no information; NB: individual strains of susceptible species may be resistant to any of these agents.

[b] Poor activity against *Proteus* spp., *Providencia* spp., and *Morganella* spp.

[c] Generally better anti-Gram-negative activity compared with other tetracyclines.

## Therapeutic use

Given its attractive qualities, it is a great pity that chloramphenicol displays one grave drawback: potentially fatal aplastic anaemia. This rare side effect has generally relegated chloramphenicol to the role of a reserve drug for use in life-threatening infections caused by bacteria resistant to safer compounds. It was once popular for the treatment of meningitis, including neonatal meningitis until another potentially fatal side effect of the antibiotic ('grey baby syndrome') may follow if the dosage is not properly adjusted. Because it is effective and cheap, chloramphenicol is still widely used in the developing world, especially for typhoid fever and meningitis. It is also commonly used as a topical agent for the treatment of bacterial conjunctivitis.

## Tetracyclines

The first tetracycline, chlortetracycline, was described in 1948 as a product of *Streptomyces aureofaciens*. Oxytetracycline and tetracycline itself (so-called because it lacks both the chlorine of chlortetracycline and the hydroxyl of oxytetracycline) quickly followed. These, and other members of the group, including demeclocycline, doxycycline, lymecycline, methacycline, and minocycline, are closely related structural variants of the same tetracyclic molecule. Tigecycline is a relatively new glycylcycline; it is a synthetic derivative of minocycline.

The tetracyclines exhibit a very broad spectrum, displaying good activity against most Gram-positive and Gram-negative bacteria (excluding *Proteus* spp., *Providencia* spp., *Morganella* spp., and *Ps. aeruginosa*), rickettsiae, chlamydiae, mycoplasmas, and spirochaetes (Table 3.2). They generally have similar antibacterial activity and are distinguished more by their pharmacokinetic behaviour. Of the older tetracyclines, doxycycline and minocycline are the most widely used. These derivatives are more completely absorbed when given orally and, unlike the others, they do not aggravate renal failure, so they can be used in patients suffering renal impairment; they also exhibit marginally better antibacterial activity and display sufficiently long serum half-lives to allow them to be given only once or twice daily. Tetracyclines should not be given to young children.

Susceptible bacteria concentrate tetracyclines by an active transport process. In the cell they interfere with the binding of aminoacyl tRNA to the A-site on the ribosome. Like chloramphenicol, the tetracyclines are predominantly bacteriostatic. The mechanism of the most common form of resistance is unusual in that a new protein is produced which appears to prevent uptake of the drug (see 'Tetracyclines' in Chapter 11). There is almost complete cross-resistance between tetracyclines, although minocycline and tigecycline may retain activity against some tetracycline-resistant strains.

Tigecycline is also active against some multiply resistant Gram-negative bacteria (e.g. *Acinetobacter* spp.), MRSA, anaerobes, and strains that are resistant to earlier compounds. It is only available as an intravenous formulation but achieves very modest blood concentrations largely because of its widespread penetration throughout the body (often referred to as a high volume of distribution; see Chapter 14).

The bacterial ribosome is the target for the tetracyclines. Binding to the 30S ribosomal subunit at the A-site blocks the entry of amino-acyl tRNA molecules into the ribosome, thus preventing the incorporation of amino acid residues into elongating peptide chains. Tigecycline binds to the 30S ribosomal subunit with higher affinity than the tetracyclines and interacts with another region of the A-site in an unusual way. These methods of action likely explain why tigecycline is active against strains with either of the two main mechanism of tetracycline resistance—ribosomal protection and drug efflux.

## Therapeutic use

The therapeutic importance of tetracyclines has declined over the years with the upsurge of resistant strains, particularly among enterobacteria and streptococci. The tetracyclines are still widely used for the treatment of respiratory infections, particularly chronic bronchitis and mycoplasma pneumonia, and in selected skin infections. Traditionally, they are the drugs of choice for rickettsial and chlamydial infections of all types, although use for the latter indication has been eroded by the newer macrolides (see 'Macrolides'). Tigecycline is used as a second or third line antibiotic to treat more difficult skin and soft-tissue or intra-abdominal infections, typically where broad-spectrum coverage is needed (but pseudomonas infection is not suspected). There is some evidence of increased mortality in patients with serious infections treated with tigecycline, which has led to it being used sometimes in combination with other antibiotics.

Tetracyclines are active against malaria parasites and some other protozoa. Doxycycline is sometimes used for antimalarial prophylaxis and in combination with quinine in the treatment of *Plasmodium falciparum* infections.

# Fusidic acid

Fusidic acid is the only therapeutically useful member of a group of naturally occurring antibiotics that display a steroid-like structure. The antibiotic prevents the translocation step in bacterial protein synthesis by inhibiting one of the substances (factor G) essential for this reaction.

Fusidic acid is active in vitro against Gram-positive and Gram-negative cocci, *Mycob. tuberculosis*, *Nocardia asteroides*, and many anaerobes; the ribosomes of Gram-negative bacilli are susceptible to the action of the drug but access is denied by the Gram-negative cell wall.

*Staphylococcus aureus* is particularly susceptible to fusidic acid, and the compound is usually regarded simply as an antistaphylococcal agent. It penetrates well into infected tissues, including bone, and it is favoured by some authorities for the treatment of staphylococcal osteomyelitis. A potential drawback is the presence in any large staphylococcal population of a small number of fusidic acid resistant variants that can proliferate during therapy. For this reason, fusidic acid is almost always administered together with another antibiotic (when given systemically), often a penicillin.

Fusidic acid is usually free from side effects when given orally. Intravenous administration of the diethanolamine salt is sometimes accompanied by a reversible jaundice. Topical preparations are available (e.g. to treat superficial skin infections) but their use is associated with the emergence of resistance.

# Macrolides

The earliest macrolide, erythromycin, was discovered in 1952 as a product of *Streptomyces erythreus*. This and related antibiotics share a similar molecular structure characterized by a 14-, 15-, or 16-membered macrocyclic lactone ring substituted with some unusual sugars. All members of the group are thought to act by causing the growing peptide chain to dissociate from the ribosome during the translocation step in bacterial protein synthesis.

Macrolides are most notable for their antistaphylococcal and antistreptococcal activity, though the spectrum encompasses other important pathogens, including chlamydiae, *Mycoplasma pneumoniae*, legionellae, and some mycobacteria; macrolides lack useful activity against enterobacteria and *Ps. aeruginosa* (Table 3.2). Resistance is common among staphylococci but less so in streptococci. However, resistant *Streptococcus pyogenes* strains are increasing in prevalence.

Macrolides have many attractive properties as well-tolerated oral compounds that display good tissue penetration. Their spectrum of activity makes them particularly suitable for the treatment of respiratory and soft-tissue disease and for infections caused by susceptible intracellular bacteria. They are also used in campylobacter enteritis if the severity of infection warrants antimicrobial treatment, and in *Legionella pneumophila* pneumonia.

## Erythromycin

Erythromycin, the oldest and most widely used macrolide antibiotic, was discovered at a time when resistance of staphylococci to penicillin was first becoming a serious problem. In the fear that its usefulness might be similarly compromised, it was at first used as a reserve antistaphylococcal agent or for streptococcal infections in patients allergic to penicillin.

Erythromycin base is broken down in the acid conditions of the stomach and it is administered in the form of enteric-coated tablets that protect the antibiotic until it reaches the absorption site in the duodenum. Alternatively, the stearate salt or esterified prodrug forms are used for oral administration. Two ester formulations are in general use: the ethylsuccinate and the estolate. Erythromycin lactobionate and erythromycin gluceptate are available for intravenous use. The estolate is generally regarded as the most toxic formulation because of its propensity to cause reversible cholestatic jaundice. However, this uncommon complication can arise with any of the preparations. Erythromycin is liable to cause nausea and abdominal cramps and this has diminished its popularity. Indeed, this side effect is used to an advantage in some patients in intensive care units to stimulate the bowel and thus to help excrete gut contents that would otherwise be retained by individuals who are paralysed and sedated.

## Erythromycin derivatives

Efforts to modify the properties of erythromycin have been more successful in generating compounds with improved pharmacological features rather than enhanced antibacterial activity. Much interest has centred on altering the molecule in such a way that the reactive groups responsible for the acid lability are modified. Such changes increase the bioavailability and often extend the plasma half-life. Any improvement in antibacterial activity is generally modest, but enhanced tissue penetration may render these compounds more effective. Acid-stable derivatives of erythromycin also appear to be less prone to cause gastrointestinal upset. Macrolides of this type include azithromycin, clarithromycin, dirithromycin, and roxithromycin.

## Azithromycin

Azithromycin has a considerably improved bioavailability and a much extended plasma half-life compared with erythromycin. The antibacterial spectrum is similar to that of erythromycin, although it is somewhat more active against some important respiratory pathogens such as *Haemophilus influenzae* and *L. pneumophila*; there is also some improvement in activity against enteric Gram-negative bacilli but this has very modest therapeutic benefit.

The most important property of azithromycin is the long terminal half-life, which enables it to be administered once a day. A single dose is effective in chlamydial and gonococcal infections of the genital tract. Increased used for these sexually transmitted infections has recently been associated with the occasional emergence of resistant *Neisseria gonorrhoeae* and *Chlamydia trachomatis* strains.

## Clarithromycin

This derivative of erythromycin is altered in the body to yield a metabolite that retains antibacterial activity but has altered pharmacokinetic properties. The activities of clarithromycin and its metabolite are similar to that of erythromycin, although concentrations required to inhibit legionellae and chlamydiae are generally lower.

There have been claims of much enhanced penetration into pulmonary sites, beneficial interactions between the parent compound and the metabolite, and other minor advantages. It is doubtful whether these translate into significantly improved therapeutic efficacy but clarithromycin is better absorbed and less prone to cause abdominal discomfort than earlier macrolides. It has been successfully used in combination regimens for the treatment of infections with *Helicobacter pylori* and some mycobacteria, notably those of the *Mycob. avium* group.

## Dirithromycin

Dirithromycin is slightly less active than erythromycin against most organisms within the spectrum but it has a much extended plasma half-life and has been successfully used for once-daily treatment of respiratory tract, skin, and soft-tissue infections.

## Roxithromycin

Roxithromycin is another erythromycin derivative and, not surprisingly, exhibits activity very similar to the older drug. It differs, however, in having an extended plasma half-life, a feature that may be related to extensive binding to plasma proteins.

## Ketolides

A new class of erythromycin derivatives, the ketolides, has been obtained by introducing a keto function into the macrolactone ring of erythromycin after removal of one of the sugars. These compounds share the Gram-positive spectrum of the earlier macrolides but retain activity against macrolide-resistant strains.

The only compound of this type presently available is telithromycin. However, its use has been restricted because of rare but serious reports of acute liver failure. Also, telithromycin may cause worsening of symptoms, including breathing problems, when taken by people with myasthenia gravis (a disease that causes muscle weakness).

## Other macrolides

Other macrolides that have been used in various parts of the world include oleandomycin (or its better absorbed derivative triacetyloleandomycin) and a series of compounds including spiramycin, josamycin, midecamycin, kitasamycin, and rokitamycin. None of these seems to offer much therapeutic advantage over erythromycin. Spiramycin is sometimes used as an alternative to pyrimethamine in infections caused by the protozoan parasite *Toxoplasma gondii*.

# Lincosamides

The original lincosamide, lincomycin, a naturally occurring product of *Streptom. lincolnensis*, has been superseded by clindamycin, which exhibits improved antibacterial activity. Lincosamides interfere with the process of peptide elongation in a way that has not been precisely defined. The ribosomal binding site is probably similar to that of erythromycin, since resistance to erythromycin caused by methylation of the ribosomal binding site also affects lincosamides.

Lincomycin and clindamycin possess good antistaphylococcal and antistreptococcal activity, and in vitro studies demonstrate reduced toxin release by producer strains even in the presence of low concentrations of clindamycin. This attribute has led to a niche use for this antibiotic, usually in combination, in serious staphylococcal and streptococcal infections thought to be mediated by toxin release (e.g. necrotizing fasciitis). Clindamycin has also proved therapeutically useful in the treatment of infections due to *Bacteroides fragilis* and some other anaerobes. Enterobacteria and

*Ps. aeruginosa* lie outside the spectrum of activity (Table 3.2). Clindamycin exhibits some activity against parasitic protozoa and has been used in toxoplasmosis, malaria, and babesiosis.

Clindamycin hydrochloride, like chloramphenicol, is extremely bitter. For oral administration, the drug is formulated in capsules or as the biologically inactive palmitate, which liberates the parent compound in vivo. Clindamycin phosphate, the soluble form used for intravenous administration, is similarly inactive in the test tube but is hydrolysed to the active drug in the body.

Patients treated with clindamycin (or lincomycin) sometimes experience diarrhoea caused by a clostridial toxin, which occasionally develops into a potentially fatal pseudomembranous colitis (see 'Antibiotic-associated diarrhoea and CDI' in Chapter 25). Other antibiotics, typically broad-spectrum penicillin, cephalosporins, and fluoroquinolones, may also cause this side effect.

## Streptogramins

Each member of the streptogramin family is not one antibiotic but two: they are produced as synergic mixtures by various species of *Streptomyces*. One of these compounds, virginiamycin, has been extensively used as a growth promoter in animal husbandry. Another streptogramin, pristinamycin, is sometimes used as an antistaphylococcal agent in some European countries but plasma concentrations after oral administration do not greatly exceed inhibitory levels, and solubility problems have militated against parenteral use. A formulation consisting of the water-soluble derivatives quinupristin and dalfopristin is, however, suitable for infusion and is now preferred for human therapy.

The two components of streptogramin antibiotics in combination are bactericidal. Component A causes distortion of the binding site for aminoacyl tRNA, thus hindering further growth of the peptide chain. It is thought that component B binds to an adjacent site and that the combined effect is to constrict the channel through which the nascent peptide is extruded from the ribosome. Protein synthesis is completely blocked and the consequences are lethal to the bacterial cell.

The activity of streptogramins is virtually restricted to Gram-positive organisms, including multiresistant staphylococci and some enterococci, notably *Enterococcus faecium*. Unfortunately, *E. faecalis*, which is more commonly encountered, is often resistant.

## Mupirocin

Mupirocin (formerly known as pseudomonic acid) is a component of the antibiotic complex produced by the bacterium *Ps. fluorescens*, and the novel structure of this inhibitor consists of monic acid with a short fatty acid side-chain. The terminal portion of the molecule distal to the fatty acid resembles isoleucine, and mupirocin inhibits protein synthesis by blocking the incorporation of this amino acid into polypeptides. The analogous process in mammalian cells is unaffected.

The spectrum of activity embraces staphylococci and streptococci but excludes most enteric Gram-negative bacilli (Table 3.2). Hopes that mupirocin might be useful in systemic therapy were thwarted by the realization that the compound is inactivated in the body. Consequently, its use is restricted to topical preparations. Mupirocin has proved particularly useful in the eradication or suppression of staphylococci (typically MRSA) from nasal carriage sites. However, resistance emergence occurs if the drug is used frequently, and especially if used on multiple occasions or for prolonged periods in patients with long-term colonization by MRSA.

## Oxazolidinones

Several oxazolidinones have attracted attention over the years owing to their activity against Gram-positive organisms, including staphylococci, pneumococci, and enterococci. They are very well absorbed by the oral route and exhibit bacteriostatic activity. They act at an early stage in protein synthesis by blocking the formation of the 70S initiation complex. A principal attraction of these compounds is that they do not show cross-resistance to other classes of drugs.

Linezolid has been available for over a decade, in both oral and intravenous formulations, and is an effective and useful agent in patients infected with multiresistant strains of staphylococci or other Gram-positive cocci. The drug is active against *Mycob. tuberculosis* and there is some evidence that it might be useful in infections with drug-resistant strains. The chief limitation of linezolid is an effect on bone marrow cells that largely limits the length of treatment to 2 weeks. Rare instances of peripheral or optic neuropathy have also been reported, typically associated with use longer than 2–4 weeks.

Resistance to linezolid has been slow to emerge and was limited to very occasional staphylococcal strains with ribosomal mutations. Resistance has been reported more commonly in coagulase-negative staphylococci and enterococci than in *Staph. aureus*. However, a worrying recent development has been reports of linezolid resistance in *Staph. aureus* strains; this resistance is mediated by the *cfr* gene, so named because it was originally noted to causes resistance to chloramphenicol and florfenicol (formerly in bacteria recovered from animals). Actually, *cfr* encodes a RNA methyltransferase that affects the binding of at least five chemically unrelated antimicrobial classes: phenicols, lincosamides, oxazolidinones, pleuromutilins (which, other than the topical agent, retapamulin, are not in clinical use at present), and streptogramin A antibiotics. As *cfr* can be transferred via plasmids, there is a risk of more widespread dissemination of this mode of resistance. Resistance to linezolid has also recently been associated with alterations to L3/L4 proteins.

Tedizolid is the most advanced (in the late stage of clinical trials) 'second generation' oxazolidinone. Tedizolid phosphate, in both oral and intravenous formulation, is a prodrug that is rapidly converted in vivo to microbiologically active tedizolid. Tedizolid interacts with the bacterial 23S ribosome initiation complex to inhibit translation and, like linezolid, is active against many Gram-positive pathogens, including linezolid-resistant *Staph. aureus*.

## Key points

- Gentamicin is a good all-purpose aminoglycoside for serious infections but streptococci, anaerobes, and intracellular organisms are not covered; plasma levels should be monitored.

- Tetracyclines still have a role in selected community-acquired respiratory tract and skin infections but must not be given to children because of teeth staining.

- Chloramphenicol is still widely used in the developing world given its low cost but has serious, albeit rare, side effects.

- Azithromycin is increasingly used as a single-dose treatment for chlamydial infections to ensure compliance.

- Linezolid is used as an oral (or intravenous) alternative to glycopeptides, particularly for the treatment of MRSA infection.

## Further reading

Finch, R.G., Greenwood, D., Norrby, S.R., and Whitley, R. J. (2010) *Antibiotic and Chemotherapy* (9th edn). London: Elsevier.

Chapter 4

# Synthetic antibacterial agents and miscellaneous antibiotics

## Introduction to synthetic antibacterial agents

Various targets other than the cell wall and ribosome are open to attack by chemotherapeutic agents. This chapter describes the properties of inhibitors of bacterial nucleic acid synthesis, compounds that act on the bacterial cell membrane, and agents used solely for the treatment of mycobacterial disease. Many of these compounds are synthetic chemicals rather than antibiotics in the strict sense.

## Inhibitors of nucleic acid synthesis

Given the universality of nucleic acid as the basis of life, it is surprising that so many antimicrobial agents have been discovered that selectively interfere with the functions of DNA and RNA. Some, like the sulphonamides and diaminopyrimidines, achieve their effect indirectly by interrupting metabolic pathways that lead to the manufacture of nucleic acids; others, of which the quinolones and nitroimidazoles are prime examples, exert a more direct action.

### Sulphonamides

The discovery of Prontosil in the 1930s was a major breakthrough in the chemotherapy of bacterial infections (see 'The foundations of modern chemotherapy' in Chapter 1). However, the emergence of resistant strains and the appearance of safer and more potent agents have relegated the sulphonamides to a minor place in therapy. Even in their traditional role, treating uncomplicated urinary infection, they are now seldom used. They are still found in combination products with trimethoprim, pyrimethamine, and other diaminopyrimidines (see 'Diaminopyrimidines').

Most bacteria synthesize folic acid and cannot take it up preformed from the environment. Mammalian cells, in contrast, use preformed folate and cannot make their own. Sulphonamides block an early stage in folate synthesis (Fig. 4.1), thus leading to a failure to synthesize purine nucleotides and thymidine. Sulphonamides have a broad antibacterial spectrum, although the activity against enterococci, *Pseudomonas aeruginosa*, and anaerobes is poor. These agents are relatively slow to act: several generations of bacterial growth are needed to deplete the folate pool before inhibition of growth occurs. Resistance emerges readily, and bacteria resistant to one sulphonamide are cross-resistant to the others.

### Diaminopyrimidines

Diaminopyrimidines inhibit dihydrofolate reductase, the enzyme that generates tetrahydrofolate (the active form of the vitamin) from metabolically inactive dihydrofolate (Fig. 4.1). Trimethoprim, the most important antibacterial agent of this type, exhibits far greater affinity for

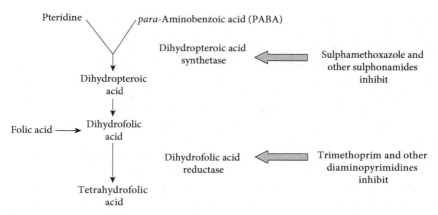

**Fig. 4.1** Mechanisms of action of sulphonamides and diaminopyrimidines.

the dihydrofolate reductase of bacteria than for the corresponding mammalian enzyme; this is the basis of the selective toxicity of the compound.

Since sulphonamides and trimethoprim act at different points in the same metabolic pathway, they interact synergically: bacteria are inhibited by much lower concentrations of the combination than by either agent alone. For this reason trimethoprim and sulphonamides have been combined in therapeutic formulations such as trimethoprim sulphamethoxazole, although trimethoprim alone is probably as effective and less toxic.

Trimethoprim is active in low concentration against many common pathogenic bacteria, although *Ps. aeruginosa* is a notable exception. Resistance is on the increase and the prevalence varies considerably between countries (see Fig. 23.3 in Chapter 23). The drug is rapidly absorbed from the gut and excreted almost exclusively by the kidneys, with a plasma half-life of about 10 hours.

The chief use for trimethoprim is in urinary tract infection. In the United Kingdom the use of this drug in combination with sulphamethoxazole (termed co-trimoxazole) declined greatly during the 1980s because of concern about life-threatening adverse effects (agranulocytosis and Stevens–Johnson syndrome). In the 1990s co-trimoxazole was principally used in pneumonia caused by the fungus *Pneumocystis carinii* (*Pne. jiroveci*; see '*P. jiroveci* (*P. carinii*)' in Chapter 8). However, co-trimoxazole has a relatively low risk of causing *Clostridium difficile* infection (see "Antibiotic-associated diarrhoea and CDI" in Chapter 25) and is available in both intravenous and oral formulations. In the past 10 years co-trimoxazole has been increasingly used in UK hospitals as an alternative to ciprofloxacin and broad-spectrum β-lactam antibiotics.

Analogues of trimethoprim, including tetroxoprim and brodimoprim, are marketed in combination with sulphonamides in some countries but offer few, if any advantages. Other diaminopyrimidines include the antimalarial agents pyrimethamine and proguanil (Chapter 9); the anti-pneumocystis agent trimetrexate; and the antineoplastic agent methotrexate.

## Quinolones

Nalidixic acid was the first representative to appear of a family of compounds that share close similarities of structure. During the 1980s a new series of quinolones were synthesized, known collectively as fluoroquinolones. These compounds, of which ciprofloxacin is a typical example, exhibit considerably enhanced activity.

All antibacterial quinolones act against the remarkable enzymes that are involved in maintaining the integrity of the supercoiled DNA helix during replication and transcription. Two enzymes are affected, DNA gyrase and topoisomerase IV, so that these drugs have a dual site of action. In Gram-negative bacilli the main target is DNA gyrase, with topoisomerase IV as a secondary site but, in *Staphylococcus aureus* and some other Gram-positive cocci, the situation is reversed. Quinolones are generally well tolerated but rashes and gastrointestinal disturbances may occur. Quinolones are antagonists of GABA (gamma-amino butyric acid) and should be used with caution in patients with epilepsy. GABA antagonism is also the mechanism for a pharmacodynamics drug interaction with non-steroidal anti-inflammatory drugs (NSAIDs), which can cause convulsions in patients with or without a history of epilepsy. These compounds affect the deposition of cartilage in experimental animals, and licensing authorities have cautioned against their use in children and pregnant women. Several promising fluoroquinolones have had to be withdrawn (e.g. temafloxacin and trovafloxacin) or have had their use restricted (moxifloxacin) because of unexpected toxicity.

All quinolones are well absorbed when taken by mouth and are more or less extensively metabolized in the body before being excreted into the urine.

Most Gram-negative bacteria, with the exception of *Ps. aeruginosa*, are susceptible to nalidixic acid and its early congeners, but Gram-positive organisms are usually resistant (Table 4.1). Susceptible bacteria readily develop resistance in the laboratory, and the emergence of resistance sometimes occurs during treatment, so these drugs are now rarely used in clinical practice. Fluoroquinolones are much more active than earlier derivatives against enterobacteria, *Ps. aeruginosa*, and many Gram-positive cocci (Table 4.1). The spectrum also includes certain problem organisms such as chlamydiae, legionellae, and some mycobacteria. Similar compounds, including enrofloxacin, danofloxacin, and sarafloxacin, have been introduced into veterinary practice and there has been considerable debate about the impact this may have had on the development of resistance.

The success of the first fluoroquinolones led to an intensive search for derivatives with further improved properties and this has borne fruit with several new agents now on the world market or at an advanced stage of development. These compounds are characterized by enhanced activity

**Table 4.1** Summary of spectrum of activity of quinolones available in the United Kingdom (as of 2013).

| Quinolone | Enterobacteria | *Pseudomonas aeruginosa* | Staphylococci | Streptococci | *Bacteroides fragilis* | Chlamydiae |
|---|---|---|---|---|---|---|
| **Narrow spectrum quinolones** | | | | | | |
| Nalidixic acid | Good | Poor | Poor | Poor | Poor | Poor |
| Norfloxacin | Very good | Good | Fair | Poor | Poor | Poor |
| **Fluoroquinolones** | | | | | | |
| Ciprofloxacin | Very good | Good | Fair | Fair | Poor | Poor |
| Levofloxacin | Very good | Good | Fair | Fair | Fair | Good |
| Moxifloxacin | Very good | Poor | Good | Good | Fair | Good |
| Ofloxacin | Very good | Good | Fair | Fair | Poor | Fair |

against Gram-positive cocci, including *Staph. aureus* and *Streptococcus pneumoniae* as well as chlamydiae and mycoplasmas; clinafloxacin, gatifloxacin, moxifloxacin, and trovafloxacin also have sufficient activity against anaerobes of the *Bacteroides fragilis* group to make treatment of infections with those organisms feasible. They are not reliably active against *Ps. aeruginosa*.

Fluoroquinolones are usually administered orally, although some, including ciprofloxacin, ofloxacin, and levofloxacin (the L-isomer of ofloxacin), can also be given by injection. Therapeutic dosages achieve relatively low concentrations in plasma but the compounds are well distributed in tissues and are concentrated within mammalian cells. The major route of excretion is usually renal, in the form of native compound or glucuronide and other metabolites, some of which retain antibacterial activity. Some fluoroquinolones, notably moxifloxacin, exhibit long terminal half-lives; these compounds are partly excreted by the biliary route and this may help to explain the long half-life.

Ciprofloxacin is the most widely used fluoroquinolone; among other indications, it is now the drug of choice for typhoid fever and other serious enteric diseases. The newer derivatives were targeted at the treatment of respiratory infections in the community and, although they are undoubtedly effective, there is no convincing evidence that they are more effective than other antibiotics. In contrast, there is growing evidence that use of fluoroquinolones in hospitals is associated with increased prevalence of *C. difficile* infection and MRSA infections. In addition, fluoroquinolone resistance is increasing rapidly in *Escherichia coli* in the community and in hospitals. Consequently many hospital and primary care antibiotic policies now restrict the use of fluoroquinolones. For primary care, European Surveillance of Antimicrobial Consumption (ESAC) has proposed that seasonal variation in fluoroquinolone use should be a quality indicator. The rationale for this is that fluoroquinolones should not be used for respiratory infections in primary care; consequently, winter use should be no greater than summer use.

## Nitroimidazoles (anaerobic infections only)

As a group, the imidazoles are remarkable in that derivatives are known which between them cover bacteria, fungi, viruses, protozoa, and helminths—in fact, the whole antimicrobial spectrum. The members of this family of compounds used as antibacterial agents are the 5-nitroimidazoles, of which metronidazole is best known. Related 5-nitroimidazoles include tinidazole and ornidazole, both of which share the properties of metronidazole but have longer plasma half-lives.

Metronidazole was originally used for the treatment of trichomoniasis and subsequently for two other protozoal infections—amoebiasis and giardiasis. The antibacterial activity of the compound was first recognized when a patient suffering from acute ulcerative gingivitis responded spontaneously while receiving metronidazole for a *Trichomonas vaginalis* infection. Anaerobic bacteria are commonly incriminated in gingivitis, and it was subsequently shown that metronidazole possesses potent antibacterial activity against strict anaerobes and also some micro-aerophilic bacteria, including *Gardnerella vaginalis* and *Helicobacter pylori*.

Metronidazole is so effective against anaerobic bacteria, and resistance to it is so uncommon, that it is now the drug of choice for the treatment of anaerobic infections. It is also commonly used for prophylaxis in some surgical procedures in which postoperative anaerobic infection is a frequent complication. It is an alternative to vancomycin in the treatment of (non-severe) antibiotic-associated colitis caused by *C. difficile* toxins (see 'Antibiotic-associated diarrhoea and CDI' in Chapter 25).

The basis of the selective activity against anaerobes resides in the fact that a reduction product is produced intracellularly at the low redox values attainable by anaerobes but not by aerobes.

The reduced form of metronidazole is thought to induce strand breakage in DNA by a mechanism that has not been precisely determined.

The 5-nitroimidazoles are generally free from serious side effects, although gastrointestinal upset is common and ingestion of alcohol induces a disulphiram-like reaction. Since these drugs act on DNA, they are potentially genotoxic and tumorigenic but there is no evidence that these problems have arisen despite widespread clinical use. Nonetheless, these compounds should not be used in pregnancy.

## Nitrofurans (nitrofurantoin)

A number of nitrofuran derivatives have attracted attention over the years, among which nitrofurantoin is much the most important. Others have very limited roles; for example, nifurtimox is only used in Chagas disease; (see 'Chagas disease' in Chapter 35).

Nitrofurantoin is the only nitrofuran derivative available in the United Kingdom. Its use is restricted to the treatment of lower urinary tract infection since it is rapidly excreted into urine after oral absorption, and the small amount that finds its way into tissues is inactivated there. It is active against most urinary tract pathogens but *Proteus* spp. and *Ps. aeruginosa* are usually resistant. The occurrence of resistant strains was uncommon but is becoming more prevalent with increasing use of nitrofurantoin. The mode of action of nitrofurantoin (or other nitrofurans) has not been precisely elucidated and is probably complex. The nitro group is reduced intracellularly in susceptible bacteria and it is likely that one effect, as with metronidazole, is the interaction of a reduction product with DNA.

## Rifamycins (rifampicin)

The clinically useful rifamycins, of which rifampicin (known in the United States as rifampin) is the most important, are semi-synthetic derivatives of rifamycin B, one of a group of structurally complex antibiotics produced by *Streptomyces mediterranei*. These compounds interfere with mRNA formation by binding to the β-subunit of DNA-dependent RNA polymerase. Resistance readily arises by mutations in the subunit. For this reason, the drugs are normally used in combination with other agents.

## Rifampicin

Rifampicin is one of the most effective weapons against two major mycobacterial scourges of mankind: tuberculosis and leprosy. It also exhibits potent bactericidal activity against a range of other bacteria, notably staphylococci and legionellae. Rifampicin is now often used in combination with other drugs in Legionnaires' disease and staphylococcal prosthetic device infections. It is also used as a single agent to eliminate meningococci from the throats of carriers and for the protection of close contacts of meningococcal and *Haemophilus influenzae* type b disease.

Rifampicin is well absorbed by the oral route, although it may also be given by intravenous infusion. Serious side effects are relatively uncommon but can be more troublesome when the drug is used intermittently, as it may be in antituberculosis regimens. Hepatotoxicity is well recognized and the antibiotic induces hepatic enzymes, thus leading to self-potentiation of excretion and the antagonism of some other drugs handled by the liver, including oral contraceptives. A potentially alarming side effect arising from the fact that rifampicin is strongly pigmented is the production of red urine and other bodily secretions; contact lenses may become discoloured. Patients should be warned of these potential problems.

Two other rifamycin derivatives (rifabutin and rifapentine) have a limited role in the treatment of infections caused by organisms of the *Mycobacterium avium* complex, which often cause disseminated disease in patients with cancer or acquired immune deficiency syndrome (AIDS).

# Macrocyclic Antibiotics

## Fidaxomicin

Fidaxomicin is a novel macrocyclic antibiotic that is licensed for the treatment of *Clostridium difficile* infection (CDI). It is poorly absorbed after oral administration and has a relatively narrow spectrum of activity that includes *Clostridia* spp. Fidaxomicin inhibits bacterial RNA polymerase but in a way that is distinct from other antibiotics. Reduced susceptibility has occasionally been described, due to mutations of RNA polymerase, but there is no evidence of cross-resistance with other antibiotics (such as rifamycins). Fidaxomicin reduces the risk of CDI recurrence from about 25% (seen after vancomycin treatment) to 13%. It is expensive to purchase but some of this higher cost may be offset by reduced recurrences. Hypersensitivity has been described in a few case reports.

# Agents affecting membrane function

## Polymyxins: pseudomonas infections only

The polymyxins are a family of compounds produced by *Bacillus polymyxa* and related bacteria. Only polymyxins B and E are used therapeutically. Polymyxin E is usually known by its alternative name, colistin. Structurally, the polymyxins are cyclic polypeptides with a long hydrophobic tail. They act like cationic detergents by binding to the cell membrane and causing the leakage of essential cytoplasmic contents. The effect is not entirely selective, and both polymyxin B and colistin exhibit considerable toxicity and so are not used for systemic therapy. They have a limited role in topical therapy such as in selective decontamination regimens (see 'Selective decontamination of the digestive tract' in Chapter 18 and 'Hospital-acquired pneumonia' in Chapter 21) and in cystic fibrosis, the latter by means of instillation of the drugs into the lungs of those suffering exacerbation of pseudomonal infection.

## Other membrane-active agents

Daptomycin, a semi-synthetic lipopeptide antibiotic not unlike the polymyxins in structure, has various effects on bacteria but the primary mode of action is thought to lie in the disruption of the cell membrane. Development of the compound in the 1980s was stopped because of fears of toxicity but the rise to prominence of multiresistant Gram-positive cocci revived commercial interest and it is now marketed for serious infections of the skin and soft tissues that are unresponsive to other agents, especially those caused by multiresistant staphylococci. Activity is restricted to Gram-positive cocci and is greatly enhanced in vitro by the presence of magnesium ions.

Antibiotics of the tyrothricin complex (gramicidin and tyrocidine), which are used in some topical preparations, are cyclic peptides that bind to the cell membrane and interfere with its function. These agents possess good activity against Gram-positive organisms but they also bind to mammalian cell membranes and are far too toxic to be used systemically in humans.

Toxicity also precludes the systemic use of the many disinfectants, including phenols, quaternary ammonium compounds, biguanides, and others, that achieve their antibacterial effect wholly or in part by interfering with the integrity of the cell membrane.

# Antimycobacterial agents

Compared with the number of agents at the disposal of the prescriber for the therapy of most bacterial infections, the resources available to treat mycobacterial disease are precariously meagre.

Part of the reason is that mycobacteria are unusual organisms with a relatively impermeable waxy coat but the fact that they are very slow growing and are able to survive and multiply within macrophages and necrotic tissue also makes them difficult targets.

In general, the development of drugs for the treatment of tuberculosis and leprosy has evolved along specialized lines but some important antimycobacterial agents, such as rifampicin and certain aminoglycosides (Chapter 3), have wider uses. Agents specifically used for the treatment of tuberculosis include isoniazid (isonicotinic acid hydrazide), pyrazinamide, ethambutol, and thiacetazone (thioacetazone). *para*-Aminosalicylic acid, which was formerly much used in antituberculosis regimens, is no longer recommended but this and other compounds with activity against *M. tuberculosis*, such as capreomycin, cycloserine, and viomycin, may be considered if first-line treatment fails. In leprosy, the most important agents (apart from rifampicin) are dapsone (or its prodrug, acedapsone) and clofazimine. The thioamides ethionamide and protionamide (prothionamide) are sometimes used but are hepatotoxic.

Some fluoroquinolones and macrolides display quite good activity against mycobacteria, including *M. leprae* and organisms of the *M. avium* complex, and these agents widen the options for treating mycobacterial disease at a time when resistance is emerging as a serious problem.

Because of the difficulties in studying mycobacteria in the laboratory, less is known about the mode of action of antimycobacterial drugs than about other antibacterial agents. Various theories have been put forward to explain the action of isoniazid. The most widely held view is that an oxidized product inhibits the formation of the mycolic acids that are peculiar to the cell walls of acid-fast bacilli. Other derivatives of nicotinic acid, including pyrazinamide, ethionamide, and protionamide, may act in the same way. Ethambutol probably inhibits the formation of arabinogalactan, a polysaccharide component of the mycobacterial cell wall. Dapsone (diaminodiphenyl sulphone) and *para*-aminosalicylic acid are related to the sulphonamides and have been assumed to share the same mode of action but this is by no means certain. The mode of action of the antileprosy agent clofazimine has not been determined but it may, like rifampicin, inhibit DNA-dependent RNA polymerase. Some puzzling aspects of the idiosyncratic spectrum of antimycobacterial agents may be explained by differences in uptake into susceptible cells.

Further information on these agents is given in the context of their use in Chapter 30.

## Key points

♦ Trimethoprim is used alone for uncomplicated cystitis.

♦ Co-trimoxazole use is increasing in some hospitals because of (1) its relatively low risk of causing *C. difficile* infection and (2) the availability of an intravenous formulation.

♦ Ciprofloxacin use is decreasing in hospitals and primary care because of concerns about growing resistance and association with *C. difficile* infection. In addition, it should not be used for community-acquired respiratory infections.

♦ Metronidazole is the drug of choice for anaerobic infections.

♦ Nitrofurantoin is useful for lower urinary tract infections and for prophylaxis against recurrent cystitis.

♦ Rifampicin is an essential component of regimens for the treatment of tuberculosis and leprosy, and also has a role in the treatment of selected staphylococcal infections.

♦ Fidaxomicin is a novel macrocyclic antibiotic that reduces the risk of CDI recurrence.

## Further reading

**Richman**, D. D., **Whitley**, R. J., **and Hayden**, F. G., **eds.** (2009) *Clinical Virology* (3rd edn). Washington, DC: ASM Press.

**Yin**, M. T., **Brust**, J. C. M., **Tieu**, H. V., **and Hammer**, S. M. (2009) 'Antiherpesvirus, anti-hepatitis virus, and anti-respiratory virus agents', in D. D. Richman, R. J. Whitley, and F. G. Hayden, eds, *Clinical Virology* (3rd edn). Washington, DC : ASM Press, pp. 217–64.

# Chapter 5

# Antiviral agents

## Introduction to antiviral agents

Viruses are almost as versatile as bacteria in the range of diseases they can cause. Vertebrates, insects, plants, and even bacteria are all open to attack. Some viruses of vertebrates (arboviruses) develop in and are transmitted by mosquitoes or other arthropods; others—rabies is a good example—can infect a wide range of mammalian hosts. In general, however, viruses are highly specific in their host range.

All viruses are obligate intracellular parasites; that is, they replicate only within living cells and cannot usually survive for long outside the host cell. Selectivity usually extends not only to the host but also to the type of cell within the host, as viruses only infect cells that express appropriate receptors on their surface. The preference of a virus for certain types of cell is known as the tropism of the virus and this often accounts for the characteristic clinical manifestations of particular viral infections. For example, some viruses preferentially infect liver cells, thereby giving rise to hepatitis.

Most viruses that infect man gain entry to the body by adsorption to superficial cells of the mucous membranes of the respiratory, intestinal, and genital tracts, or of the conjunctivae. Others may be swallowed in contaminated food or water and gain entry through the gastrointestinal tract or find their way in through damaged skin, insect bites, or direct inoculation. Intact skin is normally impermeable to viruses, although papilloma viruses are an exception, giving rise to warts.

Viruses may carry their genetic material (genome) in the form of RNA or DNA—but never both. Some antiviral drugs will only work against viruses which carry a particular type of genome, for example, drugs which act through inhibition of viral DNA polymerase enzymes will only have activity against DNA viruses. The principal types of virus causing human disease are listed, according to the nature of their genome, in Table 5.1.

## Properties of viruses

Viruses are deceptively simple. Sizes range from about 20 nm (parvovirus) to 300 nm (poxvirus); consequently, even the biggest viruses fall barely within the limits of resolution of conventional light microscopy, and the electron microscope must be used to visualize them.

Complete virus particles (virions) consist of a nucleic acid core (the viral genome), surrounded by a few proteins, and possibly a lipid envelope. The nucleic acid may be DNA or RNA (never both), single or double stranded, circular or linear, and continuous or segmented. This provides all the information needed for viral replication once it is released within the host cell. The proteins encoded by the genome serve a number of functions. The capsid, or protein coat surrounding the nucleic acid, consists of repeating structural units made up of one to three different protein molecules that are generally arranged in helical or icosahedral symmetry. The nucleic acid surrounded by its capsid is referred to as the nucleocapsid of the virus. Many viral proteins have enzymatic properties. These include polymerases and proteases that are necessary for the replication and

**Table 5.1** Principal types of virus causing human disease.

| Family | Examples | Diseases | Mode of transmission |
|---|---|---|---|
| **RNA viruses** | | | |
| Orthomyxoviruses | Influenza A and B viruses | Influenza | Respiratory |
| Paramyxoviruses | Mumps virus | Mumps | Respiratory |
| | Measles virus | Measles | |
| | Respiratory syncytial virus | Bronchiolitis (especially babies) | |
| | Human metapneumovirus | Bronchiolitis (especially babies) | |
| | Parainfluenza viruses | Croup; bronchiolitis (especially babies) | |
| Rhabdoviruses | Rabies virus | Rabies | Bite of rabid animal |
| Arenaviruses | Lassa virus | Lassa fever | Respiratory/rodent reservoir |
| Filoviruses | Ebola, Marburg | Acute haemorrhagic fever | Direct contact |
| Togaviruses | Rubella virus | German measles (rubella) | Respiratory/congenital |
| Flaviviruses | Many arboviruses | Yellow fever | Arthropod vectors |
| | Hepatitis C virus | Hepatitis | Inoculation |
| Picornaviruses | Enteroviruses: | Meningitis; paralysis; | Faecal–oral/respiratory |
| | Polio | | |
| | Echo | | |
| | Coxsackie A and B | | |
| | Hepatitis A virus | hepatitis; | |
| | Rhinoviruses | colds | |
| Hepeviruses | Hepatitis E | Hepatitis | Faecal–oral |
| Retroviruses | Human immunodeficiency viruses | AIDS | Sexual/inoculation/ vertical |
| | Human T-cell lymphotropic viruses | T-cell leukaemia; lymphoma | Inoculation/sexual/ vertical |
| Reoviruses | Rotavirus | Infantile diarrhoea | Faecal–oral |
| Caliciviruses | Norovirus (Norwalk virus) | Gastroenteritis | Faecal–oral |
| Coronaviruses | Middle East respiratory syndrome coronavirus (MERS-CoV) | Colds; lower respiratory tract infection | Respiratory |

(continued)

**Table 5.1** (continued).

| Family | Examples | Diseases | Mode of transmission |
|---|---|---|---|
| **DNA viruses** | | | |
| Poxviruses | Variola | Smallpox (now eradicated) | Mainly respiratory |
| | Vaccinia | Smallpox vaccine | Vaccination |
| | Molluscum contagiosum | Skin disease | Contact |
| | Orf | Skin disease | Contact with sheep |
| Herpesviruses | Herpes simplex virus types 1 and 2 | Cold sores; genital herpes | Saliva/contact/sexual |
| | Varicella zoster | Chickenpox; shingles | Respiratory |
| | Cytomegalovirus | Non-specific illness; congenital infection | Close contact/kissing/ transplacental |
| | Epstein–Barr virus | Glandular fever | Saliva (e.g. kissing) |
| | Human herpesvirus type 6 | Roseola infantum (sixth disease) | Saliva |
| | Human herpesvirus type 7 | Not known | Saliva |
| | Human herpesvirus type 8 | Kaposi's sarcoma | Sexual |
| Adenoviruses | Many serotypes | Conjunctivitis; pharyngitis; infantile diarrhoea | Respiratory |
| Papillomaviruses | Human papillomaviruses (HPVs) | Cervical cancer; warts | Contact |
| Polyomaviruses | JC, BK viruses | Progressive multifocal leukoencephalopathy; BK nephropathy | Faecal–oral/respiratory |
| Hepadnaviruses | Hepatitis B virus | Hepatitis | Inoculation/sexual/ vertical |
| Parvoviruses | Parvovirus B 19 | Erythema infectiosum (fifth disease) | Respiratory |

assembly of viral particles. Proteins protruding from the surface coat of the virus act as ligands that will bind to cellular receptors during the first stage of infection of a cell. The lipid envelope possessed by some viruses is derived from membranes of the host cell.

## Targets for antiviral drugs

Virus infection of and replication within cells proceeds via a number of distinct steps, each of which, theoretically, provides a possible target for attack (Fig. 5.1).

Although the exact details of these steps vary between different viruses, they can be broadly summarized as follows:

- ◆ Attachment to the cell surface. This involves a specific interaction between proteins (ligands) on the surface of the virus, with receptors on the surface of the cell. The nature of the viral ligands and cellular receptors is known in great detail for some viruses (e.g. the gp120 of

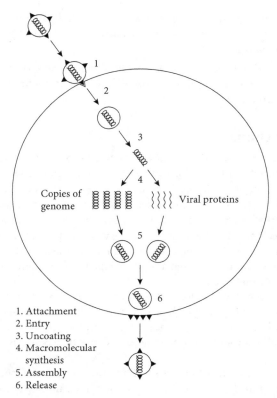

**Fig. 5.1** Schematic representation of the virus replication cycle within the host cell, showing the stages that are theoretically open to inhibition by antiviral agents.

human immunodeficiency virus (HIV) and the CD4 molecule on T lymphocytes) but not at all for others.

♦ Entry into the host cell. Some viruses can enter cells by fusion of their own outer lipid membrane with the plasma membrane of the cell, resulting in the release of the viral nucleocapsid into the cell cytoplasm. Others may be endocytosed into the cell. For some viruses, the process of translocation of the viral particle from the outside of the cell to the inside is very poorly understood.

♦ Uncoating of the viral genome. The viral nucleic acid must be released from its capsid before replication. This process may be mediated by cellular lysosomal enzymes.

♦ Macromolecular synthesis. Within the cell, multiple copies of the viral genome are made, and mRNA derived from the virus is translated into multiple copies of the proteins encoded by the viral genome. Many viruses use enzymes present within the host cell to perform these activities but some carry their own enzymes for certain synthetic processes that are not present within the host cell. A good example is HIV, which copies its RNA genome into a DNA intermediate. Since host cells are not able to convert RNA into DNA, the necessary reverse transcriptase must be encoded by the HIV genome itself, and the enzyme carried into the cell within the viral particle.

- ◆ Assembly. Before final assembly into new viral particles, viral polyproteins may be digested by viral protease enzymes, and individual proteins may be modified by host-cell processes such as glycosylation or phosphorylation.

- ◆ Release. The infected cell has by now become little more than a viral factory, and complete viral particles may be released by destruction of the cell or by continuous export via budding through the cell membrane.

## Virus–cell interactions

The viral replication cycle described above is representative of an acute viral infection: virus enters the cell, replicates, disrupts normal cellular function, and is released, often resulting in cell death. However, viruses may interact with cells in other ways. Some viruses can undergo latency within cells: the viral genome is present within the cell, usually as an episome within the cell nucleus, but no replication of the genome occurs and few, if any, viral proteins are synthesized. The latent virus may cause the cell no harm but it has the propensity, under certain conditions, to become reactivated, with consequent viral replication and damage to the cell. All herpesviruses undergo latency, one consequence of which is that, once individuals become infected with a herpesvirus, they remain infected for their lifetime.

Another form of virus–cell interaction is chronic or persistent infection. In this, there is a steady production and release of virus but the host cell is able to survive. However, host-cell function may be impaired, and the expression of viral antigens on the cell surface can lead to a chronic inflammatory state, as in chronic infection of hepatocytes with hepatitis B or C viruses leading to chronic hepatitis.

A further potential consequence of virus–cell interaction is transformation, whereby virus infection leads to uncontrolled cell division, resulting in an immortal cell line. For example, Epstein–Barr virus infection of B lymphocytes in vitro results in stimulation of cell division, and the establishment of a continuous lymphoblastoid cell line. The molecular mechanisms underlying this process, and possible means of interfering with them, are of great interest, since several viruses, including Epstein–Barr virus, have been implicated in initiating malignant change in vivo.

## Limitations of antiviral therapy

Although all stages of the cycle of virus replication are potential targets for antiviral drugs, the intimate relationship between the virus and its host cell means that the design or discovery of compounds that are selectively toxic for the virus is beset with considerable problems. Moreover, antiviral therapy may be at a disadvantage for quite a different reason: in many viral diseases, initial infection and spread is commonly asymptomatic, and the onset of illness, often at the peak of viral multiplication, occurs when the host defences have been fully mobilized. Unless the patient is immunodeficient in some way, these defences are usually quite able to deal with the infection unassisted. Consequently, initiation of antiviral therapy at the onset of symptoms may have little influence on the course of the disease.

Viruses that undergo latency pose a further problem. Unless the latently infected cells can be killed or removed, the virus cannot be eliminated from the patient. Achieving such elimination by therapeutic intervention is a daunting task, as there are no virus-specific metabolic processes occurring in those cells, and there is no expression of viral antigens on the cell surface against which an immune response could be mounted.

Despite these discouraging considerations, significant progress has been achieved in the development of antiviral compounds, and an increasing number of antiviral agents is now in regular

**Table 5.2** Principal antiviral agents in present use.[a]

| Compound | Indication | Mode of action | Route of administration |
|---|---|---|---|
| Aciclovir | Herpes simplex; varicella-zoster | Nucleoside analogue | Oral; topical; intravenous |
| Amantadine | Influenza A | Uncoating of virus | Oral |
| Brincidofovir | Cytomegalovirus | Nucleotide analogue[b] | Oral |
| Cidofovir | Cytomegalovirus | Nucleotide analogue | Intravenous |
| Famciclovir | Herpes simplex; varicella-zoster | Nucleoside analogue[b] | Oral |
| Fomivirsen | Cytomegalovirus | Antisense oligonucleotide | Intra-ocular |
| Foscarnet | Cytomegalovirus | DNA polymerase inhibitor | Intravenous |
| Ganciclovir | Cytomegalovirus | Nucleoside analogue | Intravenous |
| Palivizumab | Respiratory syncytial virus | Monoclonal anti-respiratory syncytial virus (RSV) antibody | Intramuscular |
| Ribavirin | Respiratory syncytial virus | Nucleoside analogue | Nebulizer |
| | Chronic hepatitis C | | Oral |
| Valaciclovir | Herpes simplex; varicella-zoster | Nucleoside analogue[b] | Oral |
| Valganciclovir | Cytomegalovirus | Nucleoside analogue[b] | Oral |
| Oseltamivir | Influenza | Neuraminidase inhibitor | Oral |
| Zanamivir | Influenza | Neuraminidase inhibitor | Inhalation |

[a] Other than anti-HIV agents (see Chapter 6) and agents used in the treatment of viral hepatitis (see Chapter 7).

[b] Prodrug formulation.

use (Table 5.2). Many are nucleoside analogues that interfere with viral replication but other targets have been successfully exploited. Much research emphasis has been concentrated on agents that act to inhibit the replication of HIV, and on the development of effective therapies for the treatment of chronic viral hepatitis. Antiviral drugs used in the treatment of these two conditions are discussed in Chapters 6 and 7 respectively.

## Properties of antiviral agents

### Aciclovir

Aciclovir was the first antiviral drug with selective toxicity: it inhibits the replication of certain viruses while exhibiting virtually no toxic side effects on host cells. Structurally, it is acycloguanosine (Fig. 5.2), an analogue of the purine nucleoside, guanosine, in which the deoxyribose moiety has lost its cyclic configuration. Aciclovir itself is inactive; in order to achieve its antiviral effect, it must first be phosphorylated on the 5′-hydroxyl group to the triphosphate form within the infected cell. Although the second and third phosphate groups are added by cellular enzymes, the initial phosphorylation step is accomplished by a viral thymidine kinase specified by herpes simplex and varicella zoster viruses; the cellular form of this enzyme is much less efficient in producing aciclovir monophosphate. This unique feature contributes significantly to the selective

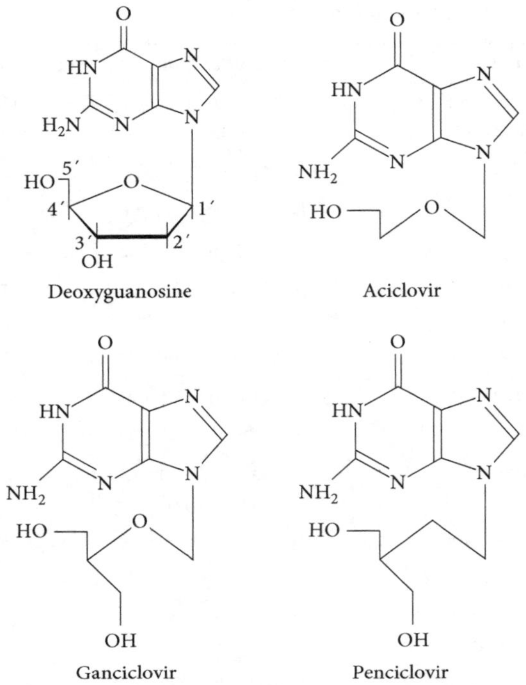

**Fig. 5.2** Structures of deoxyguanosine and three antiviral agents that act as analogues of the nucleoside: aciclovir, ganciclovir, and penciclovir.

toxicity of aciclovir, for two reasons: first, it means that the active form of the drug is produced only in virally infected cells; second, by the law of mass action, once the equilibrium

aciclovir ↔ aciclovir monophosphate

is shifted to the right within an infected cell, more free aciclovir will enter the cell from the extracellular space, thus resulting in concentration of the drug precisely where it is needed: in the infected cell.

## Mode of action

As an analogue of guanosine triphosphate, aciclovir triphosphate will compete with it for incorporation into a growing DNA chain. Incorporation results in chain termination, since it lacks the 3'-hydroxyl group necessary to form the 5'–3' phosphodiester linkage with the next base. Viral DNA polymerase enzymes bind aciclovir triphosphate with a much greater affinity than do the corresponding cellular enzymes. This preferential binding creates a third level of antiviral selectivity, as aciclovir triphosphate acts as a direct inhibitor of viral DNA polymerase.

## Resistance

It is theoretically possible for a virus to become resistant to aciclovir in several ways:

◆ viral strains that lack the thymidine kinase enzyme and which are thus known as TK⁻ variants are inherently resistant to the drug, as they cannot generate the active form;

◆ mutations in the *TK* gene may alter the thymidine kinase molecule, such that it becomes unable to perform the first phosphorylation step; and

◆ mutations in the viral DNA polymerase gene may reduce the ability of the enzyme to bind aciclovir triphosphate and thereby to escape the inhibitory properties of the drug.

All these mechanisms occur in the laboratory and in nature. However, TK⁻ strains and those with altered thymidine kinases exhibit reduced virulence, and DNA polymerase mutants are the ones that cause most clinical difficulties. These emerge particularly in immunocompromised patients, including those with HIV infection, in whom recurrent herpes simplex virus infections cause frequent and extensive disease necessitating prolonged treatment with aciclovir.

Aciclovir represents a prime example of what a good antiviral drug should be. It has potent antiviral activity but is virtually free of toxic side effects. It can be life-saving in certain infections and in others can significantly decrease morbidity (see Chapter 32). However, it is relatively poorly absorbed when given orally and, in life-threatening infection, it must be given intravenously.

## Analogues of aciclovir and other anti-herpes drugs in development

Several structural analogues of aciclovir have been developed. Valaciclovir, the L-valyl ester of aciclovir, is an oral prodrug that is well absorbed when given by mouth to release aciclovir into the bloodstream. A similar relationship exists between famciclovir and penciclovir: the former is metabolized into the latter after oral administration. Penciclovir (Fig. 5.2) exhibits antiviral activity very similar to that of aciclovir but the half-life within cells is considerably longer, so fewer doses are necessary to achieve an antiviral effect.

Despite the success of aciclovir and its derivatives, efforts have continued to develop other drugs with different modes of action. One such promising compound is pritelivir, an inhibitor of the herpes simplex helicase–primase complex, which unwinds viral double-stranded DNA, an essential step before DNA replication can occur. Extensive in vitro and animal model data showing the efficacy of this compound have now been backed up by the first clinical trial data, which show unequivocally that this drug reduces the rate of genital herpes simplex virus shedding in otherwise healthy men and women with genital herpes. Pritelivir does not require activation by phosphorylation.

Although aciclovir and its analogues are undoubtedly successful antiviral drugs, their clinical usefulness is limited by their narrow spectrum of activity. They are active only against a subgroup of herpesviruses—herpes simplex and varicella zoster viruses—that can perform the first phosphorylation step. It is particularly disappointing that these otherwise excellent drugs have no activity against cytomegalovirus, a herpesvirus that does not encode its own thymidine kinase enzyme.

## Ganciclovir

Ganciclovir (dihydroxypropoxymethylguanine (DHPG); Fig. 5.2) is a derivative of aciclovir that shows useful activity against cytomegalovirus, an opportunist pathogen that causes severe and even life-threatening disease in immunosuppressed patients such as transplant recipients and HIV-infected individuals. Ganciclovir must be activated by phosphorylation but cytomegalovirus uses a virally encoded phosphotransferase enzyme, encoded by the gene UL97, which differs from the thymidine kinase in herpes simplex or varicella zoster. Subsequent phosphorylation to the triphosphate generates a compound that acts as a viral DNA polymerase inhibitor.

Unfortunately, cellular enzymes also phosphorylate ganciclovir, so the active drug is generated in uninfected cells. Thus, the toxicity of ganciclovir is considerably greater than that of aciclovir. The most frequent unwanted effects, leucopenia and thrombocytopenia, arise from a toxic effect on the bone marrow, particularly affecting the production of neutrophils. Ganciclovir treatment can also result in a rise in serum creatinine. It is poorly absorbed (<10%) when given orally and has to be administered intravenously. The valyl ester of ganciclovir, valganciclovir, is much better absorbed orally (40%), and serum concentrations are close to those arising from intravenous ganciclovir therapy. Despite its drawbacks, ganciclovir can be sight- or life-saving in immunosuppressed patients with severe cytomegalovirus infections (see 'Cytomegalovirus' in Chapter 32).

Resistance to ganciclovir through point mutations in the UL97 phosphotransferase gene arises fairly commonly in clinical practice. Fortunately, the viral mutants remain sensitive to foscarnet (see 'Foscarnet'). Although less common, mutations in the cytomegalovirus DNA polymerase gene UL54 may also confer resistance, and such viruses may also be cross-resistant to foscarnet and cidofovir (see Cidofovir).

## Cidofovir

The difficulty in achieving the first phosphorylation step of aciclovir-like compounds is avoided by the use of acyclic nucleoside phosphonates, a class of compounds of which cidofovir (Fig. 5.3) was the first to be developed and licensed for clinical use. The phosphonate group acts as a phosphate mimetic and is attached to the acyclic nucleoside moiety through a stable P—C bond that cannot be split by cellular hydrolases. These agents need only two phosphorylation steps to reach the active triphosphate form, and cellular enzymes perform these steps. Thus, active drug may arise in both infected and uninfected cells but a selective antiviral activity is maintained since the triphosphate exhibits a higher affinity for viral DNA polymerases than for the corresponding cellular enzymes. Like aciclovir triphosphate, the drugs act as chain terminators and competitive inhibitors.

Cidofovir is an acyclic cytosine analogue, with potent activity against cytomegalovirus. It is administered by intravenous infusion in the treatment of cytomegalovirus retinitis. It has a prolonged half-life such that dosing is required only once a week or less. It is a substrate of organic ion transporter 1, which acts to concentrate the drug in renal proximal tubules, resulting in significant nephrotoxicity in a dose-dependent manner, and therefore it must be administered with probenecid to prevent irreversible renal damage. Brincidofovir, formerly known as CMX001, is a promising derivative of cidofovir which shows much greater antiviral potency in vitro. The cidofovir molecule is bound to a lipid moiety and in this form is not recognized by organic ion transporter 1, thereby reducing the risk of renal toxicity. Brincidofovir is orally bioavailable, and after cellular uptake, undergoes cleavage of the lipid moiety and phosphorylation to cidofovir triphosphate. Clinical trial data demonstrating the effectiveness of brincidofovir have recently been published.

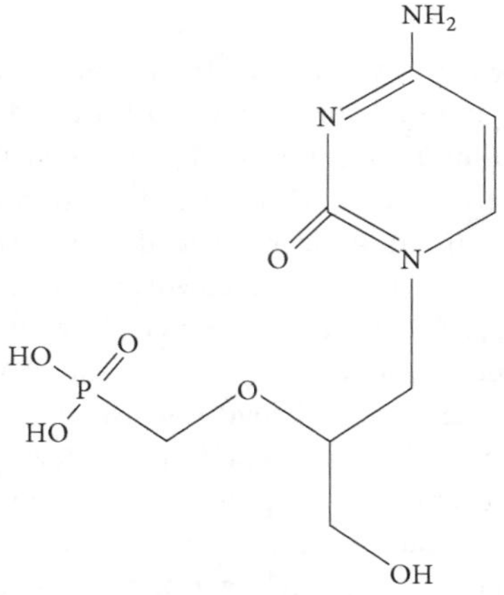

**Fig. 5.3** Structure of cidofovir.

The mechanism of action of this class of drugs raises the possibility that they may have a much broader spectrum of activity than aciclovir and its derivatives, potentially against all viruses with a DNA polymerase function. Cidofovir is indeed active against all herpesviruses, as well as adeno, polyoma-, papilloma-, and poxviruses, although clinical use in these infections is limited by drug toxicity. However, other class members such as adefovir and tenofovir have useful inhibitory activity against either or both the reverse transcriptase of HIV, and the DNA polymerase of hepatitis B virus (see 'Other nucleos(t)ide analogues' in Chapter 6 and see 'Tenofovir' and 'Adefovir' in Chapter 7). This class of drugs thus offers great promise for the treatment of a wide range of virus infections.

In theory, resistance to cidofovir and its congeners may arise through mutations in the viral DNA polymerases, and time will tell how much of a problem this will become.

## Foscarnet

Unlike the drugs discussed so far, foscarnet (Fig. 5.4) is not a nucleoside analogue; it is trisodium phosphonoformate, a derivative of phosphonoacetic acid, and is therefore a pyrophosphate analogue. It does not require phosphorylation. It forms complexes with DNA polymerases and prevents cleavage of pyrophosphate from nucleoside triphosphates, resulting in inhibition of further DNA synthesis. It shows some selective toxicity for viral rather than host-cell enzymes and is active against all the herpesviruses, including cytomegalovirus. It is used as an alternative to ganciclovir in the treatment of serious cytomegalovirus infection, as well as in the treatment of aciclovir-resistant herpes simplex infection. Like ganciclovir, oral bioavailability is poor and it has to be administered by intravenous injection. It is nephrotoxic and can cause acute renal failure. Other side effects include symptomatic hypocalcaemia, and penile ulceration.

## Fomivirsen

Fomivirsen is an oligonucleotide, 21 bases in length. It is not marketed in the European Union but is available in some countries for the treatment of cytomegalovirus retinitis by intravitreous injection. It is an antisense molecule: the mirror image of a section of cytomegalovirus-derived mRNA encoding regulatory proteins. Binding of the drug to this region prevents translation of the RNA into protein.

## Ribavirin

Ribavirin is a synthetic nucleoside in which ribose is linked to a triazole derivative (Fig. 5.5). Like other nucleoside analogues, it has to be activated intracellularly by phosphorylation. The precise mode of action has proved elusive, though there are several theories including the possibilities that it inhibits an essential step (5' capping) in the processing of viral mRNA or that it causes lethal mutations in viral nucleotides.

Ribavirin has an unusually broad spectrum of activity, against both RNA and DNA viruses, at least in vitro. Its main use is in the treatment of severe lower respiratory tract infection, caused by respiratory syncytial virus, in young children. The compound is administered via inhalation of an aerosolized solution. Oral ribavirin has also been used successfully in the treatment of Lassa fever.

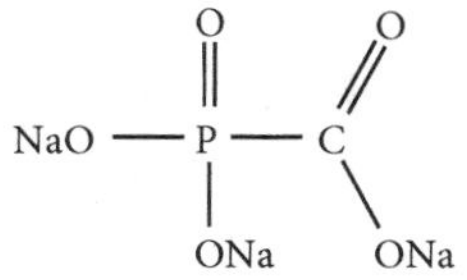

**Fig. 5.4** Structure of foscarnet.

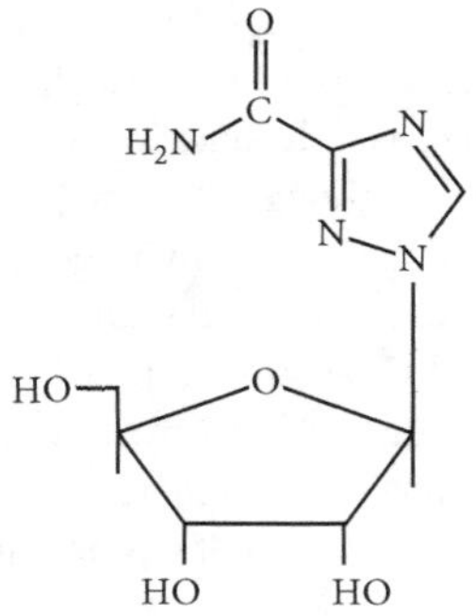

**Fig. 5.5** Structure of ribavirin.

Although ribavirin itself is ineffective in the treatment of chronic hepatitis C, combination therapy with interferon (especially peginterferon; see Chapter 7) produces a considerable improvement in response rates compared with the use of interferon alone.

The most commonly encountered serious side effect of prolonged ribavirin use is haemolytic anaemia.

## Older nucleoside analogues

Nucleoside analogues have been used for many years as antiviral agents but the older ones are very toxic and have been eclipsed by later developments. Idoxuridine and trifluridine are still available in many countries for topical application in recurrent herpes simplex infections but are no longer recommended. Cytarabine (cytosine arabinoside; ara-C) and vidarabine (adenine arabinoside; ara-A) are cytotoxic drugs of limited availability that are sometimes used as agents of last resort in life-threatening and otherwise untreatable viral infections.

## Amantadine and rimantadine

Amantadine (Fig. 5.6) is a tricyclic amine derivative of adamantane, a compound that originally aroused interest because of its symmetrical three-dimensional structure, which is composed entirely of carbon atoms and is thus related to the crystalline array of natural diamonds. The antiviral activity of amantadine was first described in 1964. Rimantadine is a closely related substance that is available in some countries.

The activity of both amantadine and rimantadine is restricted to influenza A virus. Other influenza viruses are virtually unaffected at therapeutically achievable concentrations. These compounds block a viral matrix protein ion channel, thereby interfering with the uncoating of

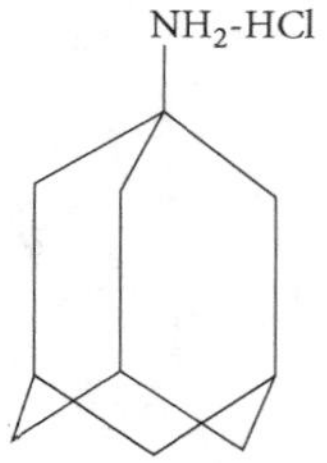

**Fig. 5.6** Structure of amantadine.

the viral nucleic acid within the infected cell. Resistance readily arises by mutation in the matrix protein, which is then unable to bind the drugs.

Amantadine has dopaminergic effects and may cause restlessness, insomnia, agitation, and confusion, especially in the elderly, one of the groups who stand to benefit most from an effective anti-influenza drug. Rimantadine gives rise to fewer side effects and is generally favoured in countries where it is available.

Combination therapy of amantadine with interferon has been used in patients with chronic hepatitis C virus infection, but ribavirin plus interferon is more effective and is now preferred. Amantadine is also licensed in the United Kingdom for use in shingles but this has few advocates.

## Oseltamivir and zanamivir

These drugs belong to a class of anti-influenza compounds that selectively inhibit viral neuraminidase, one of the two proteins (the other being haemagglutinin) present on the surface of all types of influenza viruses. Viral neuraminidase enables budding influenza virus particles to break away from an infected cell by hydrolysing the cellular sialic acid residues to which the haemagglutinin binds. It may also facilitate the passage of virus particles through mucus to reach epithelial cell surfaces, thereby aiding infection of new cells. Oseltamivir and zanamivir act extracellularly to inhibit the release and propagation of infectious influenza viruses from the epithelial cells of the respiratory tract. Unlike amantadine, they act against both influenza A and B viruses and inhibit all the known neuraminidase subtypes of influenza A viruses. Oseltamivir is administered by mouth, while zanamivir is formulated for oral inhalation. They appear to be generally safe but zanamivir occasionally causes bronchospasm in patients with underlying lung disease.

These drugs bind to the active site of neuraminidase, which is highly conserved among different strains of influenza virus. Oseltamivir has a more bulky side chain than zanamivir (see Fig. 5.7). High-level resistance to oseltamivir may arise through a single point mutation (H275Y) within its binding site, although such viruses remain sensitive to zanamivir. New neuraminidase inhibitors are in development, including peramivir.

## Interferon

Interferon (IFN) was described in 1957 as an antiviral compound in chick embryo cells. The antiviral activity is associated with a family of species-specific glycosylated proteins produced in vivo in response to viral or antigenic challenge. When IFNs were discovered, they were hailed as the antiviral equivalent of penicillin. As these substances were produced by cells as a natural defence in response to a wide range of virus infections, it seemed reasonable to imagine that, when used as therapeutic agents, they would exhibit a broad antiviral spectrum, and that their toxic effects on host cells would be minimal. However, clinical trials of IFNs as a treatment for a range of viral infections have in general been disappointing, with the notable exception of their use in the management of patients with chronic hepatitis B or C infection. IFNs are therefore discussed in more detail in Chapter 7.

# Prevention of virus infections

Prevention rather than cure plays such an important part in the control of viral diseases that an appreciation of the methods used is essential to understanding the complementary role of antiviral agents. The scourge of smallpox has been removed by appropriate use of vaccinia vaccine and

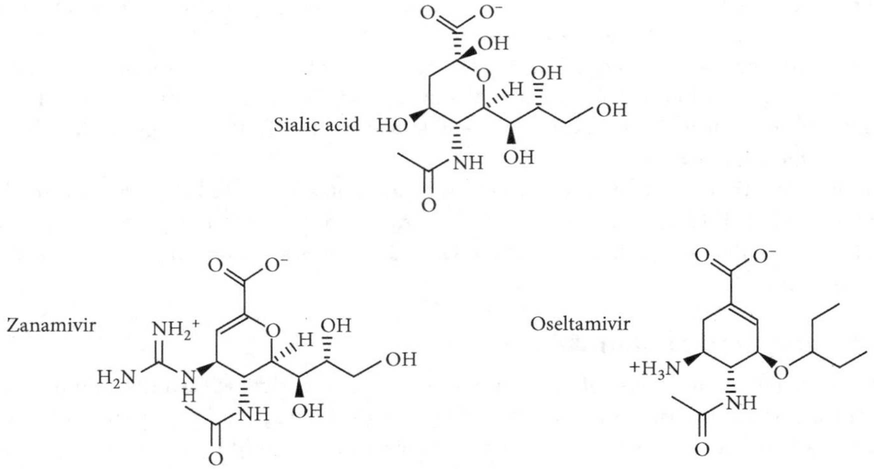

**Fig. 5.7** Structure of sialic acid, zanamivir, and oseltamivir.

Adapted from *Journal of Clinical Virology*, Volume 41, Issue 1, Ferrais O and Lina B, 'Mutations of neuraminidase implicated in neuraminidase inhibitors resistance', Copyright © 2008, with permission from Elsevier, http://www.sciencedirect.com/science/journal/13866532

certain other viral infections may be similarly eradicated. The World Health Organization campaign to eliminate polio is progressing towards a successful conclusion, and in many developed countries measles, mumps, and rubella are becoming rare.

## Passive immunization

### Immune globulin

The transfer of preformed antibodies from one individual to another can be achieved with human gamma globulin derived from the blood of healthy individuals known to have high antibody titres. In the days before an effective vaccine against hepatitis A became available, normal human immunoglobulin obtained from pooled routine blood donations was widely used for the protection of individuals visiting countries where the virus is common. Other types of immunoglobulin are obtained specifically from known hyperimmune individuals. Those in current use include immunoglobulin preparations against hepatitis B, varicella zoster, and rabies viruses.

### Monoclonal antibody

Techniques allowing the production of monoclonal antibodies with their exceptional intrinsic specificity have led to investigation of such compounds in the prevention of viral infection. The only one presently available, palivizumab, is a monoclonal antibody directed against respiratory syncytial virus. It is administered by intramuscular injection to vulnerable infants (those with underlying chronic lung disease, congenital heart disease, or immunodeficiency) at monthly intervals during the autumn and winter—seasons of greatest risk of infection with the virus.

## Active immunization

The host can be stimulated to produce a protective immune response by vaccination with a form of the infectious agent that does not cause disease. Vaccines can be alive or dead. Live vaccines consist of attenuated forms of the infectious agent. Examples include measles, mumps, rubella, and live poliovirus (Sabin) vaccines.

Dead vaccines may consist of the whole agent, grown in the laboratory and subsequently killed by some means, or of a subunit of the agent, usually prepared by recombinant DNA technology. Dead vaccines have the advantage that there is no risk of reversion to virulence. However, they are less immunogenic than live vaccines and therefore more doses need to be given to achieve a satisfactory response. Examples of such vaccines include the Salk polio vaccine (now generally preferred to the live Sabin vaccine), the rabies vaccine, and the hepatitis A and hepatitis B virus vaccines; the latter is a subunit vaccine, consisting only of the surface protein HBsAg, prepared by cloning and expressing the appropriate gene in yeast cells.

## Key points

- Viruses are obligate intracellular parasites which rely to a greater or lesser extent on host-cell functions for their replication.

- Nevertheless, a number of viral targets have been successfully exploited in the development of effective antiviral agents.

- Aciclovir and derivatives are nucleoside analogues that require initial phosphorylation by a virally encoded enzyme (thymidine kinase (TK)), and subsequently act to inhibit viral DNA polymerase (DNA pol). Resistance may arise through mutations in the gene that encodes TK or the gene that encodes DNA pol.

- Cidofovir and derivatives are nucleotide analogues which are further phosphorylated by host enzymes and act to inhibit viral DNA pol.

- Foscarnet is a pyrophosphate analogue which inhibits viral DNA pol.

- Ribavirin is a nucleoside analogue with an unknown mechanism of action but has a broad spectrum of activity in vitro.

- Zanamivir and oseltamivir are neuraminidase (NA) inhibitors and therefore prevent release of mature influenza virus particles from infected cells. Resistance, particularly to oseltamivir, may arise through point mutations in the NA gene.

## Further reading

**De Clercq,** E. (2013) Antivirals: past, present and future. *Biochemical Pharmacology,* **85**: 727–44.

**Yin, M. T., Brust, J. C. M.,Tieu, H. V., and Hammer, S. M.** (2009) 'Antiherpesvirus, anti-hepatitus virus, and anti-respiratory virus agents', in D. D. Richman, R. J. Whitley, and F. G. Hayden, eds, *Clinical Virology* (3rd edn). Washington, DC: ASM Press, pp. 217–64.

# Chapter 6

# Antiretroviral agents

## Introduction to antiretroviral agents

The first human immunodeficiency virus (HIV) was identified and characterized as a retrovirus in 1983. Long-term infection with HIV leads to inexorable destruction of the host immune system, and the development of the acquired immune deficiency syndrome (AIDS). Since that momentous discovery, considerable progress has been made in devising novel antiretroviral agents, which, by inhibiting HIV replication, can prolong the time to the development of AIDS. Unfortunately, the concept of 'curing' a patient of HIV infection remains an elusive and as yet unattainable goal.

The fact that HIV belongs to the retroviral family identified the first and most obvious target in the search for anti-HIV drugs—the enzyme reverse transcriptase. This enzyme, which copies an RNA template into DNA, is not present within host cells, which have no need to perform this 'backwards' synthetic process. The enzyme is encoded within the HIV genome, and the protein itself is an essential component of infectious viral particles.

Initially, the reverse transcriptase inhibitors were all nucleoside analogues. Subsequently, it became clear that compounds with other structures could also act as reverse transcriptase inhibitors. Further advances came with the development of drugs that target completely different steps within the viral life cycle (see Fig. 6.1), including binding of the virus particle to target cells, fusion of the viral envelope with host cell membranes leading to cell entry, integration of the proviral DNA into the host chromosome, and post-translational processing of the viral polyprotein mediated by the virally encoded protease enzyme. Thus, there are currently a number of classes of antiretroviral drugs licensed for clinical use: nucleoside and non-nucleoside reverse transcriptase inhibitors, protease inhibitors, binding-blockers, fusion inhibitors, and integrase inhibitors (Table 6.1). Various other potential targets have been identified, and it is hoped that the number of anti-HIV drugs will continue to expand.

Antiretroviral drugs are commonly formulated as combination products in the hope of suppressing the development of resistance, to simplify the often complex dosage regimens that are required for effective therapy and, in some cases, to exploit possible synergistic interactions. However, the frequent occurrence of toxic interactions between various antiretroviral compounds demands careful selection of such drug permutations. Currently available combination products include those listed in Table 6.2.

The use of antiretroviral agents may be associated with a wide range of adverse effects—these are considered below in the description of individual drugs and drug classes. Particularly worrisome are effects on fat and carbohydrate metabolism, leading to dyslipidaemia, insulin resistance (even frank diabetes mellitus), and fat redistribution (e.g. increased abdominal fat, 'buffalo humps', and breast hypertrophy), collectively known as the lipodystrophy syndrome. The frequency and pathophysiology of these reactions are unclear, as is the long-term risk of other complications such as ischaemic heart disease. The protease inhibitors have been particularly

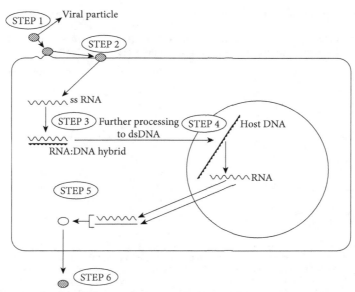

**Fig. 6.1** HIV replication cycle and targets for antiretroviral drugs. Step 1: viral binding to primary (CD4) and secondary (CCR5, CXCR4) receptors. Step 2: viral entry via fusion. Step 3: reverse transcription of single-stranded RNA (ssRNA) into an RNA–DNA hybrid. Step 4: integration of double-stranded DNA (dsDNA) provirus into host DNA. Step 5: positive ssRNA plus translated polyproteins form immature viral particles. Step 6: protease processing of polyproteins results in the maturation and release of the virus particles.

implicated but nucleoside analogue reverse transcriptase inhibitors also cause metabolic disturbances, and combinations of these drug classes may increase the risk.

# Reverse transcriptase inhibitors

There are two types of reverse transcriptase inhibitors (RTIs) described in this section: nucleos(t)ide analogues (also known as NRTIs) and non-nucleoside analogue reverse transcriptase inhibitors (also known as NNRTIs).

## Nucleos(t)ide analogues

### Zidovudine

Zidovudine (azidothymidine; often simply called AZT; Fig. 6.2) was originally investigated for use as an anticancer agent. However, when the HIV epidemic arose in the 1980s, it was tested along with many other drugs for activity against the virus. It was found to inhibit the reverse transcriptase activity of retroviruses at concentrations considerably lower than those needed to interfere with synthesis of host cell DNA.

Molecules such as zidovudine are referred to as 2′-3′-dideoxy nucleoside analogues, since they lack hydroxyl groups at both the 2′- and 3′-positions of the deoxyribose ring. Like other nucleoside analogues, these compounds are activated by phosphorylation to the triphosphate form, these steps being carried out by cellular enzymes. As with aciclovir (see 'Aciclovir' in Chapter 5),

**Table 6.1** Antiretroviral agents in clinical use in the United Kingdom and/or United States (2011).

| Nucleos(t)ide reverse transcriptase inhibitors[a] | Non-nucleoside reverse transcriptase inhibitors | Protease inhibitors | Integrase inhibitors | Other antiretrovirals |
|---|---|---|---|---|
| Abacavir (ABC) | Efavirenz | Atazanavir | Raltegravir | Enfuvirtide (fusion inhibitor) |
| Didanosine (ddI) | Etravirine | Darunavir | Elvitegravir[b] | Maraviroc (CCR5 binding inhibitor) |
| Emtricitabine (FTC) | Nevirapine | Fosamprenavir[c] | Dolutegravir | |
| Lamivudine (3TC) | Rilpirivine | Indinavir | | |
| Stavudine (d4T) | | Lopinavir[d] | | |
| Tenofovir[e] (TDF) | | Ritonavir | | |
| Zidovudine (AZT) | | Saquinavir | | |
| | | Tipranavir | | |

[a] The abbreviations shown in brackets are often used to describe these compounds and are derived from their chemical structures: the chemical structure of didanosine is 2′,3′-dideoxyinosine, the chemical structure of lamivudine is 2′-deoxy-3′-thiacytidine, the chemical structure of emtricitabine is fluoro-thiacytidine, the chemical structure of stavudine is 2′,3′-didehydro-3′-deoxythymidine, and that of zidovudine is 3′-azido-2′,3′-dideoxythymidine. Tenofovir is short for tenofovir disoproxil fumarate, a prodrug.

[b] Co-formulated with cobicistat.

[c] A prodrug formulation of amprenavir.

[d] Formulated as a combination tablet with low-dose ritonavir.

[e] A nucleotide analogue rather than a nucleoside analogue.

Source: Data taken from British National Formulary.

**Table 6.2** Currently available combination products.

| Combination product | Components |
|---|---|
| Kivexa | Abacavir + lamivudine |
| Trizivir | Abacavir + lamivudine + zidovudine |
| Truvada | Tenofovir + emtricitabine |
| Atripla | Tenofovir + emtricitabine + efavirenz |
| Eviplera | Tenofovir + emtricitabine + rilpirivine |
| Combivir | Zidovudine + lamivudine |

incorporation of the triphosphate into a growing DNA chain will result in chain termination, as there is no 3′-hydroxyl group available for formation of the next 5′–3′- phosphodiester linkage.

Non-specific side effects such as headache, anorexia, and nausea are common with zidovudine therapy but these effects often abate after two to three weeks. More serious toxicity to bone marrow cells is dose-related and hence much effort has been directed at defining the minimum dose that exhibits effective antiviral action.

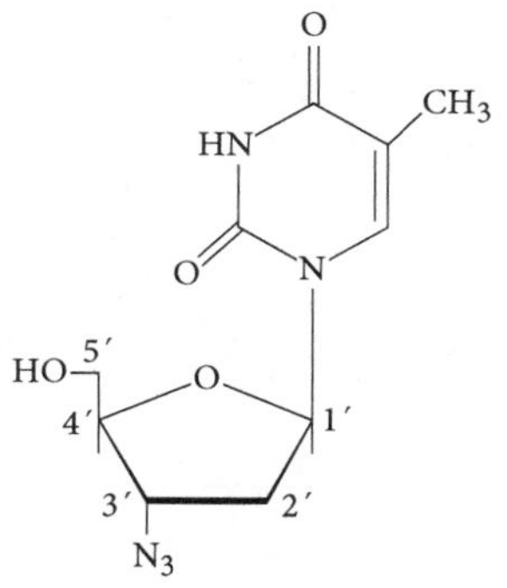

**Fig. 6.2** Structure of azidothymidine (AZT).

## Other nucleos(t)ide analogues

The success of zidovudine, albeit with limitations, at least showed that it was possible for anti-HIV drugs to be therapeutically useful. The pharmaceutical industry was therefore encouraged to design and test other potential nucleoside analogues. Currently there are six further drugs of this type licensed for use in the United States and some other countries (Tables 6.1 and 6.3). One of these compounds, tenofovir, is phosphorylated and is thus, like cidofovir (see 'Cidofovir' in Chapter 5), a nucleotide analogue rather than a nucleoside analogue but its mode of action is similar to that of true nucleoside analogues: it is converted to a triphosphate form that acts as a chain terminator and a competitive inhibitor of HIV-derived reverse transcriptase.

The most frequent adverse reaction with all of these drugs is gastrointestinal disturbance, including nausea, vomiting, abdominal pain, and diarrhoea. More serious and potentially life-threatening effects include lactic acidosis and hepatomegaly. Abacavir is associated with life-threatening hypersensitivity reactions in patients with the human leukocyte antigen (HLA) allele HLA-B*5701. Thus, the presence of this allele must be excluded before initiating abacavir therapy. Among the many side effects more commonly associated with individual compounds are peripheral neuropathy (didanosine, stavudine); pancreatitis (didanosine); elevation of liver transaminases (stavudine); increased serum phosphate levels and renal failure (tenofovir); reduced bone density (tenofovir); and pruritus (emtricitabine).

## Non-nucleoside analogue reverse transcriptase inhibitors

The recognition that compounds with a range of dissimilar structures could also act as inhibitors of reverse transcriptase led to the categorization of a new class of anti-HIV agents: the non-nucleoside analogue reverse transcriptase inhibitors. In contrast to the nucleoside analogues, these agents bind specifically to a non-substrate-binding site of reverse transcriptase located close to the substrate-binding site. These drugs inhibit the reverse transcriptase of HIV-1 but not that

**Table 6.3** Nucleos(t)ide analogues.

| Thymidine analogues | Cytosine analogues | Adenosine analogues | Guanosine analogues |
|---|---|---|---|
| Zidovudine | Lamivudine | Didanosine | Abacavir |
| Stavudine | Emtricitabine | Tenofovir | |

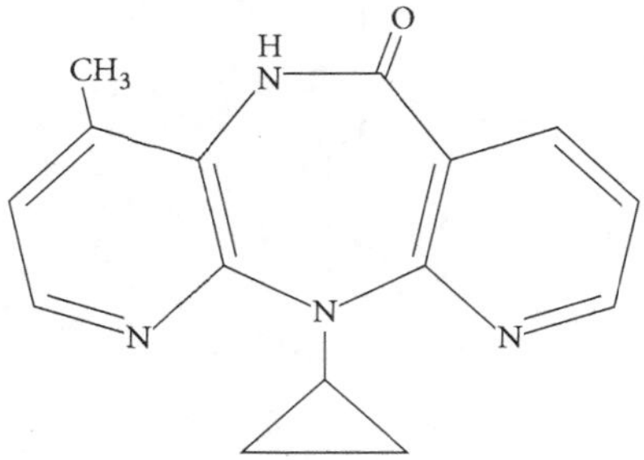

**Fig. 6.3** Structure of nevirapine.

of HIV-2. Many chemical classes of non-nucleoside compounds that act as reverse transcriptase inhibitors have been described, of which four are currently used extensively in the treatment of HIV infection: nevirapine (Fig. 6.3 shows this is clearly not a nucleoside analogue), efavirenz, etravirine, and rilpivirine.

Rashes, which can be severe (e.g. Stevens–Johnson syndrome), hepatotoxicity, and numerous other side effects of varying frequency and severity are associated with the use of this class of compounds. Efavirenz is also associated with a number of psychiatric or central nervous system adverse effects such as sleep disturbance and abnormal dreams, which can be reduced by taking the dose at bedtime.

## Protease inhibitors

The development of drugs acting on a viral target other than reverse transcriptase represented a major breakthrough in therapy for HIV-infected patients. When HIV replicates, it produces polycistronic mRNA, which is translated into a series of polyproteins that must be cleaved to yield the component proteins for infectious viral particles. This function is performed by a virally encoded aspartyl protease. Although mammalian cells also contain aspartyl proteases, these do not cleave HIV polyproteins efficiently.

Eight drugs that specifically inhibit HIV protease are currently licensed for use (Table 6.1). They are complex molecules and most are structurally related. All have important side effects. Besides gastrointestinal problems (prominent with ritonavir), the protease inhibitors are particularly associated with all manifestations of the lipodystrophy syndrome, referred to above. Second-generation protease inhibitors such as atazanavir and darunavir may be less culpable in this respect. Indinavir may cause nephrolithiasis, by precipitation in the renal tubules.

Ritonavir has the useful property of boosting the activity of other protease inhibitors by inhibiting the liver enzyme systems responsible for their metabolism. This effect is obtained with low doses of ritonavir that lack intrinsic antiviral activity.

## Fusion inhibitors

The process of fusion whereby viral particles gain entry into the CD4 T cell following the initial attachment process is an attractive target for selectively active antiretroviral drugs. Various synthetic peptides have been designed to mimic part of the viral envelope glycoprotein gp41, which is involved in the fusion of the virus to the membrane of the target cell, and several of them efficiently prevent viral infection of cells in vitro. Only one of these compounds, enfuvirtide (formerly pentafuside) has so far been approved for therapeutic use. As a peptide, enfuvirtide is digested when taken by mouth and it is therefore administered by subcutaneous injection twice daily. Enfuvirtide is licensed for use in patients who are intolerant of other antiretroviral drugs or are not responding to preferred regimens. Side effects of the drug are common but are not normally serious.

## CCR5 binding inhibitors

The primary cellular receptor for HIV is CD4. However, binding to CD4 alone is not sufficient to allow viral entry into a target cell. A number of essential co-receptors have been identified, the two most important ones being the chemokine receptors CCR5 and CXCR4. The observation that individuals homozygous for deletions in their CCR5 gene exhibit no significant clinical disease despite their lack of functional CCR5 but are highly resistant to infection with CCR5-tropic HIV led to the development of small-molecule CCR5 antagonists aimed at blocking the binding of HIV to target cells. Maraviroc is the leading agent in this class of compounds. Given this mode of action, it is necessary to confirm that a patient is infected with CCR5-(and not CXCR4-)tropic virus before prescribing this drug.

## Integrase inhibitors

The most recent target exploited for the development of antiretroviral drugs is the virally encoded integrase enzyme, which mediates integration of the DNA provirus into the host cell chromosome. Although an obvious target, it proved difficult to delineate the structure of this enzyme in order to design appropriate inhibitors, but raltegravir, the leading agent in this class of drugs, was licensed for clinical use in 2008. Elvitegravir, the next integrase inhibitor, is co-formulated with cobicistat, a molecule which has no anti-HIV activity but which inhibits the cytochrome P450 system responsible for its metabolism, thereby increasing plasma concentrations. Dolutegravir is the latest integrase inhibitor, showing considerable promise in late-stage clinical trials.

## Resistance to anti-HIV drugs

Unfortunately, optimism encouraged by the emergence of effective anti-HIV drugs has had to be tempered by the realization that the virus can rapidly acquire resistance to these agents. The enzyme reverse transcriptase is considerably more error-prone than other DNA polymerases. Thus, the generation of large numbers of viral mutants is part of the natural replication cycle of HIV: it has been estimated that, within a single patient, every possible base substitution could occur at every possible nucleotide position in the viral genome every day! Clearly, the vast majority of these mutations will be deleterious and result in non-viable virus. However, the potential is there for mutations to occur that do confer benefit to the virus, especially if those mutations result in the decreased efficacy of an antiviral drug. Experience with all anti-HIV drugs used thus far indicates that resistance is an inevitable consequence of drug usage, at least if the suppression of virus replication is not absolute.

Isolates of HIV derived from patients who have been taking zidovudine for at least six months are invariably less sensitive to the drug in vitro than isolates taken from the same patient at the initiation of therapy. This arises from mutations in the gene coding for reverse transcriptase, leading to reduced binding of zidovudine triphosphate. Resistance arises as a series of sequential point mutations within the reverse transcriptase gene, each additional mutation resulting in an increase in the dose of drug necessary to inhibit the virus. This relative resistance is of considerable clinical importance. Trials of zidovudine monotherapy conducted in the late 1980s showed early promise, increasing CD4 cell counts and prolonging survival in treated patients. However, as these patients were followed for longer periods, it became clear that the therapeutic efficacy of the drug was limited to a period of about six months, after which it was of no benefit. This loss of efficacy coincided with the emergence of highly resistant viruses in treated patients.

Resistance to other nucleoside analogues similarly arises through mutations in the reverse transcriptase gene. In general, cross-resistance between zidovudine and the other nucleoside analogues is not a problem, as the positions of the mutations conferring resistance to zidovudine differ from those giving rise to resistance to, for instance, didanosine. In contrast, mutations causing resistance to didanosine overlap with those causing lamivudine resistance.

The news concerning resistance mutations may not be all bad, however. Mutation at position 184 in the reverse transcriptase gene results in increasing resistance to lamivudine but paradoxically causes an increase in sensitivity to zidovudine in virus previously resistant. Thus, in theory at least, a combination regimen of zidovudine plus lamivudine should be of benefit, a hope reflected by the availability of a tablet that contains both agents.

Yet another set of mutations in the reverse transcriptase gene confers resistance to the non-nucleoside reverse transcriptase inhibitors, and several such changes have been reported. Some, but not all, lead to cross-resistance among the different drugs of this type but they are distinct from those leading to resistance to the nucleos(t)ide analogues.

As with the reverse transcriptase inhibitors, resistance to the protease inhibitors may arise through point mutations in the gene coding for the target protein. Various mutations in the protease gene have been described. Many of these map at similar points in the genome of virus from patients receiving different protease inhibitors, indicating that cross-resistance between these drugs is common. Continued use of a given protease inhibitor leads to the accumulation of mutations, with a concomitant increase in resistance. Tipranavir and darunavir, so-called second-generation protease inhibitors, were introduced because they are active against strains resistant to other protease inhibitors.

Although the use of combination therapy substantially reduces the chance of treatment failure due to the emergence of drug resistance, there are disturbing reports of simultaneous resistance developing to two or more classes of antiretroviral drug. The spread of multiresistant strains of the virus clearly constitutes a major threat and it is important to minimize this possibility. Tests for drug resistance on isolates from patients receiving treatment are valuable in directing appropriate changes in therapy. These usually require sequencing of the appropriate viral gene to identify drug resistance mutations. Since resistant strains may revert to susceptibility when therapy is discontinued, a prompt switch to alternative agents is often helpful.

## Anti-HIV drugs in development

Despite the clinical successes achieved by use of the above agents, there remains a need for new drugs with different sites of action, and different toxicity profiles in the fight against HIV infection. Much investigation continues into safer and more effective alternatives for existing classes of antiretroviral compounds.

Optimal therapy for patients with HIV infection may involve treatment with other drugs that do not necessarily exhibit antiviral activity. Immunomodulatory agents such as interleukin-2 have their advocates. Initially encouraging reports of the use of hydroxyurea, which blocks cellular activation necessary for viral replication in resting CD4-positive T cells, have unfortunately not been confirmed.

## Key points

- A detailed understanding of the replication cycle of HIV has led to the development of a number of classes of antiretroviral drugs acting at a number of different steps.
- Reverse transcriptase inhibitors include nucleos(t)ide analogues, referred to as NRTIs, and non-nucleoside analogues (also known as NNRTIs). These act to prevent the synthesis of proviral DNA from the genomic RNA template.
- Protease inhibitors prevent the post-translational cleavage of the HIV polyproteins generated by the polycistronic mRNA transcribed from the proviral DNA and hence prevent the maturation of nascent viral particles.
- Fusion inhibitors act to inhibit a very early step in the viral entry process. Another class of drugs acting at the viral entry stage comprises the CCR5 antagonists, which prevent binding of the viral gp120 to the CCR5 secondary co-receptor.
- Integrase inhibitors target the viral integrase enzyme responsible for integrating proviral DNA into the host cell chromosomes.
- The emergence of resistance to any of the above antiretroviral drugs may arise through spontaneous mutations within the target gene (e.g. genes encoding reverse transcriptase, protease, gp120, integrase).

## Further reading

Arts, E. J. and Hazuda, D. J. (2012) HIV-1 antiretroviral drug therapy. *Cold Spring Harbour Perspectives in Medicine*, 2: a007161.

Sobieszczyk, M. E., Taylor, B. S., and Hammer, S. M. (2009) 'Antiretroviral agents', in D. D. Richman, R. J. Whitley, and F. G. Hayden, eds, *Clinical Virology* (3rd edn). Washington, DC: ASM Press, pp. 167–216.

# Chapter 7

# Drugs used in the treatment of viral hepatitis

## Introduction to the treatment of viral hepatitis

The World Health Organization estimates that there are over 350 million individuals chronically infected with hepatitis B virus (HBV), and over 200 million chronically infected with hepatitis C virus (HCV). Another way of looking at this is to say that one in 12 inhabitants of the Earth is infected with one of these two hepatotropic viruses. Between 15 and 40 per cent of individuals with chronic viral hepatitis will develop long-term complications of the disease such as cirrhosis, with all its attendant life-threatening complications, or hepatocellular carcinoma, the fourth commonest cause worldwide of death due to malignant disease. HBV infection is thought to account for around one million deaths per year, and the toll from chronic HCV infection is likely to be of similar magnitude.

In the face of such morbidity and mortality, and in the knowledge of the huge potential market for any successful drugs generated in this area, there have been extensive efforts to develop effective therapy for patients with chronic viral hepatitis. Initial efforts to treat chronic HBV infection were focused on interferon (IFN), a naturally produced cytokine with multiple modes of action. However, a better understanding of the molecular biology of HBV replication has led to a revolution in the management of chronic HBV infection in the past 15 years. Similarly, a detailed understanding of the molecular biology of HCV has resulted in the identification of several potential targets for antiviral drugs, with several new molecules now licensed for use or in late-stage clinical trials.

## Drugs used in the treatment of chronic HBV infection

### IFN-α

There are three classes of human IFN: class 1 includes IFN-α, produced by many cell types, and IFN-β, produced by fibroblasts; class 2 comprises IFN-γ (sometimes referred to as immune IFN) produced by T lymphocytes. Class 3 includes IFN-λ 1, 2, 3, and 4. IFN-α and IFN-β share 30 per cent structural homology but they are quite distinct from IFN-γ, which shares only about 10 per cent homology in its amino acid sequence. Moreover, there are over 15 different forms of IFN-α, each differing by a few amino acids, and, possibly, 2 forms of IFN-β.

IFNs have a wide range of biological effects. They activate several different biochemical pathways within a cell, with the result that the cell is rendered resistant to virus infection. The relative importance of each of these pathways differs between different IFNs, and indeed between different cells stimulated by the same IFN. One pathway results in the activation of a ribonuclease that digests viral RNA. Another results in the phosphorylation of a protein known as an initiation factor; phosphorylation of this factor, the normal function of which is to assist in the initiation of transcription of mRNA into protein, effectively prevents the production of viral proteins.

IFNs also have various effects on cells of the immune system. As with their antiviral properties, these immunomodulatory effects vary in detail between different IFNs but they include stimulation of natural killer cells, induction or suppression of antibody production, stimulation of T-cell activity, and stimulation of expression of HLA class I and II molecules on the surface of cells. Finally, IFNs affect cell proliferation, and this property has led to their successful use in the management of certain malignant tumours.

Early studies of the efficacy of IFN therapy were hampered by difficulties in obtaining sufficient quantities of IFNs to conduct clinical trials. This problem was solved by recombinant DNA technology, which allowed cloning and expression of the relevant genes. Unexpectedly, clinical trials revealed that patients receiving IFN experienced flu-like side effects: fever, headache, and myalgia. This led to the realization that individuals suffering from influenza complain of flu-like symptoms precisely because of the induction of IFNs by the virus. Most patients become tolerant to these effects after the first few doses.

Chronic HBV infection was the first infection in which IFN-α was shown in appropriate clinical trials to be of clear therapeutic benefit. The standard regimen involved intramuscular administration three times a week for a minimum period of six months. Pegylated interferon (PEG-IFN) is a preparation in which IFN-α is covalently cross-linked to polyethylene glycol. This formulation has an extended half-life, leading to more prolonged therapeutic levels of the drug and therefore requiring only once weekly injections (Fig. 7.1). PEG-IFN is better tolerated and, most importantly, produces a much superior virological response and has therefore replaced the use of standard IFN. The evidence suggests that, in the context of chronic HBV infection, IFN exerts its therapeutic effect through immunomodulation rather than by acting directly as an antiviral agent. This is discussed further in Chapter 34.

## Nucleoside and nucleotide analogues

There has been significant progress in the management of chronic HBV infection in the past 15 years, entirely due to the emergence of detailed information about the extraordinary and unique replicative cycle of the virus. Although the virus carries a partially double-stranded DNA genome, once within the cell, a full-length RNA copy of the genome is transcribed (the RNA pre-genome), along with transcripts from the four open reading frames (surface, core, polymerase, and X open reading frames (ORFs)). The RNA pre-genome is packaged within newly synthesized

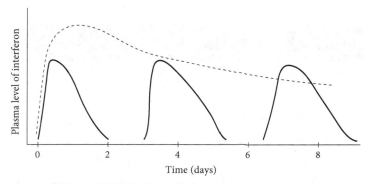

**Fig. 7.1** Plasma levels of IFN and PEG-IFN. The solid lines show the IFN concentrations achieved after three individual injections of standard interferon. The dotted line shows the levels achieved after a single injection of pegylated interferon.

core protein, together with copies of the viral polymerase enzyme. The latter has reverse transcriptase (RT) activity and copies the RNA pre-genome into single-stranded DNA, after which there is partial synthesis of the complementary DNA strand, resulting in the partially double-stranded DNA genome of the mature virus particle.

RT was formerly believed to exist only within the *Retroviridae*, so the elucidation of the convoluted replication strategy of HBV was a major surprise. The recognition of the key role of this enzymic activity within the HBV life cycle provided an obvious potential target for antiviral drugs and, thanks to the epidemic of infection with the human immunodeficiency viruses which emerged in the 1980s, a variety of RT inhibitors were already available for appropriate clinical trials. Not all anti-HIV drugs have activity against the RT of HBV, and the same is true in reverse, that is, there are some agents active against HBV but not HIV. The potency of some of these drugs in inhibiting HBV DNA production has revolutionized the management of these patients.

Historically, lamivudine and adefovir were the first two agents to be licensed for the treatment of chronic HBV infection. Telbivudine was the next, but this drug failed to achieve National Institute for Health and Clinical Excellence (NICE) approval in the United Kingdom. Due to their relative lack of potency and, more pertinently, much lower thresholds for the development of resistance, these agents have now been replaced by entecavir and tenofovir.

## Lamivudine

This agent (3-thiacytidine; Fig. 7.2), developed as a nucleoside analogue reverse transcriptase inhibitor (see Chapter 6), was the first RT inhibitor shown to inhibit HBV replication. It is

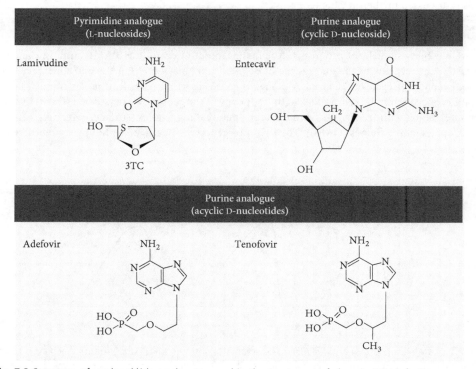

**Fig. 7.2** Structure of nucleos(t)ide analogues used in the treatment of chronic HBV infection.

triphosphorylated in the cell by cellular enzymes, and the triphosphate acts as both a chain terminator and a DNA polymerase inhibitor. While treatment results in a dramatic decline in HBV viral loads, resistance has emerged as a major problem. After five years of therapy, over 80 per cent of lamivudine-treated patients harbour resistant virus, evidenced by the rebound of HBV DNA to pretreatment levels, and the presence of specific drug resistance mutations (DRMs) within the viral polymerase gene, the most important of which result in replacement of the methionine at position 204 in the YMDD domain at the active site of the enzyme.

## Adefovir

This acyclic adenine analogue (Fig. 7.2) is formulated as the dipivoxil ester for the oral treatment of chronic hepatitis B infection. As the first phosphate group is already present on the acyclic ring, this is a phosphonate nucleotide analogue. This agent has no anti-HIV activity but does inhibit HBV replication. Although resistance does not emerge to quite the same extent as with lamivudine, nevertheless prolonged therapy does result in the induction of DRMs and loss of efficacy. The adefovir resistance mutations, most notably at positions A181 and N236, are distinct from those associated with lamivudine, so this drug is useful in patients with lamivudine resistance.

## Entecavir

Entecavir is a nucleoside analogue based on guanosine (Fig. 7.2) but differs from aciclovir and ganciclovir in that carbon replaces oxygen in the modified ribose substituent, which retains a cyclic arrangement. It is a potent inhibitor of HBV replication, several hundredfold more so than lamivudine. In treatment-naive patients receiving entecavir, emergence of resistance is very unusual, despite prolonged therapy. However, resistance is more likely to arise in patients who harbour virus containing lamivudine-resistance mutations, and therefore the dose recommended for lamivudine-experienced patients is twice the usual dose. It is administered orally.

## Tenofovir

This more potent derivative of adefovir (Fig. 7.2) is formulated as tenofovir disoproxil fumarate. Not only does it demonstrate enhanced potency in viral suppression compared to adefovir, resistance mutations to this drug have not been identified to-date, indicating a very high barrier to resistance.

## Drugs used in the treatment of chronic HCV infection

### IFN-α

Even before the identification of HCV as the causative agent of chronic non-A non-B hepatitis (NANBH), in the light of the moderate success achieved by IFN-α therapy of chronic HBV infection, such therapy was also applied to NANBH patients. This resulted in normalization of liver function tests and apparent cessation of disease progression in a minority of patients. HCV was characterized in 1989, so subsequent trials of IFN therapy were able to monitor the virological response, as opposed to the biochemical or histological responses to treatment. Standard IFN-α, given as thrice-weekly injections for a minimum period of six months, led to clearance of virus in around 10 per cent of infected patients (Fig. 7.3).

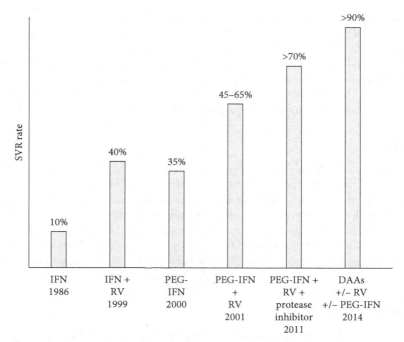

**Fig. 7.3** Response rates to evolving therapies in chronic HCV infection.

## Ribavirin

Many other antiviral agents were tested empirically as possible therapy for chronic HCV infection. Ribavirin (RV; see 'Ribavirin' in Chapter 5) used as monotherapy had very little effect on the viral load detectable in peripheral blood, although it did normalize liver function in some patients. However, trials of co-therapy consisting of RV and standard IFN-α proved to be much more successful than the use of either drug alone, and this became the standard of care for patients with chronic HCV infection from the mid-1990s onwards. The overall response rate to IFN and RV combination therapy can reach as high as 40 per cent (Fig. 7.3), although this is dependent on a number of host and viral factors (age, gender, degree of underlying liver damage, viral load, and, most especially, viral genotype) discussed in more detail in Chapter 34.

## PEG-IFNs

The next significant advance in the therapy of chronic HCV infection was the emergence of the PEG-IFNs (see 'IFN-α'). Indeed, PEG-IFNs were first trialled in the context of chronic HCV (as opposed to chronic HBV) infection. The dramatic effect that pegylation has on the maintenance of plasma levels of IFN, compared with standard IFN, is shown in Fig. 7.1.

PEG-IFN-α alone, given as once weekly injections for at least six months, achieved viral clearance rates similar to those from standard IFN-α plus RV combination therapy (Fig. 7.3).

## PEG-IFN/RV combination therapy

Given the improvement in response rates seen with PEG-IFN, the natural next step was to set up clinical trials of PEG-IFN/RV combination therapy. Overall response rates increased yet again, to around 50 per cent (Fig. 7.3), the exact figure again being dependent on the particular characteristics of the treated population, especially the infecting viral genotype. This regimen therefore replaced standard IFN/RV as the standard of care from 2001 onwards.

Both drugs are associated with adverse effects. IFN injections result in fever, myalgia, and headache. This can be controlled by paracetamol use, and after the first few doses, patients become tolerant to these effects. More serious effects include bone marrow suppression (neutropaenia, thrombocytopaenia), and depression which may result in suicidal ideation—patients may require psychiatric assessment before commencing therapy, and ongoing support with antidepressives. Autoimmune manifestations may emerge on therapy, particularly autoimmune thyroid disease. RV causes a haemolytic anaemia. Combination therapy is therefore difficult, and patients may require extensive support and help in order to complete their course—especially in genotype 1 infection, for which 12 months of therapy is recommended. Patient compliance is a problem—all clinical trials report at least a 10 per cent patient dropout rate.

It should be noted that although PEG/RV combination therapy can cure around half of all patients with chronic HCV infection, the mode of action(s) of either drug in this context remains unknown. The biochemical response to IFN therapy in chronic HCV infection is different from that in chronic HBV and therefore it is unlikely that the action is entirely due to immunomodulation. There are a number of theories as to how RV might potentiate the response to IFN but none have thus far been proven.

Genotype 1 virus is undoubtedly more resistant to PEG/RV therapy than any of the other genotypes (see 'What should patients be treated with?' in Chapter 34), but in the absence of any understanding of how the drugs work, it has not been possible to discern at the molecular level why this should be, or what viral sequences in which genes confer resistance/sensitivity to either IFN or RV. An 'interferon sensitivity determining region' in the non-structural gene 5a has been reported in the literature, although this is controversial, and there is no practical benefit to be gained from sequencing the virus before therapy.

There has been much recent interest in identifying host genetic factors linked with response/non-response to PEG/RV therapy. Genome-wide association studies have identified a number of single nucleotide polymorphisms (SNPs) on chromosome 19 close to the gene encoding interleukin (IL)-28B (also known as IFN-$\lambda$ 3) which define responder and non-responder phenotypes, especially for genotype 1 infection. The distribution of these polymorphisms differs in populations of different ethnic origins, which explains the clinical observations that African Americans have much lower overall response rates than do European Americans—as the latter group has a much higher prevalence of the good-responder alleles (over 80%) than does the latter (around 50%). In the search to provide a functional explanation for the association between IL-28B SNPs and PEG-IFN responsiveness, more recent studies have identified a novel polymorphism upstream of the IL-28B gene, comprising either a single deletion ($\Delta G$) or a TT insertion. The $\Delta G$ deletion, which is associated with lower response rates to PEG/RV therapy, results in the creation of an ORF encoding the protein IFN-$\lambda$ 4. Endogenous production of this cytokine may underlie the relative failure of patients to respond appropriately to the administration of exogenous IFN-$\alpha$. Even more recently, a SNP within the IFN-$\lambda$4 gene resulting in an amino acid change at position 70 has been shown to correlate even better with treatment response.

## Directly acting antivirals (DAAs)

In the 20 years or so since HCV was first characterized and sequenced, understanding of the molecular biology of the virus has increased dramatically. A number of potential viral (and host)

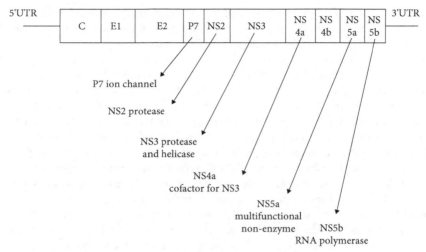

**Fig. 7.4** HCV genome structure, and potential targets for DAAs.

targets within the viral replication cycle have been identified and a wide range of drugs designed to act at those targets are undergoing clinical trials. This has led to the concept of treating patients with DAAs. A detailed map of the HCV genome is shown in Fig. 7.4, illustrating the known functions of the various components of the genome, and the potential targets for DAAs.

## Drugs

The most clinically advanced DAAs are targeted against the products of the NS3, NS5a, and NS5b genes. The nomenclature associated with these new drugs is explained in Table 7.1. While monotherapy with any of these agents induces a considerable decline in viral load within a few days of onset, viral rebound occurs associated with specific DRMs in the target gene. The clinical trials of these molecules have therefore been conducted as triple therapy, with the DAA being added to a PEG/RV backbone. However, with the emergence of different drug classes inhibiting different virally encoded functions, the concept of 'interferon-free' therapy has now arisen, involving the use of multiple DAAs in combination, with or without RV (see 'Which drugs should be used?' in Chapter 34).

## NS3 protease inhibitors

The first-generation NS3 protease inhibitors (PIs) telaprevir and boceprevir were licensed for clinical use in 2011. These agents are genotype specific, essentially having clinical utility only against genotype 1 viruses. In genotype 1 infection, where response rates to PEG and RV dual therapy

**Table 7.1** Nomenclature for the directly acting antiviral agents used to treat hepatitis C virus.

| Gene target | Function of gene | Suffix of directly acting antiviral agent drug names | Examples |
| --- | --- | --- | --- |
| NS3 | Protease | -previr | Telaprevir, boceprevir, simeprevir |
| NS5a | Non-enzymatic | -asvir | Daclatasvir, ledipasvir |
| NS5b | RNA polymerase | -buvir | Sofosbuvir, dasabuvir |

are around 45 per cent, the addition of a first-generation PI increases the response to 65–70 per cent. Similar response rates to triple therapy have been reported in patients who have previously failed PEG/RV therapy. These drugs may cause severe adverse effects in a minority of patients— both may cause anaemia, thereby exacerbating the effect of RV on haemoglobin levels; telaprevir is particularly associated with development of a rash which may be severe and life-threatening; boceprevir may result in dysgeusia, an unpleasant metallic taste in the mouth. On the plus side, the added antiviral effect of these agents may mean that even for genotype 1 infection, the course of PEG and RV may only be necessary for 6 rather than 12 months. Resistance to these drugs arises through the acquisition of a series of DRMs within the NS3 gene, for example, at positions 36, 54, 55, 80, 155, 156, and 168. Some of these DRMs may exist pretreatment in a small percentage of patients. Sequence differences between HCV genotype 1a and 1b viruses at some of these key positions means that it is easier for a 1a virus to acquire these DRMs than it is for a 1b virus, that is, genotype 1b has a higher barrier to resistance. This is reflected in better response rates for patients infected with genotype 1b virus compared to those with 1a virus.

There are a number of second-generation PIs in late-stage clinical trials—simeprevir was licensed in late 2014. The advantages of these agents over the first-generation PIs are increased potency and much better side-effect profiles. Other PIs with broader pan-genotypic activity are in development.

## NS5b inhibitors

As with the HIV RT inhibitors, there are a number of different classes of NS5b inhibitors. Nucleos(t)ide analogue inhibitors bind to the active site of the enzyme, while non-nucleoside inhibitors may bind to a number of different sites in the enzyme. The former class have a high barrier to resistance—while a key resistance mutation (S282T) has been described, such a mutation comes at a considerable fitness cost to the virus, and emergence of this DRM occurs very rarely. Resistance to the non-nucleosides arises much more easily and frequently. Sofosbuvir (a pyrimidine nucleotide analogue) is the most advanced of the NS5b inhibitors. Clinical trial data show this to be an extraordinarily effective antiviral, with sustained response rates in excess of 90 per cent against all genotypes when added to a PEG/RV backbone in triple therapy. It also has an excellent safety profile, with no major side effects thus far described. Approval for clinical use in the United Kingdom is expected in 2015.

## NS5a inhibitors

The product of the viral NS5a gene is a multifunctional protein, essential for successful execution of several steps within the viral replication cycle, but it is not an enzyme. NS5a inhibitors are the most potent antiviral agents available—a single dose of daclatasvir results in over a 3-log drop in viral load within 24 hours. The barrier to resistance for the NS5a inhibitors is higher than for the PIs but lower than for the nucleoside polymerase inhibitors, with one or two key DRMs (e.g. at Q30 and Y93) having been identified.

## Other drug targets

Other targets include the p7 protein, which is thought to act as an ion channel that is important in viral uncoating and/or production of mature virus particles, the NS2 protease, the NS4b protein (which forms the membranous web within the cell that acts as a scaffold for viral replication), and the internal ribosomal entry site (IRES) within the 5′-non-coding region (NCR). A new concept of 'host-targeted therapy' has also emerged in recognition of the fact that HCV replication is dependent on a number of host cellular factors. For instance, NS5a is known to bind to cyclophilin A, a host cell molecule. Alisporivir is a cyclophilin antagonist which inhibits HCV replication by interfering with NS5a binding. Similarly, a host factor, microRNA-122 (miR-122) is known to be an essential cofactor for proper IRES binding, and an antisense RNA molecule, miravirsen, which targets miR-122 has shown some promise in reducing viral load in a chimpanzee model of infection. A theoretical advantage of these agents is that, as they act on host, rather than viral, molecules, it will be difficult for the virus to generate mutations resulting in resistance.

The management of chronic HCV infection has already undergone several seismic shifts since the virus was first identified in 1989. We are now on the verge of another major paradigm change—the use of all oral combinations of potent, well tolerated, DAAs in IFN-(and hopefully also RV-)free regimens, perhaps for as little as 12 weeks, without serious side effects, and sustained virological response rates for all genotypes in excess of 95 per cent. Such astounding clinical trial data are already in the literature from late phase 3 trials. The next 5–10 years will be a time of intense study and interest, with the likely outcome of a dramatic improvement in the prognosis for HCV-infected patients.

## Key points

- The management of chronic HBV and HCV infections has changed dramatically in the last 10 years, concomitant with an increased understanding of the replication cycles of both viruses.

- There are two modes of therapy for chronic HBV infection—immunomodulation with IFN-α (now available in pegylated form), or inhibition of the viral RT activity by nucleos(t)ide analogues such as lamivudine, adefovir, entecavir, and tenofovir.

- The nucleos(t)ide analogues differ in both potency and their genetic barrier to the development of resistance. Tenofovir and entecavir have superseded lamivudine and adefovir, as they are more potent drugs and have high genetic barriers to resistance.

- Treatment of chronic HCV infection has evolved from standard IFN alone, to combination therapy with PEG-IFN and RV. The latter combination achieves sustained viral clearance in around 50 per cent of patients.

- DAAs are in late stages of development for the treatment of chronic HCV infection. First-generation NS3 PIs were licensed in 2011. Second-generation PIs, nucleoside and non-nucleoside NS5b inhibitors, and NS5a inhibitors will be licensed in 2015.

- Long-term, combination, all-oral DAA therapy will obviate the need for the PEG/RV backbone, will require shorter duration of therapy, will be better tolerated, and will achieve treatment response rates in excess of 95 per cent.

## Further reading

Balagopal, A., Thomas, D. L., and Thio, C. L. (2010) IL28B and the control of hepatitis C virus infection. *Gastroenterology*, **139**: 1865–76.

Halegoua-De Marzio, D. and Hann, H. W. (2014) Then and now: the progress in hepatitis B treatment over the past 20 years. *World Journal of Gastroenterology*, **20**: 401–13.

Poordad, F. and Dieterich, D. (2012) Treating hepatitis C: current standard of care and emerging direct-acting antiviral agents. *Journal of Viral Hepatitis*, **19**: 449–64.

# Chapter 8

# Antifungal agents

## Introduction to antifungal agents

Fungi may cause benign but unsightly infection of the skin, nail, or hair (dermatophytosis), relatively trivial infection of mucous membranes (thrush), or systemic infection causing progressive, often fatal disease. The taxonomy of fungi is highly complex but for medical purposes they are commonly considered to comprise four morphological groups:

- yeasts that reproduce by budding (e.g. *Cryptococcus neoformans*);
- yeasts that produce a pseudomycelium (e.g. *Candida albicans*);
- filamentous fungi (moulds) that produce a true mycelium (e.g. *Aspergillus fumigatus*); and
- dimorphic fungi that grow as yeasts or filamentous fungi, depending on the cultural conditions (e.g. *Histoplasma capsulatum*).

In addition, *Pneumocystis jiroveci*—formerly *P. carinii*, an important opportunist pathogen, especially of patients with AIDS—is now regarded as a fungus.

Fungi are eukaryotic organisms, and antibacterial agents are generally ineffective against them. Specialized antifungal agents must therefore be used, and some are quite toxic. In order to minimize problems of toxicity, superficial lesions are usually treated by topical application but deep mycoses, which are serious life-threatening infections, need vigorous systemic therapy. The polyene amphotericin was formerly the mainstay; the choice of agents to use also includes flucytosine, griseofulvin, azole derivatives (mainly triazoles), allylamines, and a group of semi-synthetic antibiotics, the echinocandins. *P. jiroveci* is not susceptible to conventional antifungal agents, and so alternative treatment regimens (e.g. co-trimoxazole) are used.

The differential activity of the main antifungal agents in common use is summarized in Table 8.1. Precise assessment of the activity of antifungal agents in vitro is beset with methodological difficulties, and susceptibility tests are not generally available, except in reference centres.

## Polyenes

The polyenes are naturally occurring compounds exhibiting a complex macrocyclic structure. All act by binding to sterols in the fungal cell membrane, thereby interfering with membrane integrity and causing leakage of essential metabolites. The only one that can be administered parenterally is amphotericin. Among related polyenes available for topical treatment in some countries are nystatin, natamycin (pimaricin), and trichomycin (hachimycin).

The activity of the polyenes embraces a variety of pathogenic fungi; yeasts are particularly susceptible. Nystatin has been extensively used for treating *Candida* infections of the mucous membranes but has largely been replaced by imidazoles and triazoles (see 'Imidazoles' and 'Triazoles'). Most polyenes are restricted to topical use but intravenous amphotericin remains an important agent for the treatment of systemic fungal infections, including disseminated candidiasis, cryptococcosis, aspergillosis, and deep mycoses caused by dimorphic fungi. Amphotericin can also

**Table 8.1** Summary of the differential activity of antifungal agents against the more common pathogenic fungi.[a]

| Fungus | Principal diseases caused | Polyenes (e.g. amphotericin) | Flucytosine | Griseofulvin | Azoles[b] | Allylamines (e.g. terbinafine) | Echinocandins (e.g. caspofungin) |
|---|---|---|---|---|---|---|---|
| **Yeasts** | | | | | | | |
| Cryptococcus neoformans | Meningitis | + | + | – | + | – | – |
| Candida albicans | Thrush; systemic candidiasis | + | + | – | + | +/– | + |
| **Filamentous fungi (moulds)** | | | | | | | |
| Trichophyton spp. | Infection of skin, nail or hair ('ringworm') | – | – | + | (+)[c] | + | – |
| Microsporum spp. | | | | | | | |
| Epidermophyton floccosum | | | | | | | |
| Aspergillus fumigatus | Pulmonary aspergillosis | + | – | – | (+/–)[c] | + | + |
| **Dimorphic fungi** | | | | | | | |
| Histoplasma capsulatum | Histoplasmosis | + | – | – | (+/–)[c] | – | ? |
| Coccidioides immitis | Coccidioidomycosis | + | – | – | (+/–)[c] | – | ? |
| Blastomyces dermatitidis | Blastomycosis | + | – | – | (+)[c] | – | ? |

[a] +, useful activity; –, no useful activity; +/–, variable activity; ?, clinical efficacy not established.

[b] Imidazoles (e.g. clotrimazole, miconazole, and ketoconazole) and triazoles (e.g. itraconazole, fluconazole, and voriconazole).

[c] Itraconazole, voriconazole, and posaconazole are the only azoles active against moulds; itraconazole is the only agent approved for treatment of dimorphic fungi, although case reports indicate voriconazole is effective.

be administered orally for the treatment of oral, oesophageal, and intestinal candidiasis but azole derivatives are now preferred.

Toxicity is a major problem in systemic therapy with amphotericin and it needs to be used with care. The drug is highly insoluble and for parenteral use is normally formulated in a surfactant vehicle. Various ways have been tried to minimize toxicity problems. Lipid-complexed colloidal formulations exhibit improved safety. Alternatively, phospholipid vesicles (liposomes) are used as carriers of the drug. Packaged in this way, the drug is delivered to the site of infection and this allows the use of higher doses without compromising safety. The combination of amphotericin with flucytosine improves the outcome for cryptococcal meningitis.

## Flucytosine (5-fluorocytosine) — Combination therapy for severe yeast infections only

Flucytosine is a pyrimidine analogue originally developed as an anticancer drug but found to have considerable activity against yeasts; it has no useful activity against filamentous fungi. The activity depends on its being converted intracellularly to 5-fluorouracil, which is incorporated into fungal RNA. The drug can be given orally or parenterally but resistance develops readily and sometimes emerges during treatment. For this reason, flucytosine is normally administered in combination with amphotericin, especially for the treatment of HIV-associated cryptococcal meningitis, for which it enhances fungal clearance from the cerebrospinal fluid and thus improves the clinical outcome.

Flucytosine is usually well tolerated but marrow toxicity can occur, particularly if the drug is allowed to accumulate in patients with impaired renal function. Adjustment of dosage according to the results of drug assays is therefore indicated.

## Griseofulvin — Dermatophyte infections only

Griseofulvin was the first antifungal antibiotic to be described. It is well absorbed when administered orally, particularly if a fine-particle formulation is used, and serious side effects are uncommon. It is ineffective topically. The mode of action has not been definitively established but activity appears to be directed against the process of mitosis, perhaps by interfering with the microtubules of the mitotic spindle. Use of griseofulvin is confined to the treatment of dermatophyte infections of the skin, nail, or hair. In the case of nail infections, treatment is prolonged. The failure rate is high, so alternative drugs, especially terbinafine (see 'Allylamines') are usually preferred. It induces the hepatic metabolism of some drugs and should not be taken with alcohol because it can cause flushing and vomiting (antabuse-type reaction).

## Azoles

Many imidazole and triazole derivatives display antifungal activity and, in fact, these compounds offer the nearest approximation to broad-spectrum antifungal agents. They act selectively against fungi (and some protozoa) by interfering with the demethylation of lanosterol during the synthesis of ergosterol, which is the principal sterol in the fungal cell membrane.

## Imidazoles — Topical use only

Antifungal imidazoles are most widely used for topical application in superficial fungal infections and vaginal candidiasis. Indeed, these are virtually the only useful roles for bifonazole, butoconazole, clotrimazole, econazole, fenticonazole, isoconazole, miconazole, oxiconazole, sulconazole, and terconazole, all of which have very similar properties and indications. One antifungal imidazole, tioconazole, is also available in a formulation that is painted on infected nails, but is unlikely to be effective alone in severe nail infections, for which better treatment is available.

The only imidazole to be used in the oral therapy of systemic fungal infections is ketoconazole. This derivative achieves therapeutic concentrations for several hours after oral administration. However, early enthusiasm for ketoconazole waned when it was realized that it was occasionally implicated in fatal hepatotoxic reactions. It has been largely replaced by triazoles for the treatment of systemic mycoses. It should not be used for trivial dermatophyte infections.

## Triazoles   For serious systemic mycoses

The triazoles fluconazole, itraconazole, voriconazole, and posaconazole are well absorbed after oral administration. They have many properties in common, but also display some distinctive features:

+ fluconazole and voriconazole achieve higher plasma concentrations than itraconazole and penetrate into cerebrospinal fluid in therapeutically useful concentrations;

+ itraconazole, voriconazole, and posaconazole exhibit much better activity than fluconazole against *Aspergillus* spp. and against *Can. krusei* and *Can. glabrata*, which are yeasts that are seen with increasing frequency in immunocompromised patients and are often resistant to fluconazole;

+ fluconazole, itraconazole, and posaconazole have long plasma half-lives (20–35 hours), properties that make them suitable for once-daily administration; and

+ fluconazole is less extensively metabolized and protein bound than the other triazoles and is less prone to side effects.

Triazoles are used in many forms of systemic mycosis. Fluconazole is widely used in the treatment of systemic *Candida* infections and, because of its ability to penetrate into cerebrospinal fluid, cryptococcal meningitis. It is also widely used in chemoprophylactic regimens in patients vulnerable to systemic mycoses. Itraconazole has been largely superseded by the newer agents voriconazole and posaconazole, although it is still considered the agent of choice for the endemic dimorphic fungi (e.g. histoplasmosis, coccidiomycosis, and blastomycosis). Voriconazole is the preferred agent to treat infections with *Aspergillus* spp. and is a reserve drug for yeasts resistant to fluconazole.

Fluconazole can be used to treat superficial *Candida* infections if oral therapy is thought to be necessary or more acceptable than, for example, vaginal pessaries. Oral itraconazole is also effective in dermatophyte infections, including those involving nails.

Side effects are not as common with the azoles as with amphotericin B but life-threatening liver toxicity can arise with long-term use. The severe liver toxicity noted with ketoconazole has been less problematic with the newer triazoles. Other side effects include nausea and vomiting. Drug interactions are a potential problem between azoles and other drug classes, as they inhibit the hepatic metabolism of many drugs, including cyclosporin, warfarin, anti-epileptics, and oral hypoglycaemic drugs.

Resistance to triazoles is increasing, and extensive use of these compounds could compromise their value in the long term.

## Allylamines   Dermatophyte infections only

Allylamines, like the antifungal azoles, interfere with ergosterol synthesis but act at an earlier stage by inhibiting the formation of squalene epoxide, a precursor of lanosterol. The most important compound of this type, terbinafine, exhibits broad-spectrum antifungal activity and is almost completely absorbed when given orally. It accumulates in keratin, where it persists after treatment is stopped. This is particularly important in dermatophyte infections of the toenails, which are notoriously refractory to therapy.

*Can. albicans* is more susceptible in the mycelial phase than in the yeast form and, whereas the drug is generally fungicidal, the action against *Candida* is fungistatic. Terbinafine is the drug of choice for fungal infections of the toenail and offers an alternative to griseofulvin and azoles for the treatment of other dermatophyte infections if systemic therapy is indicated. An earlier allylamine, naftifine, is insufficiently active to be useful systemically but is marketed in some countries for topical use.

## Echinocandins   Severe systemic mycoses only

Caspofungin was the first of this new class of antifungal drugs—the echinocandins. It was soon followed by the related compounds micafungin and anidulafungin. The echinocandins have recently become available for the treatment of systemic and invasive candidiasis resistant to the azoles and amphotericin. They are cyclic lipopeptides and interfere with fungal cell wall synthesis. While resistance is uncommon among *Candida* spp., when it occurs, such strains are generally cross-resistant to all echinocandins. *Aspergillus* spp. are also inhibited by these agents.

Clinical experience with echinocandins is now extensive and these agents have found a place in the treatment of systemic mycoses; echinocandins have become the preferred agent for invasive candidiasis and for the salvage treatment of invasive aspergillosis.

## Topical antifungal agents

Apart from the azole, polyene, and allylamine derivatives that are available for topical use, a range of other agents is available in some countries for the treatment of ringworm and other superficial fungal infections. These include tolnaftate, haloprogin, and ciclopirox. None of these agents exhibits useful activity against *Candida* spp. A variety of ointments containing benzoic acid (e.g. Whitfield's ointment: benzoic acid and salicylic acid in an emulsifying base) have been used traditionally for treating dermatophyte infections of the skin. Though old-fashioned and a little messy, they are cheap and effective. The monounsaturated fatty acid, undecylenic (undecenoic) acid is also widely used in proprietary preparations for conditions such as 'athlete's foot'.

A morpholine derivative, amorolfine, which is active against *Candida* and the dermatophytes, is marketed for the topical treatment of fungal infections of the skin and, in the form of a lacquer, for application to infected nails. Its action is said to persist so that it needs to be applied to infected nails only once or twice a week.

### *P. jiroveci (P.carinii)*

Originally encountered as a rare cause of interstitial pneumonia in infants, *P. jiroveci* (formerly *P. carinii*) was later recognized as an infection of severely immunocompromised individuals, in whom it can cause a life-threatening pneumonia, most notably in individuals suffering from HIV/AIDS. The incidence of pneumocystis pneumonia has declined among these patients since the advent of highly active antiretroviral therapy (see 'HIV/AIDS' in Chapter 31). Prophylaxis, usually with the antibacterial agent, co-trimoxazole (see 'Diaminopyrimidines' in Chapter 4) has also been successful in reducing the incidence of this disease.

Co-trimoxazole is the drug of choice for treatment of established pneumocystis infection but patients suffering from AIDS are often intolerant of the high doses used. Other combinations that have found favour in some units are trimethoprim with the antileprosy drug dapsone or clindamycin with the antimalarial agent primaquine. The diamidine derivative, pentamidine isethionate is also active against *P. jiroveci* but the intravenous infusion carries problems of toxicity, which may be severe, and the drug is sometimes (at least in prophylactic use) administered directly into the lungs by nebulizer in an effort to reduce systemic toxicity. Atovaquone appears to be a safe alternative to co-trimoxazole and pentamidine and is sometimes used in patients intolerant of the older drugs.

The use of these agents in the treatment and prophylaxis of pneumocystis infection is discussed in Chapter 31.

## Key points

## Antifungal agents: prescribing choices

♦ Topical imidazoles are effective for treating mild fungal infections of skin and mucous membranes.

♦ Oral terbinafine is the first choice for treating infections of finger- and toenails and more widespread dermatomyoses.

♦ Triazoles are oral and parenteral agents suitable for systemic mycoses treatment: fluconazole is active against yeasts, not moulds; itraconazole is active against yeasts, moulds, and dimorphic fungi but is being superseded by the newer azoles voriconazole and posaconazole.

♦ Amphotericin is active against yeasts, many moulds, and dimorphic fungi; lipsomal formulations are expensive but less toxic.

♦ Echinocandins are used for first-line therapy against severe, invasive *Candida* infections and for salvage therapy for invasive mould infections.

## Further reading

Hay, R. (2013) Superficial fungal infections. *Medicine*, **41**(12): 716–18.

Pappas, P. G., Kauffman, C. A., Andes, D., et al. (2009) Clinical practice guidelines for the management of candidiasis: 2009 update by the Infectious Diseases Society of America. *Clinical Infectious Diseases*, **48**(5): 503–35.

Perfect, J. R., Dismukes, W. E., Dromer, F., et al. (2010) Clinical practice guidelines for the management of cryptococcal disease: 2010 update by the Infectious Disease Society of America. *Clinical Infectious Diseases*, **50**(3): 291–322.

Walsh, T. J., Anaissie, E. J., Denning, D. W., et al. (2008) Treatment of aspergillosis: clinical practice guidelines of the Infectious Diseases Society of America. *Clinical Infectious Diseases*, **46**(3): 327–60.

# Chapter 9

# Antiprotozoal and anthelminthic agents

## Introduction to antiprotozoal and anthelminthic agents

Pathogenic protozoa and helminths are among the most important causes of morbidity and mortality in the world (see Chapter 35). An estimated 700 million people suffer from malaria, filariasis, and schistosomiasis alone, and two-thirds of the world's population live in conditions in which parasitic diseases are unavoidable.

Some parasitic diseases were among the first to be treated by specific remedies; indeed, cures for malaria, amoebic dysentery, and tapeworm infection have been known for centuries. Nevertheless, the therapeutic armamentarium for parasitic infection remains severely restricted. Many of the antiparasitic drugs that are available leave much to be desired in terms of efficacy and safety, and a few parasitic infections remain for which there is no effective remedy at all.

## Antiprotozoal drugs

Protozoa are unicellular organisms. Those of medical importance are conveniently classified into four groups: amoebae, flagellates, sporozoa, and 'others' (Table 9.1). The agents used for treatment are very varied and often specific to the particular organism involved. Consequently, antiprotozoal agents defy formal classification and are best considered in the context of the organisms against which they are used. Their mode of action is often poorly characterized.

### Antimalarial agents

#### Artemisinins

The artemisinins are highly effective antimalarial agents extracted from the leaves of the shrub *Artemisia annua*. Formulations include the water-soluble artesunate and dihydroartesunate, and the oil-soluble artemether and artemotil. Artesunate is the most widely used formulation and can be given intravenously, by mouth, and rectally. They should never, however, be given as monotherapy.

The mechanism of action of the artemisinins is unknown but they are highly effective drugs against all species of malaria. In particular, they have activity against all stages of the parasite, including the sexual stages (gametocytes), which means they can also reduce transmission. Large, randomized controlled trials performed in Asia and Africa have demonstrated their superiority over quinine for the treatment of severe falciparum malaria. Indeed, the artemisinins—in combination with another antimalarial—are now the recommended first-line therapy for acute and severe falciparum malaria worldwide. The WHO currently recommends five artemisinin combination treatments (ACTs): artesunate–amodiaquine, artesunate–sulphadoxine–pyrimethamine, artesunate–mefloquine, artesunate–lumefantrine, and dihydroartemisinin–piperaquine. The use of the first three of these ACTs is restricted by resistance to the partner drug in some geographic regions; the last two ACTS are, at present, effective everywhere.

**Table 9.1** Principal pathogenic protozoa infecting man, and the drugs commonly used in treatment.

| Species | Diseases caused | Useful drugs |
|---|---|---|
| **Amoebae** | | |
| *Entamoeba histolytica* | Amoebic dysentery; liver abscess | Metronidazole (diloxanide furoate) |
| *Naegleria fowleri* | Meningoencephalitis | Amphotericin |
| *Acanthamoeba* spp. | Amoebic keratitis | Propamidine (topical) |
| **Flagellates** | | |
| *Trypanosoma brucei* ssp. | Sleeping sickness | Melarsoprol; eflornithine[a] (pentamidine; suramin) |
| *Tryp. cruzi* | Chagas disease | Nifurtimox; benznidazole |
| *Leishmania* spp. | Leishmaniasis (cutaneous/mucocutaneous/visceral) | Sodium stibogluconate; miltefosine; liposomal amphotericin |
| *Trichomonas vaginalis* | Vaginitis | Metronidazole |
| *Giardia lamblia* | Diarrhoea; steatorrhoea | Metronidazole |
| **Sporozoa** | | |
| *Plasmodium* spp. | Malaria | Quinine, artesunate, chloroquine, primaquine, and many others |
| *Toxoplasma gondii* | Toxoplasmosis | Pyrimethamine + sulfadiazine; spiramycin |
| *Cryptosporidium parvum* | Diarrhoea | Nitazoxanide; (azithromycin; paromomycin) |
| *Cyclospora cayetanensis* | Diarrhoea | Co-trimoxazole |
| **Others** | | |
| *Balantidium coli* | Balantidial dysentery | Tetracycline; metronidazole |
| *Babesia* spp. | Babesiosis | Clindamycin + quinine |
| Microsporidia | Microsporidiosis | Albendazole |

[a] Eflornithine is not active against *Trypanosoma brucei rhodesiense*; drugs shown in brackets have limited usefulness.

Toxicity from the artemisinins is remarkably rare. Approximately 1 in 3,000 treatments results in a type 1 hypersensitivity reaction but few other reactions have been reported. The recent emergence in South East Asia of *Plasmodium falciparum* parasites with reduced susceptibility to artemisinins is a major concern.

## Quinine

Quinine is extracted from the bark of the cinchona tree and has been used in the treatment of malaria for centuries. It has oral and intravenous formulations. It is a highly effective antimalarial drug and, prior to the advent of artemisinins, its intravenous preparation was the first-line therapy for severe falciparum malaria. Unlike the artemisinins, however, its activity is restricted to the mature trophozoite (red cell) stage of parasite development; it has no activity on the younger stages or the sexual stages of *Pla. falciparum*, the latter being responsible for ongoing transmission to mosquitoes. The complications of quinine treatment include hypoglycaemia (which can be severe), tinnitus, and reversible deafness. Quinine also prolongs the QT interval by around 10 per cent at therapeutic concentrations and can, therefore, predispose to cardiac arrhythmias. This effect is even greater in children under 2 years of age. Intravenous quinine should always be given with careful monitoring of cardiac rhythm and blood glucose. Oral quinine is given in a dose of 10 mg/kg three times daily for seven days followed by either doxycycline or clindamycin. Combination therapy is the rule rather than the exception now in all antimalarial drug treatment.

## Chloroquine

Chloroquine is a 4-aminoquinoline which is highly active against mature malarial parasites in red cells. It can be given by almost any route (oral, intravenous, subcutaneous, rectal), is safe in pregnancy and young children, and was used on a massive scale worldwide until the widespread development of resistant falciparum parasites more than 30 years ago. Other than *Pla. vivax* in South East Asia, which has high rates of chloroquine resistance, the drug remains the first-line agent against non-falciparum malaria. The commonest side effect is pruritus, which can lead to patients believing they are allergic to the drug and refusing subsequent treatment with either chloroquine or quinine.

Amodiaquine is a closely related 4-aminoquinoline but with activity against chloroquine-resistant parasites, although amodiaquine resistance is increasing. It is only given orally and often paired with artesunate. The major side effects are agranulocytosis and hepatotoxicity, which have limited its use as a prophylactic agent.

## Primaquine

The 8-aminoquinolines primaquine and tafenoquine (an investigational compound with an extended half-life) are selectively active against the hypnozoites ('sleeping' liver stages responsible for late relapses) of *Pla. vivax* and the gametocytes (sexual stage) of *Pla. falciparum*. They are, therefore, used to either prevent relapse of *Pla. vivax* (following treatment of the blood stages by chloroquine) or to prevent transmission of *Pla. falciparum* to mosquitoes. The principal toxicity is oxidant haemolysis, especially in those with glucose-6-phosphate dehydrogenase (G6PD) deficiency. The degree of haemolysis is related to the degree of deficiency and the dose of primaquine. G6PD status should always be checked prior to using primaquine.

## Antifolates

A group of compounds collectively known as 'antifolates' are also used, usually in combination, especially for antimalarial prophylaxis. These include pyrimethamine, proguanil (and chlorproguanil), the long-acting sulphonamides sulfadoxine and sulfalene (sulfametopyrazine), and dapsone (see 'Antimycobacterial agents' in Chapter 4). Pyrimethamine, a dihydrofolate reductase inhibitor related to trimethoprim (see 'Sulphonamides' in Chapter 3), exhibits a selectively high affinity for the plasmodial form of the enzyme and interacts synergistically with sulphonamides. Proguanil and chlorproguanil are biguanides that are metabolized in the body to compounds closely related to pyrimethamine and have an identical mode of action. Surprisingly, some pyrimethamine-resistant mutants retain susceptibility to these closely related compounds. Chlorproguanil (Lapudrine) combined with dapsone—'lapdap'—is being promoted in parts of Africa as a relatively cheap treatment for malaria with a reduced propensity to generate resistance. Proguanil itself is used solely for prophylaxis, usually together with chloroquine. A combination with atovaquone (a hydroxynaphthoquinone that acts on the respiratory chain of some protozoa), called 'Malarone', is available for treatment and prophylaxis. It is well tolerated, safe, and effective.

## Other important antiprotozoal agents

### Metronidazole

Metronidazole is active against anaerobic bacteria and some protozoa. It is commonly used in the treatment of *Trichomonas vaginalis*, *Entamoeba histolytica*, and *Giardia lamblia*. It can be given orally, intravenously, or rectally and is well tolerated. Common adverse reactions include nausea, diarrhoea, and a metallic taste in the mouth. Longer term use can lead to peripheral neuropathy. Consumption of alcohol with metronidazole can lead to a disulphiram-like reaction, with flushing, tachycardia, nausea, and vomiting.

### Amphotericin B

Amphotericin B is a macrocyclic, polyene antifungal antibiotic produced by *Streptomyces nodosus*. Its primary role is in the treatment of severe fungal infections and it is thought to act by binding to sterols in the fungal cell membrane, with a resulting change in membrane permeability, allowing leakage of a variety of small molecules from the fungal cell. However, it is also an effective treatment for visceral leishmaniasis. The drug is available in its plain form or as a liposomal formulation which facilitates delivery of the drug into cells and reduces side effects. Liposomal amphotericin is the recommended treatment for visceral leishmaniasis. Serious side effects, especially from the plain intravenous preparation, are well described and include sudden hypotensive episodes with rigours immediately following infusions, nephrotoxicity and hepatitis, hypokalaemia and hypomagnesaemia, and anaemia and leucopenia.

## Antimonials and other antileishmania agents

Two related and effectually interchangeable antimonial compounds, sodium stibogluconate and meglumine antimonate, are traditionally used for the treatment of leishmaniasis. Resistance has, however, become a problem in many parts of the world. More recently, most success has been achieved with amphotericin (see 'Polyenes' in Chapter 8), especially when administered in the liposomal formulation that carries the drug into macrophages. The antifungal azoles (see 'Azoles' in Chapter 7), the aminoglycoside paromomycin, and pentamidine also exhibit some activity against leishmania and offer alternatives in recalcitrant cases. Much hope for leishmaniasis sufferers rests with an oral phosphocholine analogue, miltefosine, which has undergone successful trials in visceral leishmaniasis in India and also shows signs of benefit in cutaneous forms of the disease.

## Arsenicals and other antitrypanosomal agents

Organic arsenicals, though extremely toxic, have been used for many years to treat all forms of sleeping sickness. Melarsoprol (Mel B) is the derivative usually used. Melarsoprol affects glycolysis and also forms a complex with trypanothione, which replaces glutathione in these organisms. Resistance may occur and is thought to be due to reduced uptake of the drug.

*Tryp. brucei gambiense* infection responds to eflornithine (α-difluoromethyl-ornithine), which has shown to be effective in the late stages of the disease complicated by meningoencephalitis, but *Tryp. brucei rhodesiense* is resistant. Eflornithine is an irreversible inhibitor of ornithine decarboxylase, an essential enzyme in polyamine synthesis. Differences in enzyme turnover have been proposed to account for the differential activity on the two *Tryp. brucei* subspecies. If treatment can be started before the trypanosomes invade the central nervous system, suramin—which, like melarsoprol, interferes with glycolysis—may be curative. Because of toxicity, it is often used in a two to three dose regimen before melarsoprol in *Tryp. brucei rhodesiense* meningoencephalitis. The diamidine pentamidine is also effective in the early stages of *Tryp. brucei gambiense* infection but ineffective in *Tryp. brucei rhodesiense*. Various targets have been proposed for this drug but its primary site of action has proved elusive.

## Other agents

Clindamycin is a lincosamide antibiotic with a broad spectrum of activity which includes Gram-positive bacteria and some protozoa. It can be used in combination with chloroquine or quinine to treat falciparum malaria, and in combination with primaquine is effective in the treatment of non-severe *Pneumocystis jiroveci* pneumonia. It can also be used to treat *Toxoplasma gondii* infections, although spiramycin (a macrolide antibiotic) is probably more effective.

Nitazoxanide, a nitrothiazole derivative, which is converted in the body to the active form, tizoxanide, may offer effective therapy against *Cryptosporidium parvum* infections if antimicrobial treatment is necessary. Infections with *Isospora belli* and *Cyclospora cayetanensis* respond to co-trimoxazole, although antimicrobial therapy is seldom required.

## Anthelminthic drugs

Helminths are parasitic worms. They often have a complex life cycle involving a period of development outside the definitive host, either in soil or in an intermediate host. Helminths of medical importance fall into three major groups: nematodes (roundworms), trematodes (flukes), and cestodes (tapeworms; see Chapter 35 and Table 9.2).

Many of the human anthelminthic drugs have emerged through the application of drugs originally intended for the treatment of animals. Despite this, a wide variety of compounds is available but three compounds—ivermectin, praziquantel, and albendazole—between them cover virtually the whole helminthic spectrum. Resistance to these agents is known to occur in animals and there are reports of failures of treatment in humans but difficulties in in vitro susceptibility testing limit knowledge of the prevalence of resistance or its mechanisms.

Information on the means by which anthelminthic agents achieve their effect is also relatively limited. The neuromuscular system of worms seems to be peculiarly susceptible to chemotherapeutic attack: many important anthelminthic agents, including piperazine, praziquantel, ivermectin, levamisole, and pyrantel appear to act by paralysing the worms. In contrast, the benzimidazoles interfere with the polymerization of tubulin in the formation of microtubules in the cytoskeleton of the worm.

### The benzimidazoles: albendazole and mebendazole

The benzimidazoles are active against most intestinal roundworms. The first of the benzimidazoles to be introduced into human medicine was tiabendazole (thiabendazole) but this has now been largely abandoned because of its side effects and replaced by albendazole and mebendazole. Albendazole exhibits the broadest spectrum of activity and is the drug of choice for the elimination of intestinal roundworms. It is the most active benzimidazole against *Strongyloides stercoralis*. Orally administered albendazole is poorly absorbed from the gastrointestinal tract and extensively metabolized by the liver; the sulphoxide metabolite may be responsible for most of the drug's in vivo anthelminthic effects. Adverse effects are usually mild and transient and include nausea and vomiting. Mebendazole is also sometimes used and is effective against adult worms and larval stages but is less active than albendazole against hookworm and *Stro. stercoralis*.

**Table 9.2** Principal helminth parasites of man, and the drugs commonly used in treatment.

| Species | Intermediate host | Human disease | Geographical distribution | Useful drugs |
|---|---|---|---|---|
| **Nematodes (roundworms)** | | | | |
| *Wuchereria bancrofti* | Mosquito | Filariasis | Tropical belt | |
| *Loa loa* | *Chrysops* spp. | Filariasis | Tropical Africa | Diethylcarbamazine; albendazole; ivermectin + doxycycline |
| *Brugia malayi* | Mosquito | Filariasis | South East Asia | |
| *Onchocerca volvulus* | *Simulium* spp. | River blindness | Tropical Africa, Central America | Ivermectin |
| *Dracunculus medinensis* | *Cyclops* spp. (water flea) | Guinea worm | Tropical Africa, Yemen | Benzimidazoles |
| *Trichinella spiralis* | Pigs and other wild animals | Trichinellosis | Worldwide | Benzimidazoles |
| *Ancylostoma duodenale* | None (soil) | Hookworm | Tropics and subtropics | |
| *Necator americanus* | None (soil) | Hookworm | Tropics and subtropics | |
| *Ascaris lumbricoides* | None (soil) | Roundworm | Worldwide | |
| *Trichuris trichiura* | None (soil) | Whipworm | Worldwide | Albendazole (see Table 35.1) |
| *Strongyloides stercoralis* | None (soil) | Strongyloidiasis | Tropics and subtropics | |
| *Enterobius vermicularis* | None | Threadworm | Worldwide | |
| **Trematodes (flukes)** | | | | |
| *Schistosoma mansoni* | Snail | Schistosomiasis or 'bilharzia' | Africa, West Indies, South America | |
| *S. haematobium* | Snail | Schistosomiasis | Africa | Praziquantel |
| *S. japonicum* | Snail | Schistosomiasis | Far East | |
| *Fasciola hepatica* | Snail, vegetation | Liver fluke | Worldwide | Triclabendazole |
| *Clonorchis sinensis* | Snail, freshwater fish | Liver fluke | Far East | |
| *Paragonimus westermani* | Snail, crab, crayfish | Lung fluke | Far East, West Africa, South America | Praziquantel |
| *Fasciolopsis buski* | Snail, water chestnut | Fasciolopsiasis | Far East | |

**Table 9.2** (continued).

| Species | Intermediate host | Human disease | Geographical distribution | Useful drugs |
|---|---|---|---|---|
| **Cestodes (Tapeworms)** | | | | |
| *Echinococcus granulosus* | Sheep, human | Hydatid disease | Worldwide | Albendazole |
| *Taenia saginata* | Cattle | Beef tapeworm | Worldwide | |
| *Tae. solium* | Pig | Pork tapeworm | Worldwide | Niclosamide, praziquantel |
| *Hymenolepis nana* | None | Tapeworm | Mainly tropics and subtropics | |
| *Diphyllobothrium latum* | *Cyclops* spp., fish | Fish tapeworm | Mainly northern Russia, Finland | |

As with albendazole, it is relatively poorly absorbed and has a similar side-effect profile. Occasionally, however, it can stimulate *Ascaris* worms to emerge from the mouth and nostrils; this can be very alarming if the patient is not forewarned.

## Praziquantel

Praziquantel is the drug of choice for the treatment of all species of *Schistosoma* infection. Praziquantel appears to cause schistosomes to release their hold within the venules, and to expose surface antigens that are normally protected from host attack. It is also very effective in other trematode infections (e.g., clonorchiasis and paragonimiasis) and in cestode infections cause by *Taenia solium*, *Tae. saginata*, and *Diphyllobothrium* and *Echinococcus* spp. (which cause hydatid disease). Praziquantel is not, however, effective against the liver fluke *Fasciola hepatica*. Praziquantel can only be given orally and is very well tolerated. It is well absorbed from the gastrointestinal tract and is metabolized by the hepatic cytochrome P450 pathway; hence drugs which inhibit (e.g. antifungal azoles) or induce (e.g. rifampicin) this pathway should be given with caution.

## Ivermectin

Ivermectin was originally developed for use in animals and is still used extensively in veterinary practice, together with related derivatives, including doramectin. It is extensively used for the treatment and control of onchocerciasis, filariasis, and strongyloidiasis. It is active against many of the arthropod ectoparasites and is effective in the treatment of human scabies. It has limited activity against hookworm and *Trichuris trichiura*. It can be given topically, orally, or occasionally by intravenous injection. Ivermectin is usually given in one or two doses only and is well tolerated, although neurotoxicity (with confusion, ataxia, and coma) has been reported. Ivermectin should not be given to children under 5 years of age.

## Piperazine

Piperazine is an effective treatment for *Ascaris lumbricoides* and *Enterobius vermicularis* infections. It acts by paralysing parasites, thus enabling them to be expelled by the host. Pyrantel, another anthelminthic drug, acts in a similar way, although the two drugs are antagonistic and should not be given together.

## Diethylcarbamazine

A relative of piperazine, diethylcarbamazine has been used for many years in filariasis but its use has been steadily eroded by ivermectin. Use of ivermectin does not seem to be accompanied by the severe side effects (Mazzotti reaction) associated with the administration of diethylcarbamazine, and a further bonus is the concomitant expulsion of some intestinal worms.

---

### Key points

### Anthelminthic drugs: notes for prescribers

- Albendazole is used to treat most intestinal worms.
- Piperazine is used as an alternative treatment for threadworm or ascaris.
- Praziquantel is used to treat fluke infections and tapeworms.
- For all other worm infections, leave the choice of treatment to the experts.

---

## Further reading

Checkley, A. M., Chiodini, P. L., Dockrell, D. H., et al. (2010) Eosinophilia in returning travellers and migrants from the tropics: UK recommendations for investigation and initial management. *Journal of Infection*, **60**(1): 1–20.

Lalloo, D. G., Shingadia, D., Pasvol, G., Chiodini, P. L., Whitty, C. J., Beeching, N. J., Hill, D. R., Warrell, D. A., and Bannister, B. A., for the HPA Advisory Committee on Malaria Prevention in UK Travellers. (2007) UK malaria treatment guidelines. *Journal of Infection*, **54**(2): 111–21.

# 2

# **Resistance to antimicrobial agents**

# Chapter 10

# The problem of resistance

## What is resistance?

Bacterial isolates have been categorized as being susceptible or resistant to antibiotics ever since they became available. Some of the criteria on which this categorization has been based are discussed in Chapter 12, where the concepts of the minimum inhibitory concentrations (MIC) and the minimum bactericidal concentration of an antibiotic are described. Unfortunately, making accurate judgements about microbial susceptibility or resistance is somewhat less straightforward than this traditional working definition, since there is usually no simple relationship between the MIC (or minimum bactericidal concentrations) of an antibiotic and clinical response. Therapeutic success depends not only on the concentration of the antibiotic achieved at the site of infection (i.e. its pharmacokinetic behaviour) and its activity against the infecting organisms encountered there (i.e. its pharmacodynamic behaviour) but also on the contribution of the host's own defences towards clearance of the offending microbes. Furthermore, it is clear that, particularly in life-threatening infections, outcome is worse if antibiotic therapy is not commenced within 1–4 hours of the onset of symptoms.

The decision as to whether a given bacterial isolate should be termed susceptible or resistant depends ultimately on the likelihood that an infection with that organism can be expected to respond to treatment with a given drug; however, microbiologists and clinicians have become accustomed to the idea that an organism is 'resistant' when it is inhibited in vitro by an antibiotic concentration that is greater than that achievable in vivo. Importantly the concentration of antibiotic that is achievable will vary according to the site of infection, dosage, and route of administration. For example, some antibiotics such as trimethoprim are excreted primarily via the kidneys and therefore achieve, in the context of urinary tract infections, advantageously high concentrations in urine. Furthermore, the intrinsic activity of an antibiotic against some bacteria (e.g. staphylococci) may be greater than for others (e.g. *Escherichia coli*) because of the effect of cell envelope structure on achievable intracellular antibiotic concentrations. These issues mean that several different thresholds (breakpoint concentrations) are often used to define susceptibility to an antibiotic. For example, an *E. coli* strain for which the MIC of ampicillin is 32 mg/l might be classed as susceptible if isolated from the urine of a patient with presumed urinary tract infection, while the same bacterium causing a bloodstream infection would be classified as ampicillin resistant. These differences in definition of susceptibility relate to the variations in achievable concentrations at the site of infection: thus, an ampicillin concentration of 32 mg/l can reliably be achieved in urine but not in blood.

## Intrinsic resistance

If whole bacterial species are considered, rather than individual isolates, it is apparent immediately that they are not all intrinsically susceptible to all antibiotics (Table 10.1); for example, a coliform infection would not be treated with erythromycin, or a streptococcal infection with

**Table 10.1** Effective antimicrobial spectrum of some of the most commonly used antibacterial agents.[a]

| Organism | Penicillins | Cephalosporins | Aminoglycosides | Tetracyclines | Macrolides | Chloramphenicol | Fluoroquinolones | Sulphonamides | Trimethoprim | Metronidazole | Glycopeptides |
|---|---|---|---|---|---|---|---|---|---|---|---|
| **Gram-positive bacteria** | | | | | | | | | | | |
| Staphylococcus aureus | V | (S) | (S) | (S) | (S) | (S) | V | (S) | (S) | R | S |
| Streptococcus pyogenes | S | S | R | (S) | S | S | V | (S) | S | R | S |
| Other streptococci | S | S | R | (S) | S | S | V | (S) | S | R | S |
| Enterococci | V | R | R | (S) | S | S | V | (S) | (S) | R | (S) |
| Clostridium spp. | S | S | R | S | S | S | V | (S) | R | S | S |
| **Gram-negative bacteria** | | | | | | | | | | | |
| Escherichia coli | V | V | (S) | (S) | R | (S) | (S) | (S) | (S) | R | R |
| Other enterobacteria | V | V | (S) | (S) | R | (S) | (S) | (S) | (S) | R | R |
| Pseudomonas aeruginosa | V | V | V | R | R | R | (S) | R | R | R | R |
| Haemophilus influenzae | V | V | R | (S) | S | S | S | (S) | (S) | R | R |
| Neisseria spp. | V | S | R | (S) | S | S | (S) | (S) | R | R | R |
| Bacteroides spp. | Ft | V | R | (S) | S | S | V | (S) | R | S | R |
| **Other organisms** | | | | | | | | | | | |
| Mycobacteria | R | R | V | R | R | R | (S) | R | R | R | R |
| Chlamydiae | R | R | R | S | S | S | S | S | R | R | R |
| Mycoplasmas | R | R | R | S | S | S | S | R | R | R | R |
| Fungi | R | R | R | R | R | R | R | R | R | R | R |

[a] S, usually considered susceptible; R, usually considered resistant; (S), strain variation in susceptibility; V, variation among related drugs and/or strains.

an aminoglycoside, since the organisms are intrinsically resistant to these antibiotics. Similarly, *Pseudomonas aeruginosa* and *Mycobacterium tuberculosis* are intrinsically resistant to most of the agents used to treat more tractable infections. Such intrinsically resistant organisms are sometimes termed non-susceptible, with the term resistant reserved for variants of normally susceptible species that acquire mechanism(s) of resistance (Chapter 11). Actually, the terms resistant and non-susceptible are often used interchangeably.

A microbe will be intrinsically resistant to an antibiotic if it either does not possess a target for the drug's action or is impermeable to the drug. Thus, bacteria are intrinsically resistant to polyene antibiotics such as amphotericin B as sterols that are present in the fungal but not bacterial cell membrane are the target for these drugs. The lipopolysaccharide outer envelope of Gram-negative bacteria is important in determining susceptibility patterns, since many antibiotics cannot penetrate this barrier to reach their intracellular target. Fortunately, intrinsic resistance is therefore often predictable and should not pose problems, provided that informed and judicious choices of antibiotics are made for the treatment of infection. Of greater concern is the primarily unpredictable acquisition or emergence of resistance in previously susceptible microbes, sometimes during the course of therapy itself.

## Acquired resistance

Introduction of clinically effective antibiotics has been followed invariably by the emergence of resistant strains of bacteria among species that would normally be considered to be susceptible. Acquisition of resistance has seriously reduced the therapeutic value of many important antibiotics but is also a major stimulus to the constant search for new and more effective antimicrobial drugs. However, while the emergence of resistance to new antibiotics is inevitable, the rate of development and spread of resistance is not predictable.

The first systematic observations of acquired drug resistance were made by Paul Ehrlich between 1902 and 1909 while using dyes and organic arsenicals to treat mice infected experimentally with trypanosomes. Within a very few years of the introduction of sulphonamides and penicillin (in 1935 and 1941, respectively), microorganisms originally susceptible to these drugs were found to have acquired resistance. When penicillin came into use, less than 1 per cent of all *Staphylococcus aureus* strains were resistant to its action. By 1946, however, under the selective pressure of this antibiotic, the proportion of penicillin-resistant strains found in hospitals had risen to 14 per cent. A year later, 38 per cent were resistant, and today, resistance is found in more than 90 per cent of all *Staph. aureus* strains. In contrast, over the same period, an equally important pathogen, *Streptococcus pyogenes*, has remained uniformly susceptible to penicillin, although there is no guarantee that resistance will not spread to *Str. pyogenes* in future years. It is possible that some such examples of limited or no resistance emergence are because resistant mutant cells cannot survive and/or proliferate (i.e. the bacteria are not 'fit').

There is no clear explanation for the marked differences in rate or extent of acquisition of resistance between different species. Possession of the genetic capacity for resistance does not always explain its prevalence in a particular species. Even when selection pressures are similar, the end result may not be the same. Thus, although about 90 per cent of all strains of *Staph. aureus* are now resistant to penicillin, the same has not happened to ampicillin resistance in *E. coli* under similar selection pressure. At present, apart from localized outbreaks involving epidemic strains, about 50 per cent of *E. coli* strains are resistant to ampicillin, and this level has remained more or less steady for a number of years. However, since an increasing incidence of resistance is at least partly a consequence of selective pressure, it is not surprising that the withdrawal of an antibiotic from clinical use may often result in a slow reduction in the number of resistant strains encountered in a particular environment. For example, fluoroquinolone resistant strains of *P. aeruginosa* that emerged in some hospitals as ciprofloxacin or levofloxacin were used more frequently were replaced by more susceptible strains following the restriction or removal of these drugs. Conversely, sulphonamide resistant *E. coli* strains that became commonplace when the sulphonamide-containing combination drug co-trimoxazole was widely used are still prevalent. This is probably because the selection pressure still exists for other antibiotics, such as ampicillin, and the genes coding for sulphonamide and ampicillin resistance are often closely linked on plasmids; hence, use of one antibiotic can select or maintain resistance to another.

The introduction of new antibiotics has also resulted in changes to the predominant spectrum of organisms responsible for infections. In the 1960s semi-synthetic 'β-lactamase stable' penicillins and cephalosporins were introduced which, temporarily, solved the problem of staphylococcal infections. Unfortunately, Gram-negative bacteria then became the major pathogens found in hospitals and rapidly acquired resistance to multiple antibiotics in the succeeding years. In the 1970s the pendulum swung the other way, with the first outbreaks of hospital infection with multiresistant staphylococci that were resistant to nearly all antistaphylococcal agents. Outbreaks of infection caused by such organisms have occurred subsequently all over the world.

Gram-negative bacteria are once again assuming greater importance, particularly in hospitals. Resistance to newer cephalosporins—mediated by extended-spectrum β-lactamases—and fluoroquinolones in *E. coli* and other enterobacteria has increased or is continuing to increase, depending on geographical locale, rendering these commonly used antibiotics less effective. Multiresistant Gram-negative bacteria (such as *Acinetobacter* spp.) have emerged that are resistant to most and, occasionally, all approved antibiotics. The recent emergence of carbapenemase-producing enterobacteria is a most worrying development given the 'last line of defence' status of the carbapenem class of antibiotics. Some Gram-negative bacilli may produce both drug-inactivating enzymes and altered porins and thus become resistant to carbapenems because of a combination of antibiotic cleavage and reduced cell penetration.

## Types of acquired resistance

Two main types of acquired resistance may be encountered in bacterial species that would normally be considered susceptible to a particular antibacterial agent: mutational resistance and transmissible resistance.

### Mutational resistance

In any large population of bacterial cells, a very few individual cells may spontaneously become resistant (see Chapter 11). Such resistant cells have no particular survival advantage in the absence of antibiotic but, after the introduction of antibiotic treatment, susceptible bacterial cells will be killed, so that the (initially) very few resistant cells can proliferate until they eventually form a wholly resistant population. Many antimicrobial agents select for this type of acquired resistance in many different bacterial species, both in vitro and in vivo. The problem has been recognized as being of particular importance in the long-term treatment of tuberculosis (TB) with anti-TB drugs.

### Transmissible resistance

A more spectacular type of acquired resistance occurs when genes conferring antibiotic resistance transfer from a resistant bacterial cell to a sensitive one. The simultaneous transfer of resistance to several unrelated antimicrobial agents can be demonstrated readily, both in the laboratory and the patient. Exponential transfer and spread of existing resistance genes through a previously susceptible bacterial population is a much more efficient mechanism of acquiring resistance than the development of resistance by mutation of individual susceptible cells.

Mechanisms by which transfer of resistance genes takes place are discussed in Chapter 11. Notably, however resistance appears in a hitherto susceptible bacterial cell or population, it will only become widespread under the selective pressures produced by the presence of appropriate antibiotics. In addition, the development of resistant cells does not have to happen often or on a large scale. A single mutation or transfer event can, if the appropriate selective pressures are operating, lead to the replacement of a susceptible population by a resistant one. Without selective pressure, antibiotic resistance may be a handicap rather than an asset to a bacterium.

## Cross-resistance and multiple resistance

These terms are often confused. Cross-resistance involves resistance to a number of different members of a group of (usually) chemically related agents that are affected alike by the same resistance mechanism. For example, there is almost complete cross-resistance between the different tetracyclines (although not necessarily the closely related tigecycline; see 'Tetracyclines' in Chapter 3) because tetracycline resistance results largely from an efflux mechanism that affects all members of the group. The situation is more complex among other antibiotic families. Thus, resistance to aminoglycosides may be mediated by any one of a number of different drug-inactivating enzymes (see Table 11.3) with different substrate specificities, and the range of aminoglycosides to which the organism is resistant will depend on which enzyme it produces. Cross-resistance can also be observed occasionally between unrelated antibiotics. For example, a change in the outer membrane structure of Gram-negative bacilli may concomitantly deny access of unrelated compounds to their target sites.

In contrast, multiple drug (multidrug) resistance involves a bacterium becoming resistant to several unrelated antibiotics by different resistance mechanisms. For example, if a staphylococcus is resistant to penicillin, gentamicin, and tetracycline, the resistances must have originated independently, since the strain destroys the penicillin with a β-lactamase, inactivates gentamicin with an aminoglycoside-modifying enzyme, and excludes tetracycline from the cell by an active efflux mechanism.

It is, however, not always clear whether cross-resistance or multiple resistance is being observed. Genes conferring resistance to several unrelated agents can be transferred en bloc from one bacterial cell to another on plasmids (see Chapter 11), thereby giving the appearance of cross-resistance. In such cases, detailed biochemical and genetic analysis may be required to prove that the resistance mechanisms are distinct (multiple resistance), although the genes conferring resistance are linked and transferred together on one plasmid. The end result may be the same (i.e. resistance to multiple agents) but the risk of the spread is greater for plasmid mediated resistance.

## The clinical problem of drug resistance

Concerns about resistance have been raised at regular intervals since the first introduction of antimicrobial chemotherapy but awareness of the antibiotic resistance problem has probably never been greater than it is today. For example, a 2013 report estimated that in the United States alone at least two million people acquire serious infections with bacteria that are resistant to one or more antibiotics of potential use in such cases. Furthermore, there are at least 23,000 deaths each year as a direct result of these antibiotic-resistant infections, with many other deaths indirectly related to resistance. Indeed, some have suggested that antibiotic resistance threatens to return some settings to a 'pre-antibiotic era'. It is important not to understate or overstate the problem; the situation is presently becoming serious but is not yet desperate, since most infections are still treatable with several currently available agents. This may, however, mean that the only antibiotics that are still active are more toxic or less effective (or both) than those to which bacteria have acquired resistance. For example, it is generally accepted that glycopeptide antibiotics are less effective in the treatment of *Staph. aureus* infection than are antistaphylococcal penicillins (e.g. flucloxacillin); since the latter cannot be used against methicillin-resistant *Staph. aureus* (MRSA), this may partly explain the poorer outcome, including increased risk of death, that is seen in such cases in comparison with infection caused by methicillin-susceptible strains.

There is good evidence that if the antibiotic regimen chosen is subsequently shown to be inactive against the pathogens causing infection, then patient outcome is worse (Fig. 10.1). This means that clinicians are likely to opt for unnecessarily broad-spectrum therapy, particularly in critically ill patients. Unfortunately, repeated use of such regimens against bacteria that harbour resistance genes intensifies the selective pressure for further resistance development, notably in hospitals, where the most vulnerable patients are managed.

In many less-developed countries of the world, the therapeutic options may be severely restricted for economic reasons. There is no doubt that the problem of antibiotic resistance is a global issue, and in future years there is a real possibility that physicians will be faced increasingly with infections for which effective treatment is not available. There are many examples of the intercontinental spread of resistant pathogens, and so the judicious use of antibiotics has global as well as local relevance. Some of the organisms in which resistance is a particular problem are summarized below.

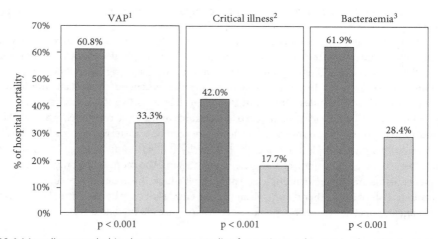

**Fig. 10.1** Mortality recorded in three separate studies for patients who received antibiotic treatment that was subsequently shown to be inactive (dark grey) or active (light grey) against pathogens isolated. VAP, ventilator-associated pneumonia.

Source: data from: 1Kollef MH, Ward S., The influence of mini-BAL cultures on patient outcomes: implications for the antibiotic management of ventilator-associated pneumonia, *Chest*, Volume 113, Number 2, pp. 412–20, Copyright © 1998; 2Kollef MH et al., Inadequate antimicrobial treatment of infections: a risk factor for hospital mortality among critically ill patients, *Chest*, Volume 115, Number 2, pp. 462–474, Copyright © 1999; and 3Ibrahim EH et al., The influence of inadequate antimicrobial treatment of bloodstream infections on patient outcomes in the ICU setting, *Chest*, Volume 118, Number 1, pp. 146–155, Copyright © 2000.

# Enteric Gram-negative bacteria

The prevalence of resistance in hospital strains of enteric Gram-negative bacteria has been rising steadily for the past 40 years, particularly in large units. Although cephalosporins, quinolones, and aminoglycosides have been developed to cope with the problem, resistance to these newer compounds has increased in most countries. Outbreaks of infection caused by multiresistant *Klebsiella* strains and extended-spectrum β-lactamase-producing enterobacteria in general are reported increasingly often, both in high dependency areas of hospitals and in urinary tract isolates from patients in the community. The latter phenomenon is consistent with more wide-spread dissemination of these strains and their carriage in faecal flora. While absolute numbers of carbapenemase-producing Gram-negative enteric bacteria (e.g. NDM-1 and KPC) are still low, there has been an exponential increase in reported isolates in the United Kingdom in recent years. Multiple different types of carbapenem-resistant bacteria (CRB), often *Klebsiella* spp., have now emerged and indeed have become endemic in some hospitals or countries, including Greece, India, Israel, Italy, and the United States. There is evidence that such strains have spread between countries, particularly in patients undergoing hospital treatment in multiple settings. CRB represent a major threat given the paucity, and sometimes lack, of suitable alternatives. While clonal spread is clear, it remains unclear what factors have driven the increase in CRB. Prior exposure to carbapenems is common in patients with CRB, but use of other (more frequently prescribed) antibiotics, including β-lactams, may also have provided a selection pressure in this case.

Widespread resistance in enteric bacteria is a particular problem in less-developed areas, where heavy and indiscriminate use of antibiotics may combine with a high prevalence of drug-resistant bacteria in the faecal flora or even in the environment, poor standards of sanitation, and a high incidence of diarrhoeal disease to encourage the rapid emergence and spread of multiresistant strains of enteric bacteria. Epidemics of diarrhoeal disease caused by multiresistant strains of intestinal pathogens, including *Vibrio cholerae*, shigellae, salmonellae, and toxin-producing strains of *E. coli*, have occurred around the world.

## *Acinetobacter*

These organisms cause hospital-acquired infections, especially in patients in intensive care units, for example, in patients with ventilator-associated pneumonia. Such infections are usually extremely difficult to treat because of the multiple classes of antibiotic resistance found in these bacteria. Very few antibiotics are now reliably effective for the treatment of acinetobacter infections. Even with carbapenems such as imipenem or meropenem, resistance has emerged. Colistin, a relatively toxic old antibiotic that has largely been abandoned for systemic administration, is used to treat some strains that are resistant to all other licensed antibiotics. Some multiresistant *Acinetobacter* spp. strains are susceptible to tigecycline, although again resistance to this agent has already become more common. Faced with the most resistant acinetobacter strains, typically occurring in patients who have often already been exposed to multiple antibiotics, increasingly 'experimental' combinations of antimicrobial agents are being used to attempt to obtain a therapeutic response.

## Staphylococci and enterococci

The epidemiology of MRSA varies markedly across the world but these bacteria have a particular propensity to spread in hospitals and nursing homes. The proportion of *Staph. aureus* isolates that cause serious sepsis such as bloodstream infection and which are resistant to methicillin reached 40–50 per cent in the United Kingdom and some countries in southern Europe, although recent improvements in infection control practice have markedly reduced their prevalence in some (e.g. United Kingdom) but not all (e.g. United States, Asia, Far East) settings. Some MRSA strains have a propensity to spread primarily in health-care institutions (e.g. EMRSA 15, EMRSA 16), while others emerged in community settings (e.g. USA 300, USA 400), typically causing skin sepsis, and then have become established in hospitals. MRSA infections have often been treated with glycopeptides but isolates with low-level resistance to these antibiotics can be found; thus, there is some doubt about whether these antibiotics are effective in some patients, notably those with serious infections. Very occasional MRSA strains with high-level resistance to glycopeptides have also been reported. More recent antibiotics, including linezolid, daptomycin, and tigecycline, are active against these strains but resistance to these also occasionally occurs.

Coagulase-negative staphylococci and enterococci are often multiresistant and cause infections typically in patients with indwelling prosthetic material, such as catheters, vascular grafts, joints, and heart valves. A combination of antibiotics may be required to treat serious enterococcal infections but the emergence of high-level aminoglycoside resistance may seriously limit this option. Enterococci carrying genes conferring high-level resistance to glycopeptides have emerged (Chapter 10). Linezolid has been used successfully to treat infection caused by such strains, but resistance has some occurred in patients receiving long courses of therapy, particularly if the focus of infection has not been removed.

## Str. pneumoniae

Another major problem concerns the emergence of resistance in *Str. pneumoniae*, the most common cause of community-acquired pneumonia and other respiratory infections. This organism used to be combated easily by treatment with penicillin and its derivatives. Unfortunately, isolates with resistance to most antibiotics can now be found in most countries of the world. Such infections are often treated with broad-spectrum cephalosporins, which can attain sufficient tissue concentrations to exceed the raised MIC for these strains. The prevalence of macrolide-resistant pneumococci tends to correlate with how often these antibiotics are used, especially in the community, where most respiratory tract infections are treated. Newer fluoroquinolones such as moxifloxacin have increased activity against pneumococci. Some resistance emergence has developed in units where these agents have been used commonly.

## Neisseria spp.

Decreased levels of susceptibility of *Neisseria meningitidis* to penicillin have been seen in many countries but high-level resistance is exceptionally rare. The emergence of resistance to penicillin in *N. meningitidis* has important strategic implications because of the need for immediate treatment of the life-threatening infections caused by these organisms. Currently, penicillin is still used empirically in some cases of suspected meningococcal infection. The cephalosporins cefotaxime or ceftriaxone are often favoured for the empirical treatment of meningitis because the antibiotic concentration achieved in the cerebrospinal fluid more reliably exceeds the MIC for the pathogen in both meningococcal and pneumococcal infection.

*N. gonorrhoeae* have progressively become resistant to successive antibiotics (e.g. penicillin, ciprofloxacin, cefixime) recommended to treat patients with sexually transmitted infections (Chapter 24). Ironically, treating all gonococcal infections with one particular (presumed) active antibiotic may actually hasten the emergence of resistance, via selective pressure, to that agent. Occasional *N. gonorrhoeae* strains have also recently been reported that are resistant to the more recently preferred antibiotics (ceftriaxone and azithromycin).

## TB

Strains of *M. tuberculosis* that are resistant to two or more of the first-line drugs—isoniazid, ethambutol, rifampicin, and streptomycin—are increasingly common, particularly in HIV-infected patients. Multidrug-resistant TB (MDR-TB) is caused by bacteria that are resistant to the most effective anti-TB drugs (isoniazid and rifampicin). MDR-TB results from either primary infection or may develop in the course of a patient's treatment. Extensively drug-resistant TB (XDR-TB) is a form of TB caused by bacteria that are resistant to isoniazid and rifampicin (i.e. MDR-TB) as well as any fluoroquinolone and any of the second-line anti-TB intravenous antibiotics (amikacin, kanamycin, or capreomycin). These forms of TB do not respond to the standard six-month treatment with first-line anti-TB drugs and can take two years or more to treat with drugs that are less potent, more toxic, and much more expensive. The resistant bacteria can be transmitted, for example, in hospitals, in prisons, and in the community and represent a major public health issue. The emergence of resistance is associated with poor compliance with antituberculosis medication. Directly observed therapy is advocated therefore for patients in whom compliance may be unreliable (see Chapter 30).

The World Health Organization estimates that there were 450,000 new MDR-TB cases and 170,000 deaths in 2012, with nearly half of all the world's cases occurring in China, India, and the Russian Federation. The prevalence of MDR-TB is extremely variable: in parts of north-west Russia, 1 in 4 new TB patients diagnosed have MDR-TB, as compared with 1 in 50 in London. As of September 2013, 92 countries have reported at least 1 case of XDR-TB. About 10 per cent of MDR-TB cases have XDR-TB, and about 25,000 of the latter are estimated to develop each year. Only an estimated 7 per cent of all MDR-TB patients are diagnosed and notified as such. Nevertheless, approximately 60 per cent of people with MDR-TB who are enrolled on treatment programmes are successfully treated.

## Key points

- The extent of antibiotic resistance does not reverse in some cases when antibiotics stop being used.
- There is no clear explanation for the marked differences in rate or extent of acquisition of resistance between different bacterial species.
- The prevalence of MRSA has declined in many but not all European countries; MRSA remains very common in other parts of the world, including the United States and Asia/Far East.
- Widespread resistance has emerged to each of the successive antibiotics used to treated gonorrhoea.
- The continuing spread of carbapenemase-producing enterobacteria is a serious threat given the 'last line of defence' status of the carbapenems.
- MDR-TB is caused by bacteria that are resistant to the most effective anti-TB drugs (isoniazid and rifampicin) and may occur because of poor compliance; directly observed therapy of TB is preferred when compliance is uncertain.
- XDR-TB is defined asMDR-TB plus resistance to any fluoroquinolone and any of the second-line anti-TB intravenous antibiotics (amikacin, kanamycin, or capreomycin) and is increasing rapidly.

## Further reading

**British Society for Antimicrobial Chemotherapy.** (2014) *British Society for Antimicrobial Chemotherapy.* <http://www.bsac.org.uk/>, accessed 24 November 2014.

**Centers for Disease Control and Prevention.** (2014) *Antibiotic/Antimicrobial Resistance: Threat Report 2013.* <http://www.cdc.gov/drugresistance/threat-report-2013/>, accessed 24 November 2014.

**Department of Health, Public Health England and Department for Environment, Food, and Rural Affairs.** (2014) <https://www.gov.uk/government/collections/antimicrobial-resistance-amr-information-and-resources >, accessed 5 December 2014.

**World Health Organization.** (2014) *Antimicrobial Resistance. Fact Sheet 194.* <http://www.who.int/mediacentre/factsheets/fs194/en/>, accessed 24 November 2014.

**World Health Organization.** (2014) *Tuberculosis (TB).* <http://www.who.int/tb/challenges/mdr/en/>, accessed 24 November 2014.

Chapter 11

# The genetics and mechanisms of acquired resistance

## Introduction to the genetics and mechanisms of acquired resistance

The mechanisms discussed in the second part of this chapter illustrate the diversity of ways that microbes can become resistant to the drugs deployed against them. However, attempts to limit the spread of drug resistance require not only knowledge of the mechanisms themselves, but also an understanding of the genetic factors that control their emergence and continued evolution.

## Genetics of resistance

All the properties of a microbial cell, including its antibiotic resistance and virulence determinants, are determined ultimately by the microbial genome. The genome comprises the three possible sources of genetic information: the chromosome, plasmids, and bacteriophages. Resistance of bacteria to antibiotics may be either intrinsic or acquired (see Chapter 10). Intrinsic resistance is the 'natural' resistance possessed by a bacterial species and is usually specified by chromosomal genes. An example of a bacterial species with a high degree of intrinsic resistance is *Pseudomonas aeruginosa*. By contrast, acquired resistance occurs in formerly susceptible cells, either following alterations to the existing genome or by transfer of genetic information between cells. Thus, a basic knowledge of microbial genetics is essential to understand the development and spread of resistance to antimicrobial drugs.

The heritable information that specifies a bacterial cell and passes to daughter cells at cell division, is carried in bacteria, as in all living cells, as an ordered sequence of nucleotide pairs along molecules of DNA. The process of transcription of this information into messenger RNA, and its subsequent translation into functioning proteins by ribosomes, is also similar in bacteria and in other cells.

## The bacterial chromosome

Each bacterial cell has a single chromosome, which is the main source of genetic information and usually comprises a closed circular DNA molecule. In *Escherichia coli*, the organism studied most intensively, this single DNA molecule comprises about $4 \times 10^3$ kb (kilobases) and is about 1.4 mm in length. Considering the average cell is about 1–3 mm in length, only by 'super-coiling' the DNA can the chromosome fit inside the bacterium. Enzymes known as DNA gyrases control the process of super-coiling DNA. Conversely, DNA uncoiling, which is necessary for messenger RNA production or chromosome replication, is controlled by DNA topoisomerases. The chromosome is found in the cytoplasm of the cell, not separated from it by a nuclear membrane. Transcription of DNA and translation of the resulting messenger RNA can therefore proceed simultaneously. Most bacterial chromosomes contain sufficient DNA to encode for 1,000–3,000 different genes. Not all of these genes need to be expressed at any one time, and indeed it would be wasteful for the cell to do so. Gene regulation is therefore necessary and can occur at either the transcriptional or translational level.

## Chromosomal mutations to antibiotic resistance

Mutations result from rare mistakes in the DNA replication process and occur at the rate of between $10^{-4}$ and $10^{-10}$ per cell division. They usually involve deletion, substitution, or addition of one or only a few base pairs and thus alter the amino acid composition of a specific protein. Such mistakes are random and spontaneous. They occur continuously in cell genes and are independent of the presence or absence of antibiotics. The vast majority of mutations are repaired by the cell without any noticeable effect. In the presence of an antibiotic, some of these occasional spontaneous antibiotic-resistant mutants that are present among a predominantly susceptible population of bacteria may be selected. In such a situation, the susceptible cells will be killed or inhibited by the antibiotic, whereas the resistant mutants will survive and proliferate to become the new predominant type. Most chromosomal resistance mutations result in alterations to permeability or specific antibiotic target sites but some result in the enhanced production of an inactivating enzyme or bypass mechanism. The latter types are mutations at the transcriptional or translational level in gene regulatory mechanisms.

Chromosomal mutations causing antibiotic resistance can be divided into single-step and multistep types.

## Single large-step mutations

With these mutations, a single mutational change results in a large increase in the minimum inhibitory concentration of a particular antibiotic and may lead to treatment failure if this drug is used alone. In some Gram-negative bacilli, mutations in the genetic regulatory system for the normally low-level chromosomal β-lactamase may result in a vast overproduction (sometimes referred to as 'derepression') of this enzyme with resulting slow hydrolysis of compounds such as cefotaxime and ceftazidime that are normally considered to be β-lactamase stable.

## Multistep (stepwise) mutations

These are sequential mutations that result in cumulative gradual stepwise increases in the minimum inhibitory concentration of a particular antibiotic. They are clinically quite common, especially in situations where only low concentrations of antibiotic can be delivered to the site of an infection.

## Plasmids

Many, perhaps all, bacteria carry, in addition to the chromosome, DNA molecules (usually 2–200 kb in size) known as plasmids. These normally replicate independently of the bacterial chromosome. Plasmids can carry genes that confer a wide range of properties on the host cell and, while such properties are usually not essential for survival, they offer a survival advantage in unusual or adverse conditions. Examples of such properties are

- fertility (the ability to conjugate with and transfer genetic information into other bacteria; see 'Transfer of genetic information');
- resistance to antibiotics;
- the ability to produce bacteriocins (proteins inhibitory to other bacteria that may be ecological competitors);
- exotoxin production;
- immunity to some bacteriophages; and
- the ability to use unusual sugars and other substrates as foods.

'Compatible' plasmids can coexist in the same host cell, while 'incompatible' plasmids cannot and so tend to be unstable and displace one another. There are at least 20 incompatibility groups within the plasmids found in enteric Gram-negative bacilli, and similar incompatibility schemes are used to subdivide staphylococcal plasmids and those found in *Pseudomonas* spp.

## Bacteriophages

The third possible source of genetic information in a bacterial cell is a bacteriophage. Bacteriophages (phages) are viruses that infect bacteria. Most phages will attack only a relatively limited range of bacteria, and can be divided into two main types:

- virulent phages, which inevitably destroy by lysis any bacteria that they infect, with the consequent release of numerous new phage particles from the lysed cell; and

- temperate (lysogenic) phages, which may either lyse or lysogenize infected bacterial cells.

For the latter class of phages, during the lysogenic cycle, the phage nucleic acid is replicated in a stable and dormant fashion within the infected cell, often following insertion into the host cell chromosome. Such a dormant phage is known as a prophage. However, while in the prophage state, some prophage genes may be expressed and may confer additional properties on the cell. Once in every few thousand cell divisions, a prophage becomes released from the dormant state and enters the lytic cycle, with subsequent destruction of its host cell and release of new phage particles into the surrounding medium.

Naturally occurring phages have been used in limited settings (for example, the countries formerly part of the Soviet Union) for the treatment of some infections (phage therapy). Some companies are exploring such treatment modalities in response to the threat posed by antibiotic-resistant pathogens.

## Transfer of genetic information

There are three ways in which genetic information can be transferred from one bacterial cell into another: transformation, transduction, and conjugation.

- Transformation involves the lysis of a bacterial cell and the subsequent release of naked DNA into the surrounding medium. Under certain circumstances, intact bacterial cells in the vicinity can acquire some of this DNA. This process has been much studied in the laboratory but there are few convincing demonstrations of its occurrence in vivo. The process depends crucially on whether the recipient cells are competent for uptake of free DNA.

- Transduction involves the accidental incorporation of bacterial DNA, either from the chromosome or a plasmid, into a bacteriophage particle during the phage lytic cycle. The phage particle then acts as a vector and transfers the bacterial DNA to the next cell that it infects.

- Conjugation involves physical contact between two bacterial cells. The cells adhere to one another, and DNA passes from one cell, termed the donor, into the other, the recipient. The ability to conjugate depends on carriage of an appropriate plasmid or transposon (see 'Transposons') by the host cell.

These transfer mechanisms mean that bacteria do not have to rely solely on a process of mutation and selection for their evolution. They can, therefore, acquire and express blocks of genetic information that have evolved elsewhere. A bacterial cell can, for example, acquire by conjugation a plasmid that carries genes conferring resistance to several different antibiotics. As a result, within a very short time following the receipt of such a plasmid by a susceptible cell, the bacteria in a given niche may change from being predominantly susceptible to being resistant to multiple drugs. Of course, the ability to transfer genes in this way does not eliminate the need for these to evolve; however, once they have evolved, it ensures their eventual widespread dissemination under appropriate selection pressures.

## Evolution of new resistance gene combinations

The distinction between chromosomal and plasmid genes is not absolute. Where appropriate regions of DNA homology exist, classic ('normal' or 'homologous') recombination can occur, both between different plasmids and between plasmids and the chromosome. Although this process can lead to the formation of new antibiotic resistance gene combinations, it is relatively uncommon in bacteria because there are few regions of sequence homology between the bacterial chromosome and plasmids that can be exploited for this purpose. Homologous recombination is used by researchers to create 'knockout' cells in which the function of a specific gene is disrupted. A more important mechanism by which antibiotic resistance genes can pass naturally from one bacterial replicon to another is the 'illegitimate' recombination process known as transposition.

### Transposons

Transposition depends on the existence of specific genetic elements termed transposons. These elements are discrete sequences of DNA capable of translocation (transposition) from one replicon (plasmid or chromosome) to another. Unlike the DNA in classic ('normal') recombination, transposons do not share extensive regions of homology with the replicon into which they insert. In many cases, transposons consist of individual resistance genes, or groups of genes, bounded by DNA sequences that are either direct or inverted repeats; that is, a sequence of bases at one end of the transposon also appears, either in direct or reverse order, at the other end. These repeats may be relatively short, often of the order of 40 base pairs, but longer examples have been identified. It is likely that these DNA sequences provide highly specific recognition sites for certain enzymes (transposases) that catalyse the movement of transposons from one replicon to another, without the need for extensive regions of sequence homology. Depending upon the transposon involved, insertion may occur at only a few or at many different sites on the host replicon. Transposons may carry genes conferring resistance to many different antibiotics, as well as other metabolic properties, and most likely explain how a single antibiotic resistance gene can become disseminated over a wide range of unrelated replicons.

Isolated DNA sequences analogous to the terminal sequences of transposons can also move from one replicon to another or be inserted in any region of any DNA molecule. Such insertion sequences appear to contain only genes that are related to insertion functions; however, in principle at least, two similar insertion sequences could bracket any assemblage of genes and convert it into a transposon. Thus, theoretically, all replicons are accessible to transposition, and all genes are potentially transposable. This theory is of crucial evolutionary importance since it explains how genes of appropriate function can accumulate on a single replicon under the impact of selection pressure. Transposons and insertion sequences therefore play a vital part in plasmid evolution.

### Integrons

Transposons may contain combinations of genes conferring resistance to various different antibiotics. An important question concerns the mechanism by which new combinations of antibiotic resistance genes are formed. It is now apparent that special molecular structures, termed integrons, may enable the formation of new combinations of resistance genes within a bacterial cell, either on a plasmid or within a transposon, in response to selection pressures.

Integrons appear to consist of two conserved segments of DNA located either side of inserted antibiotic resistance genes. Individual resistance genes seem to be capable of insertion or removal as 'cassettes' between these conserved structures. The cassettes can be found inserted in different orders and combinations. Integrons also act as an expression vector for 'foreign' antibiotic resistance genes by supplying a promoter for the transcription of cassettes derived originally from completely unrelated organisms. Integrons lack many of the features associated with transposons, including direct or inverted repeats and functions required for transposition. They do, however, possess site-specific integration functions, notably, a special enzyme termed an integrase.

Integrons can spread via site-specific insertion, following insertion into a transposon or via plasmids. The precise role of integrons in the evolution and spread of antibiotic resistance genes remains to be determined but they have been found, together with their associated antibiotic resistance gene cassettes, in many different Gram-negative bacteria. Notably, unrelated clinical isolates from different worldwide locations have been shown to carry the same integron structures and it appears that these structures play a key role in the formation and dissemination of new combinations of antibiotic resistance genes.

## Genotypic resistance and spread

The process of evolution and spread of antibiotic resistance genes continues. The origin of resistance genes carried by integrons, transposons, or plasmids, or even the origin of these elements themselves, is generally not known but it has been possible to observe a steady increase in the numbers of resistant bacterial strains following the introduction of successive chemotherapeutic agents into clinical use. For example, the *qnrA* genes that encode plasmid-mediated quinolone resistance are embedded in complex integrons. Similar genes have been identified in the water-borne species *Shewanella algae*, emphasizing the potential for the spread of resistance mechanisms from environmental bacteria. Furthermore, the discovery of a variant gene encoding an aminoglycoside-modifying (acetyltransferase) enzyme that can mediate quinolone resistance highlights the plasticity of resistance mechanisms. In this case, the new mechanism is all the more startling given that antimicrobial-modifying enzymes have traditionally been antibiotic-class specific.

Chromosomal and plasmid-mediated types of resistance may be equally important in the antibiotic management of an individual patient. However, the plasmid-encoded variety has achieved greater notoriety because of the spectacular fashion in which bacteria may acquire resistance to a number of unrelated agents by a single genetic event. Furthermore, the potential for the spread of plasmid-borne resistance to other species or genera highlights the importance of controlling pathogens that are antibiotic resistant by virtue of such plasmid genes. Nevertheless, mutational resistance involving the bacterial chromosome is also a common cause of treatment failure with some compounds. Antibacterial agents for which resistance is not known to be encoded on plasmids (e.g. rifampicin and fusidic acid) generally suffer from mutational resistance problems instead.

## Phenotypic resistance

Phenotypic resistance is due to changes in the bacterial physiological state. Bacteria in the stationary phase (e.g. in biofilms) or in spore form are good examples of cells that are not actively dividing and thus relatively non-susceptible to antibiotics. By contrast, although daughter cells released from a biofilm may be readily inactivated by antibiotics, the biofilm 'source' remains viable: once the antibiotics are removed, biofilm bacteria may then continue to release daughter cells and thus cause infection recrudescence. The extent of phenotypic resistance to antibacterial agents is unclear, particularly as it is not always possible to be sure that phenotypic changes brought about in the micro-environment of a lesion do not contribute to insusceptibility of bacteria. In the laboratory, phenotypic resistance can sometimes be induced; for example, varying the conditions of growth of *P. aeruginosa* can alter the outer envelope and thus affect susceptibility to polymyxins.

Another example is the failure of penicillins and cephalosporins to kill 'persisters' (those cells in a bacterial population that survive exposure to β-lactam agent concentrations that are lethal to the rest of the culture). This does not result from a genetic event, since the resistance is not heritable, and it is probable that the 'resistant' bacteria are caught in a particular metabolic state at the time of first encounter with the drug.

A peculiar form of phenotypic resistance is observed with mecillinam, a β-lactam antibiotic which, unusually, does not affect bacterial cell division. In susceptible Gram-negative bacilli, mecillinam induces surface changes which generally lead to cell death by osmotic rupture (see 'Extension of spectrum' in Chapter 2). However, those cells in the population that happen to have low internal osmolality survive and, as mecillinam lacks the ability to prevent growth and division, such bacteria continue to grow in a morphologically altered form. On withdrawal of the drug, the bacteria resume their normal shape and, in due course, revert to the same mixed susceptibility as the original parent culture.

## The influence of antibiotic selection pressure

Antibiotic resistance genes, and the genetic elements that carry them, existed before the introduction of antibiotics into human medicine. However, it is clear that the emergence and survival of predominantly resistant bacterial populations is due to the selective pressure associated with the widespread use of antibiotics. Resistant cells survive in a given niche at the expense of susceptible cells of the same or other species. In some cases, however, there is a fitness cost to resistant bacterial cells that may mean that they are less able to compete once the selective pressure imparted by the antibiotic is removed. In such cases, any antibiotic susceptible progeny cells that remain may be counterselected in preference to these unfit mutants. Individual cells may lose their plasmids, and chromosomal mutations may revert to being antibiotic susceptible. The implications of this process for efforts to control and limit the spread of bacterial drug resistance are discussed in Chapter 11.

## Mechanisms of acquired resistance

Three conditions must be met in order that a particular antimicrobial agent can inhibit susceptible bacteria:

◆ the antibiotic must be able to reach the target in sufficient concentration and be metabolically active (e.g. optimal pH, redox potential);

◆ the antibiotic must not be inactivated before binding to the target; and

◆ a vital target susceptible to the action of the antibiotic must exist in the bacterial cell.

The targets of individual antibiotics are often enzymes or other essential proteins. Most antimicrobial agents have to pass through the cell wall and outer membrane to reach their target, and many are carried into the cell by active transport mechanisms that usually transport sugars and other beneficial substances. Some of the differences in susceptibility of bacterial species are therefore related to differences in cell wall structure. For example, the cell envelope of Gram-negative bacteria is a more complex structure than the Gram-positive cell wall (see Chapter 2) and offers a relatively greater barrier to many antibiotics, including penicillins, glycopeptides, and macrolides. Polymyxins exert their effects at the cell surface by disrupting the Gram-negative cell membranes from the outside in a way that resembles the action of some detergents.

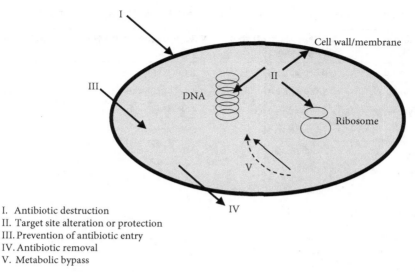

I. Antibiotic destruction
II. Target site alteration or protection
III. Prevention of antibiotic entry
IV. Antibiotic removal
V. Metabolic bypass

**Fig. 11.1** Mechanisms of antimicrobial drug resistance.

The mechanisms by which resistance may occur can be divided into the following major groups:

- destruction or inactivation of the antibiotic (Fig. 11.1, I);

- alteration or protection of the target site to reduce or eliminate binding of the antibiotic to the target (Fig. 11.1, II);

- reduction in cell surface permeability, or blockage of the mechanism by which the antibiotic enters the cell (Fig. 11.1, III) or is removed from the cell (efflux; Fig. 11.1, IV); and

- acquisition of a replacement for the metabolic step inhibited by the antibiotic (Fig. 11.1, V).

It is worth emphasizing that certain resistance mechanisms overlap within these groups. Furthermore, bacteria can become resistant to an antibiotic by several different mechanisms; for example, drug efflux, target protection, target alteration, and enzymatic inactivation may each afford resistance to tetracyclines.

Some of the known mechanisms of antibiotic resistance are summarized in Table 11.1.

## Inactivation or modification mechanisms

Inactivation or modification mechanisms are probably the most important resistance mechanisms in clinical practice since they include the common modes of resistance to penicillins and cephalosporins, the therapeutic agents of widest use.

### β-Lactam antibiotics

There are many different agents in this group (see Chapter 2), and a correspondingly large number of β-lactamases that catalyse hydrolysis of the β-lactam ring to form an inactive product. In addition, varying levels of β-lactamase production, variable properties of the enzymes, notably the breadth of activity, and differences in the permeability of the Gram-negative cell envelope determine the differential susceptibilities of bacteria to these antibiotics.

**Table 11.1** Important known resistance mechanisms for the major groups of antibiotics.

| Inactivation or modification | Altered or protected target site | Reduced permeability or access | Metabolic bypass |
|---|---|---|---|
| β-Lactam antibiotics | β-Lactam antibiotics | Tetracyclines[d] | Trimethoprim |
| Chloramphenicol | Streptomycin | β-Lactam antibiotics | Sulphonamides |
| Aminoglycosides[a] | Chloramphenicol | Chloramphenicol | |
| | Erythromycin[b] | Quinolones[d] | |
| | Fusidic acid | Aminoglycosides | |
| | Quinolones | | |
| | Rifampicin | | |
| | Glycopeptides[b] | | |
| | Tetracyclines[c] | | |

[a] Resulting in reduced drug uptake.

[b] Resulting from enzymic modification.

[c] Resulting from ribosomal protection.

[d] Resulting from an increased efflux.

All bacteria appear to contain enzymes capable of hydrolysing β-lactam antibiotics. Indeed, it has been suggested that the normal function and evolutionary origin of β-lactamases is to break a β-lactam structure that is a transitory intermediate in cell wall synthesis. These constitutive enzymes are encoded by the bacterial chromosome and are normally bound closely to the cell membrane. In general, they are produced only in small amounts, they attack cephalosporins more readily than penicillins, and they act relatively slowly. In certain organisms, notably *Enterobacter* spp., *Acinetobacter* spp., *Citrobacter* spp., and *P. aeruginosa*, gross overproduction of these chromosomal enzymes has been associated with treatment failure, even with so-called 'β-lactamase-stable' cephalosporins and carbapenems. Resistance seems to result from a combination of the slow enzyme-mediated hydrolysis, and cell wall mutations that partially impede antibiotic entry into the bacterial cell.

The classification of β-lactamases has become extremely complex as more and more examples of these enzymes (now numbering more than 200), some differing from one another by only one or a few amino acids, have been described. Various characteristics are used to distinguish the different enzymes, including substrate profile, and the action of enzyme inhibitors such as clavulanic acid and the ion-chelator ethylenediaminetetraacetic acid (EDTA). Substrate profile refers to the hydrolytic activity of a β-lactamase preparation against a number of β-lactam substrates, often expressed as the ratio to a value for a reference substrate such as benzylpenicillin. Methods based on DNA–DNA hybridization or the polymerase chain reaction (PCR) to identify specific genes have been used to distinguish newly recognized enzymes. A simplified classification of the common bacterial β-lactamases is shown in Table 11.2.

Gram-negative bacteria produce a greater variety of β-lactamases than Gram-positive bacteria do. From a clinical point of view, most interest centres on the large number of plasmid-encoded enzymes, particularly given their potential for widespread dissemination. Plasmid-encoded enzymes are the major cause of bacterial resistance to penicillins and cephalosporins in clinical isolates. Some are located on transposons (see 'Transposons'), thus allowing movement of genes

**Table 11.2** Simplified categorization of the most common bacterial β-lactamases.

| Group | Molecular class | Preferred substrates | Inhibited by | | Representative enzymes |
|-------|-----------------|----------------------|--------------|------|------------------------|
| | | | Clavulanic acid | EDTA[a] | |
| 1 | C | Cephalosporins | No | No | Gram-negative chromosomal enzymes |
| 2a | A | Penicillins | Yes | No | Staphylococcal β-lactamases |
| 2b | A | Penicillins; cephalosporins | Yes | No | TEM series; SHV series; CTX-M |
| 2c | A | Penicillins; carbenicillin | Yes | No | PSE series |
| 2d | D | Penicillins; cloxacillin | Variable | No | OXA series |
| 2e | A | Cephalosporins | Yes | No | Proteus cephalosporinase |
| 2f | A | Carbapenems | Yes | Yes | IMI-1, KPC-2, SME-1 |
| 3 | B | Most β-lactam antibiotics | No | Yes | Metallo-enzymes (carbapenemases; e.g. IMP-1, VIM-1) |

[a] EDTA, ethylenediaminetetraacetic acid.

Adapted from the scheme of Bush K, Jacoby GA, Medeiros AA, A functional classification scheme for beta-lactamases and its correlation with molecular structure, *Antimicrobial Agents and Chemotherapy*, Volume 39, Number 6, pp. 1211–1233, Copyright © 2005, and Bush K, Jacoby GA, Updated Functional Classification of β-Lactamases, *Antimicrobial Agents and Chemotherapy*, Volume 54, Number 3, pp. 969–976, Copyright © 2010, by permission of the American Society for Microbiology.

between plasmids and the chromosome. This means that the distinction between plasmid-encoded and chromosome-encoded enzymes sometimes is blurred.

Among Gram-positive cocci, plasmid-encoded β-lactamases of clinical significance are found almost exclusively in staphylococci. These enzymes rapidly hydrolyse benzylpenicillin, ampicillin (see 'Extension of spectrum') and cephalosporins. Staphylococcal β-lactamases are inducible exo-enzymes that are usually related closely. In streptococci, β-lactamases are usually absent, and these bacteria have consequently remained, with few exceptions, susceptible to benzylpenicillin.

The most widely distributed of the plasmid-mediated enzymes is TEM-1, which is encoded by many different plasmids (see 'Plasmids') and transposons (see 'Transposons'). The resultant genetic promiscuity, coupled with sustained selective pressure from antibiotic prescribing, probably explains the widespread distribution of this and closely related enzymes. Following the first recognition of TEM-1 in *Esch. coli* in 1965, it was detected in *Haemophilus influenzae* and *Neisseria gonorrhoeae* in the mid-1970s, and in *N. meningitidis* in 1989.

There are more than 100 genetic TEM variants, some of which have an altered substrate spectrum. Some produce β-lactamases that can hydrolyse a wide variety of penicillins and cephalosporins (extended-spectrum β-lactamases). Extended-spectrum enzymes unrelated to TEM have also been described, notably, the plasmid-encoded cefotaxime-hydrolysing class of β-lactamases known as the CTX-M enzymes, which are found in some *Klebsiella* spp., in *Esch. coli*, and in salmonellae. They have become much more prevalent in the United Kingdom and other European countries, in particular causing urinary tract infections or septicaemia. The laboratory detection of these enzymes is not straightforward and relies on a combination of clues obtained from the results of routine susceptibility testing and additional tests based on cephalosporin-induced β-lactamase production in vitro.

Other types of β-lactamases that are encountered in Gram-negative bacilli include SHV-1 and its many variants—of which there are now more than 50—that are common in *Klebsiella* spp.; the OXA group of enzymes, which can hydrolyse methicillin and isoxazolylpenicillins; and the PSE group, which hydrolyse carbenicillin at least as fast as they hydrolyse benzylpenicillin and which were thought originally to be confined to *P. aeruginosa*.

Control of the resistance caused by TEM-1 and some other β-lactamases produced by Gram-negative organisms is afforded by 'β-lactamase-stable' cephalosporins and the use of β-lactamase inhibitors such as clavulanic acid. However, some plasmid-encoded β-lactamases inactivate even the newer 'β-lactamase-stable' β-lactam agents. Many of these novel enzymes seem to be derived by mutation from the widely distributed TEM-1 and SHV-1 β-lactamases.

Most β-lactamases have serine at the active site and are often referred to as serine β-lactamases. However, some β-lactamases require zinc and thus are known as metallo-β-lactamases; these enzymes are inhibited by the chelating agent EDTA. Metallo-β-lactamases are found in diverse organisms including *Acinetobacter* spp., *P. aeruginosa*, and the *Bacteroides* group. They hydrolyse virtually all β-lactam compounds, including the carbapenems (see 'Other β-lactam agents' in Chapter 2), and enzyme inhibitors such as clavulanic acid do not offer protection (Table 11.3). Serine β-lactamases that inactivate carbapenems have also been described. Fortunately, strains that elaborate such enzymes are still relatively uncommon, although they are now being reported with increasing frequency from many different countries. Increasing numbers of outbreaks are reported involving multiresistant *Klebsiella* strains that have also acquired a carbapenemase, leaving very few therapeutic options.

## Aminoglycosides

Resistance to aminoglycosides results largely from interference with the drug transport mechanism following modification of the antibiotic by one or more of a series of enzymes produced by the resistant bacteria. Such aminoglycoside-modifying enzymes are often plasmid-encoded but have been associated increasingly with the presence of transposons (see 'Transposons') and integrons (see 'Integrons'). They are classified according to the precise type of modification performed and by the site of modification on the aminoglycoside molecule. Over 30 such modifying enzymes and their variants have been identified by biochemical or nucleic acid-based methods, and these can be divided into three main groups: aminoglycoside acetylating enzymes, nucleotidyltransferase enzymes, and phosphorylating enzymes. Various patterns of cross-resistance can

**Table 11.3** Examples of carbapenemases and their most common host bacteria.

| | Pseudomonas | Acinetobacter | Enterobacteria |
|---|---|---|---|
| KPC | – | – | +++ |
| OXA | – | +++ | + |
| GES | + | – | + |
| VIM[a] | ++ | +/– | + |
| IMP[a] | ++ | +/– | + |
| SPM[a] | +++ | – | – |
| NDM* | – | – | ++ |

[a] Metallo-β-lactamases; others are serine β-lactamases.

be shown by bacteria that produce different enzymes but these patterns are complicated further because many clinical isolates produce more than one enzyme at any one time. Susceptibility or resistance to any one agent cannot be predicted reliably from results obtained for another; thus, susceptibility tests must be performed with the agent that is to be used therapeutically.

Although aminoglycosides exhibit poor activity against enterococci, they interact synergistically with β-lactam antibiotics to achieve a more rapid and complete bactericidal action. Unfortunately, plasmid-mediated high-level aminoglycoside resistance, which abolishes synergy, has become much more prevalent in enterococci, thus removing the possibility of synergistic β-lactam–aminoglycoside therapy in serious enterococcal infection caused by such strains.

When the aminoglycoside-modifying enzymes were first described, they were considered to be examples of drug-inactivating enzymes analogous to those responsible for resistance to β-lactam antibiotics and to chloramphenicol. However, aminoglycoside-modifying enzymes mediate resistance by modifying only small amounts of antibiotic. They are strategically placed near the inner cytoplasmic membrane where they are accessible to acetyl coenzyme A and adenosine triphosphate. As soon as a few molecules of drug are modified, all further transport of drug into the cell becomes blocked.

## Chloramphenicol

Resistance to chloramphenicol in both Gram-positive and Gram-negative bacteria is normally associated with the production of an enzyme, chloramphenicol acetyltransferase, which converts the drug to either the monoacetate or the diacetate. The acetylated drug will not bind to the bacterial ribosome and so cannot block protein synthesis. Several different acetyltransferases have been described. Some appear to be genus and species specific; others, usually plasmid or transposon associated, are more widespread. This variety is a little surprising since chloramphenicol has been used less widely than many other antibiotics because of its rare, but serious, toxic side effects.

# Alteration or protection of the target site

Resistance arising from the selection of rare, pre-existent mutants from within an otherwise susceptible bacterial population has been described for many antibiotics. The mutations usually affect the drug target and often confer high-level resistance in a single step. The emergence of this type of resistance during therapy is an important cause of treatment failure with certain drugs, including rifampicin, the older quinolones, fusidic acid, and various antituberculosis drugs. Use of combinations of antibiotics can prevent the emergence of such resistance during therapy, since the likelihood of independent mutations conferring resistance to two or more unrelated antibiotics appearing simultaneously in the same cell is very small. This strategy has been crucial in antituberculosis therapy. Similarly, monotherapy of staphylococcal infection with rifampicin or fusidic acid should not normally be used.

Variants exhibiting low levels of resistance to almost any antibiotic can be isolated readily from most bacteria. In contrast to single-step mutants, they usually develop in a stepwise fashion and may exhibit other phenotypic changes (e.g. slower growth rate, colonial variation on solid media, reduced virulence). These 'fitness costs' become more marked as the degree of resistance increases. It is likely that the shifts in penicillin susceptibility of gonococci and pneumococci that have occurred over the years result from such cumulative changes.

## β-Lactam antibiotics

The major mechanism of resistance to β-lactam antibiotics is enzymic inactivation (see 'β-Lactam antibiotics' in 'Inactivation or modification mechanisms') but mechanisms involving target site modification also occur. *Streptococcus pneumoniae* strains with reduced susceptibility to penicillin exhibit alterations in the target penicillin-binding proteins (PBPs; see 'Mode of action of β-lactam agents' in Chapter 2) that result in a reduced ability to bind penicillin. Similarly, methicillin resistance in staphylococci is associated with the synthesis of a modified PBP (PBP 2′), which exhibits decreased affinity for methicillin and other β-lactam antibiotics. Low-level resistance to penicillin in *N. gonorrhoeae* has also been associated with alterations to PBPs. Such resistance appears to have developed by rare mutational events and to have become disseminated as a result of considerable antibiotic selection pressure.

## Glycopeptides

Resistance to vancomycin and teicoplanin first emerged in enterococci only after the antibiotic had been available for 30 years. Expression of resistance depends on the presence or absence of several genes and two enzymes (a ligase and a dehydrogenase), which probably originated in non-human pathogens and were transferred to enterococci. The net effect of these is target site alteration. Glycopeptides bind to the D-alanyl-D-alanine terminus of the muramyl pentapeptide of peptidoglycan (see 'Cell wall construction' in Chapter 2). Enterococci that exhibit high-level resistance to glycopeptides produce a new dipeptide terminus, either D-alanyl-D-lactate or D-alanyl-D-serine. Such substitutions allow cell wall synthesis to continue in the presence of one or both of the currently available glycopeptides, vancomycin, and teicoplanin. Several different glycopeptide resistance phenotypes have been described (Table 11.4). Glycopeptide resistance is usually inducible in those strains that possess the necessary genes and enzymes, but some essentially non-pathogenic enterococci (e.g. *Enterococcus gallinarum*, *Enteroc. casseliflavus*, and *Enteroc. flavescens*) are constitutively resistant to low to moderate levels of vancomycin.

The mechanism of the low-level resistance to glycopeptide antibiotics that has emerged in some *Staphylococcus aureus* and coagulase-negative staphylococci has not been completely elucidated but appears to be associated with the overproduction of peptidoglycan precursors that thus require increased amounts of drug to saturate them. Very rare strains of *Staph. aureus* that are highly resistant (minimum inhibitory concentration > 128 mg/l) to vancomycin and teicoplanin have been described. So far these have all possessed the *vanA* gene that confers the VanA glycopeptide resistance phenotype in enterococci. Some years before these clinical isolates were first seen, *vanA* was successfully transferred from an enterococcal strain into *Staph. aureus* in vitro. It now appears that enterococci can also transfer the genes coding for high-level glycopeptide resistance to *Staph. aureus* in vivo. The hope is that such occurrences remain rare and that highly glycopeptide resistant strains do not spread widely.

## Streptomycin

Streptomycin binds to a protein (S12) in the smaller (30 S) ribosomal subunit in bacteria. A single amino acid change in the structure of this protein can prevent the binding of streptomycin entirely, thus rendering bacteria resistant to very high concentrations of the drug. The alteration is so specific that other aminoglycosides such as gentamicin are unaffected by the change.

## Erythromycin and chloramphenicol

Changes in the proteins of the larger (50 S) ribosomal subunit have been implicated in resistance to chloramphenicol and macrolides such as erythromycin. However, erythromycin resistance in staphylococci and streptococci results more usually from methylation of the 23 S ribosomal RNA subunit by an inducible plasmid-encoded enzyme. Methylation of the ribosomal RNA also renders the bacteria resistant to other macrolides, lincosamides (see 'Lincosamides' in Chapter 3),

**Table 11.4** Types of glycopeptide resistance in enterococci.[a]

| Phenotype | | VanA | VanB | VanC | VanD | VanE | VanG |
|---|---|---|---|---|---|---|---|
| Susceptibility to | vancomycin | R (high) | R (low or high) | R (low) | R (high) | R (low) | R (low) |
| | teicoplanin | R | S | S | S or R | S | S |
| Expression | | Inducible | Inducible | Constitutive or inducible | Constitutive | Inducible | Unknown |
| Gene location | | Plasmid or chromosome | Plasmid or chromosome | Chromosome | Chromosome | Chromosome | Chromosome |
| Species commonly affected | | *Enterococcus faecalis, E. faecium* | *E. faecalis, E. faecium* | *E. gallinarum, E. casseliflavus, E. flavescens* | *E. faecium* | *E. faecalis* | *E. faecalis* |

[a] R, resistant; S, susceptible.

and streptogramins (see 'Streptogramins' in Chapter 3) by reducing ribosomal binding of these drugs. Since erythromycin is a specific inducer of the methylating enzyme, bacteria carrying a plasmid encoding this property are resistant to the other drugs only in the presence of erythromycin. This phenomenon is known as dissociated resistance. Because of a similarity in the sites of action of macrolides and lincosamides, lincosamide resistance is more likely to emerge during the treatment of infections caused by strains that are initially erythromycin resistant.

## Fusidic acid

Fusidic acid inhibits the translocation of the growing polypeptide chain. Resistance occurs via point mutations in *fusA*, so that the structure of elongation factor G, the protein that regulates translocation, is altered, or via the expression of proteins that protects the drug target (FusB and FusC classes).

## Quinolones

Intermediate levels of resistance to quinolones in Gram-negative rods are usually caused by chromosomal-encoded structural alterations to a subunit of the DNA gyrase target (see 'The bacterial chromosome'). High levels of resistance are associated with additional mutations in the secondary target, topoisomerase IV. In Gram-positive cocci, the situation is reversed, since topoisomerase IV is the primary target. In general, mutations that confer reduced susceptibility to older quinolones ('first stage mutations') may not reduce the effectiveness of newer more active versions, unless additional ('second' or 'third stage') mutations occur, an example of stepwise resistance. There is some evidence that quinolones differ in their propensity to select for resistance mutations. This observation has led to the concept of a 'mutant protection concentration'; that is, the concentration that prevents the growth of the least susceptible single-step mutant present in a bacterial population. It has been suggested that these differences between quinolones, related to their achievable tissue concentrations, may influence the likelihood of resistant mutant selection during therapy.

Quinolone resistance can be transferred by plasmids that may additionally code for resistance to other antibiotic classes. Two types of plasmid resistance occur with variable prevalence. One is mediated by the *qnr* gene, which encodes a protein that protects DNA gyrase and DNA topoisomerase from the action of quinolones. The other is a more recently discovered bifunctional aminoglycoside acetyltransferase variant, AAC(6′)-Ib, which catalyses the acetylation of fluoroquinolones and aminoglycosides.

## Rifampicin

Resistance to rifampicin is invariably the result of a structural alteration in *rpo*, which encodes the β-subunit of RNA polymerase and is thus involved in the transcription of DNA to mRNA; this alteration reduces the binding affinity of the protein for rifampicin. The location of the *rpo* mutation is usually within a well-defined small area; molecular tests (Chapter 12) are now available for the direct detection of this gene (for example, in *Mycobacterium tuberculosis* strains).

## Linezolid

This oxazolidinone antibiotic inhibits protein synthesis at the stage of ribosomal assembly (see 'Introduction to inhibitors' in Chapter 3). A ribosomal mutation leads to linezolid resistance in both staphylococci and enterococci. More recently, some strains have acquired a plasmid-mediated *cfr* gene, so named because it causes resistance to chloramphenicol and florfenicol. This gene encodes an RNA methyltransferase and affects the binding of at least five chemically unrelated antimicrobial classes: phenicols, lincosamides, oxazolidinones, pleuromutilins, and streptogramin A antibiotics. Linezolid resistance is currently very uncommon in *Staph. aureus* and is only occasionally seen in enterococci; it is usually associated with prolonged therapy, and failure to remove or drain a focus of infection.

## Interference with drug transport and accumulation

In addition to reduced drug accumulation resulting from enzymic modification of aminoglycosides (see 'Aminoglycosides' in 'Inactivation or modification mechanisms'), interference with transport of drugs into the bacterial cell is of proven clinical importance as a cause of resistance to tetracyclines, β-lactam antibiotics, and quinolones.

### Tetracyclines

Uptake of tetracyclines into cells normally involves an active transport mechanism that uses energy and results in the accumulation of the drug inside the cell. Plasmid or transposon-mediated resistance to tetracyclines is common in both Gram-positive and Gram-negative bacteria. Generally, there is complete cross-resistance, so a strain that is resistant to one tetracycline is resistant to all the others; exceptions to this rule may be found with minocycline. Tigecycline, which is related to minocycline, retains activity against bacteria that are resistant to other tetracyclines, possibly because of higher affinity binding to the ribosome.

Tetracycline resistance is often associated with the synthesis of a membrane protein that mediates the rapid efflux of antibiotic by an active mechanism; thus, the drug entering the cell is removed almost simultaneously and so fails to reach an inhibitory level. Such resistance is normally inducible, and full expression of resistance is obtained only after cells have been exposed to subinhibitory concentrations of the drug.

Some bacteria produce a cytoplasmic protein that appears to have the function of protecting ribosomes from tetracycline attack. In addition, tetracycline resistance in *Helicobacter pylori* is mediated by a modification to the ribosomal target.

### β-Lactam antibiotics

The outer membranes of Gram-negative bacilli vary greatly in permeability to various penicillins and cephalosporins. Most β-lactam agents reach their targets in Gram-negative bacilli by passing through porins, which are water-filled pores that extend across the outer membrane bilayer. The rate of permeation is governed largely by the physical size of a particular β-lactam molecule in comparison with the size of the porin but ionic charge also plays a part. In some bacteria, resistance can result from changes to the size or function of the porins so that passage of the antibiotic is prevented. In a few instances, genes carried on plasmids encode non-specific changes in cell permeability to β-lactam antibiotics; these changes seem to affect the overall outer membrane structure of the cell. Resistance to carbapenems can be caused by loss of porins, sometimes exacerbated by β-lactamase production (e.g. imipenem resistance in *P. aeruginosa*).

### Chloramphenicol

A few strains of chloramphenicol-resistant Gram-negative bacilli possess a plasmid that appears to confer the property of impermeability to chloramphenicol upon the host cell.

### Quinolones

Gram-negative bacteria have been described in which resistance to quinolones is caused by impermeability associated with a decrease in the amount of the OmpF outer membrane porin protein. Such strains may simultaneously acquire resistance to β-lactam antibiotics and some other agents that gain access through the OmpF porin. Resistance caused by active efflux also occurs in some Gram-negative bacilli and staphylococci. This can be mediated by efflux pumps that are specific for quinolones, or by non-specific transporter pumps.

### Aminoglycosides

A mechanism of resistance to aminoglycosides, unrelated to enzymic modification, is associated with alterations in membrane proteins that affect active transport of the antibiotic into the cell.

## Metabolic bypass

Most common resistance mechanisms can be accommodated in one or other of the three major groups described already. However, there are two known examples in which a plasmid or transposon provides the cell with an entirely new and drug-resistant enzyme that can bypass the susceptible chromosomal enzyme that is also present unaltered in the cell.

### Sulphonamides

Sulphonamides exert their bacteriostatic effect by competitive inhibition of dihydropteroate synthetase. Sulphonamide-resistant strains of Gram-negative bacilli synthesize an additional dihydropteroate synthetase that is unaffected by sulphonamides. The additional enzyme allows continued functioning of the threatened metabolic pathway in the presence of the drug. At least two such enzymes are widespread in Gram-negative bacilli throughout the world.

### Trimethoprim

Trimethoprim blocks a later step in the same metabolic pathway by inhibiting the dihydrofolate reductase enzymes in susceptible bacteria. Resistant strains synthesize a new, trimethoprim-insensitive dihydrofolate reductase as well as the normal drug-susceptible chromosomal enzyme. At least 14 groups of trimethoprim-insusceptible dihydrofolate reductases have been described in Gram-negative bacilli, and a further example is found in multiresistant isolates of *Staph. aureus*.

# Resistance to antiviral agents

Most of the antiviral agents (see Chapters 5 and 6) act by inhibiting a virus gene product, which is usually (but not always) a protein with enzymatic function (e.g. DNA polymerase, reverse transcriptase, protease) that is essential to viral replication. Such inhibition prevents production of mature virus particles, thereby halting the spread of infection and hopefully buying time for the host immune system to eliminate the pathogen. The emergence of resistance to antiviral agents is an example of Darwinian evolution. Randomly distributed mutations may arise as the viral genome is copied but those that confer a survival advantage in the face of selective pressure (presence of an antiviral drug) will emerge in new viral particles. Thus, a mutation which alters the structure of a target viral protein such that the antiviral agent no longer binds to its target, or does so with lower affinity, will be advantageous to the virus, allowing the essential process mediated by the target protein to go ahead despite the presence of the inhibitor, that is,. the virus will become resistant to the drug.

Drug resistance arising from a single point mutation in the target gene is not usually an all or none phenomenon—the drug may still exert some inhibitory activity but increased concentrations of the drug will be needed to achieve its purpose. This can be quantified in vitro by measuring the concentration of the drug necessary to achieve 50 per cent inhibition of virus replication—referred to as an $IC_{50}$ (or an $IC_{90}$ if inhibiting 90%) value. However, the appearance of further mutations within the target gene may have a cumulative effect. A good example is that of azidothymidine (AZT) and HIV, where resistance arises through a series of mutations, each one resulting in a stepwise increase in $IC_{50}$ values, until the gene contains a complete set of mutations, and the reverse transcriptase is effectively completely resistant to the drug.

Just as with bacteria, mutations may have a fitness cost which, if too great, may not confer a selective advantage and will therefore not persist in progeny virus. A good example of this is the S282 mutation within the hepatitis C virus (HCV) RNA polymerase enzyme. This single point mutation confers high-level resistance in in vitro assays to nucleos(t)ide analogue polymerase inhibitors such as sofosbuvir; however, the fitness cost to the virus is so great that this mutation has not been described thus far in any patients who have received the drug.

Mutations which directly alter drug binding are referred to as primary resistance mutations. However, other (secondary) mutations may arise which, although by themselves do not alter the interaction between drug and target protein, may nevertheless have significant effects on the emergence of antiviral resistance. Thus, a secondary mutation at a distant site may increase the stability of a protein structure rendered less stable by the primary resistance mutation(s). Secondary mutations may also result in restoration of some or all of the enzymatic function otherwise lost due to the change in shape of the active site of the enzyme induced by the primary resistance mutation(s). In other words, secondary mutations may lessen the fitness cost arising from primary resistance mutations, thereby enhancing the chances of the emergence of resistance.

The occurrence of multiple mutations within a target gene does not necessarily always increase drug resistance. For instance, if an HIV reverse transcriptase gene containing a full set of AZT resistance mutations subsequently acquires a mutation at position M184, then the consequent change in structure of the molecule is such that the enzyme becomes more, not less, sensitive to the inhibitory effects of AZT. The M184 mutation is the key primary resistance mutation to lamivudine (LMV). These in vitro observations are important, as they introduce some logic to the choice of multidrug regimens. The combination of AZT and LMV has been shown to be particularly effective in vivo because, as the virus mutates to become resistant to LMV, it paradoxically becomes more sensitive to AZT. AZT/LMV combination therapy was therefore the recommended backbone of antiretroviral regimens for many years.

The possibility of a fitness cost to the virus raises the concept of the 'barrier to resistance'. This describes the ease or otherwise with which a virus may acquire the mutation(s) necessary to confer significant resistance to an antiviral drug. Lamivudine is an effective inhibitor of the polymerase of the hepatitis B virus (see 'Lamivudine' in Chapter 7). However, the drug has a very low barrier to resistance, that is, the mutations which confer resistance to LMV come with very little fitness cost to the virus and therefore are very easily accommodated. This is evidenced by the fact that over 75 per cent of patients who are prescribed lamivudine for their chronic hepatitis B virus (HBV) infection will develop lamivudine resistance after 4 years of continuous therapy. In marked contrast, the nucleotide polymerase inhibitor tenofovir has a very high barrier to resistance—such that resistance mutations to tenofovir have not yet been described despite this drug being prescribed to very large numbers of patients for many years.

## Resistance to antifungal agents

Polyenes and azoles act on the fungal cell membrane, echinocandins disrupt the fungal cell wall, and flucytosine (5FC) acts as an antimetabolite to interfere with DNA and RNA synthesis. Yeast resistance to polyenes is very uncommon. Proposed mechanisms of polyene resistance in moulds include decreased access to the drug target due to altered membrane ergosterol content, accumulation of other sterols and reduced intercalation, and increased catalase activity, which leads to a reduction in oxidative damage. Resistance of yeasts to 5FC is mediated by enzymatic modifications that interfere with either drug uptake into the cell or the metabolism of 5FC.

Four major mechanisms of resistance to azoles have been described in *Candida* spp. and, if multiple of these are present, additive effects can be seen; the first two of those listed below are believed to be more prevalent:

- the induction of efflux pumps that lead to decreased drug concentration at the enzyme target within the fungal cell;
- the acquisition of point mutations in the gene encoding for the azole target enzyme (lanosterol 14-α-sterol-demethylase in yeasts, and 14-α-sterol-demethylase in moulds), resulting in an altered target with reduced affinity for drug binding;
- overexpression or upregulation of the altered target enzyme; and
- the development of bypass pathways that negate the membrane-disruptive effects of azoles.

Echinocandin resistance in yeasts is mediated via point mutations resulting in target modification, and a similar mechanism appears to be operative in emerging echinocandin resistance in moulds.

## Key points

- Resistance genes located on plasmids have the greatest potential for spread within and between bacterial species.
- Co-location of resistance genes, especially on plasmids, means that bacteria can become resistant to multiple antibiotic classes.
- The widespread use of β-lactam antibiotics has led to the development of hundreds of different types of enzymes capable of rendering these drugs inactive.
- Carbapenemases (enzymes that destroy carbapenems) were once rare but in some places are now becoming a common cause of resistance, particularly in Gram-negative bacilli.
- Efflux systems can either be specific for an antibiotic or may eject multiple different classes of antimicrobial agents from the bacterial cell.
- Resistance to antiviral agents arises from mutations within the genes encoding the viral proteins targeted by the drugs.

## Further reading

Nature Publishing Group. (2014) *Nature Reviews Genetics*. <www.nature.com/nrg/index.html>, accessed 25 November 2014.

Nature Publishing Group. (2014) *Nature Reviews Microbiology*. <www.nature.com/nrmicro/index.html>, accessed 25 November 2014.

Pfaller, M. A. (2012) Antifungal drug resistance: mechanisms, epidemiology, and consequences for treatment. *The American Journal of Medicine*, **125** (Suppl): S3–13.

3

# General principles of usage of antimicrobial agents

# Chapter 12

# Laboratory investigations and the treatment of infection

## Introduction to laboratory investigations

This chapter covers the basic principles and limitations of using a microbiology laboratory to obtain information on the selection and control of antimicrobial therapy. It is not a comprehensive account of clinical laboratory microbiology. The examples used refer primarily to bacteriological practice but the principles apply to the investigation of any infection.

In the diagnostic microbiology laboratory, the aim is to identify the presence of pathogens as rapidly as possible and to provide, where applicable, antimicrobial susceptibility data to the clinician. A wide range of techniques, including microscopy, culture, antigen or antibody detection, and nucleic acid detection methods are used in the diagnostic laboratory. There is an increasing trend to standardize the protocols used to detect microorganisms and their antimicrobial susceptibility. In addition, the use of automation is increasing markedly in microbiology laboratories and this offers the opportunity for more rapid diagnosis of infection. A key issue will be demonstrating that speedier diagnosis translates into more effective treatment and, of course, outcome.

## The importance of clinical details

When using laboratory services, it is important to provide appropriate clinical details (e.g. travel history, antibiotic therapy) on the request form; without these, the optimal use of diagnostic methods cannot be guaranteed. Clinical details (e.g. travel history, exposure to infection, antimicrobial treatment) may dictate the tests used and/or influence the interpretation of the result; for example, in a patient treated for endocarditis with penicillin and gentamicin, the optimal serum aminoglycoside concentration is lower than that required in other infections.

Crucially, many diagnostic methods, in particular those involving microbial culture, are prone to biological variability, which may hinder the interpretation of results. Clinical details can play a key part in the correct interpretation of the microorganisms recovered from samples; for example, knowing that a patient has symptoms of a urinary tract infection (as opposed to being asymptomatic) and whether the sample was collected as a clean catch specimen (rather than via a catheter) shifts the interpretation towards the result being a clinically significant pathogen. Bacteria commonly colonize foreign bodies, such as catheters, drains, breathing tubes, and other sites such as surgical wounds and ulcers. In the absence of specific symptoms of infection, recovered microorganisms may simply reflect 'normal' flora at that site.

Interpretation of the results of specimens taken from areas of the body that have a resident microbial flora, which may sometimes assume a pathogenic role, is particularly difficult. Culture results from respiratory sources are often the most difficult to interpret, given that sputum has to traverse sites with their own flora (e.g. the mouth) before reaching the specimen pot. *Candida albicans* is often a harmless commensal, although it can cause serious disease in immunocompromised patients. The ability of some organisms to strike while the host defences are down has given them the title 'opportunist pathogens'. However, merely by looking at cultures of these opportunists, it is impossible to say in a particular case whether or not they are adopting a pathogenic role. The interpretation of their detection can be influenced by ancillary findings (e.g. presence or absence of pus, numbers of organisms isolated), possibly by their repeated detection, and most importantly by clinical information provided on the request card. If the latter is absent, non-contributory, or misleading, the report issued may be valueless. Conversely, demonstration of some microorganisms (e.g. *Mycobacterium tuberculosis*), is always significant and, even in the absence of clinical disease, the patient must be further examined and treated.

Although many diseases have a well-defined microbial aetiology, the clinical information and the results of specimen examination are often insufficient to form a definitive opinion as to the microbial cause in an individual case. Most patients with infection survive, and many improve so rapidly that the significance of microbes isolated is never known. Thus, although we know from historical and epidemiological evidence that *Streptococcus pyogenes* causes tonsillitis and is involved in the aetiology of rheumatic fever, when an individual patient presents with joint pains following a sore throat, we cannot be absolutely sure that the *Str. pyogenes* in the throat is the cause of the illness or represents the chance finding of asymptomatic colonization in someone with disease due to another cause. In such situations, additional investigations (such as raised antistreptolysin O antibodies in the serum, in this case) may be needed in order to establish a causal relationship.

In the absence of sufficient supportive information, the laboratory can adopt one of two approaches: report any microbe isolated regardless of any possible significance, or report only common pathogens and dismiss all the others as 'normal flora'. The importance of this to antimicrobial therapy is that, if the isolate is not considered 'significant', no further work (including antimicrobial susceptibility tests) will be carried out. The corollary is that many susceptibility tests may be carried out, some unnecessarily. This occurs more commonly than is usually admitted. In turn, patients may be prescribed unnecessary and potentially toxic antimicrobial drugs because commensal bacteria isolated from a badly taken specimen were considered significant and susceptibility results issued. Sometimes a great deal of effort and expense is put into treating colonizing organisms that are merely filling a vacuum left by the normal flora and would quietly disappear if antimicrobial chemotherapy were withheld.

## Specimen collection

Clinical laboratories rely on the quality of the specimens they receive; none more so than microbiology departments, where the final result may depend on the degree of care observed in taking the specimen. A single contaminating bacterium introduced into a blood culture during collection may result in a patient being incorrectly diagnosed as having bacteraemia. Similarly, extraneous nucleic acid contaminating a sample can cause a false-positive result, for example in midstream samples from women tested for chlamydial or gonococcal infection. Such an error could have profound consequences.

Some of the more common problems are listed below.

- Inappropriate specimen: saliva is submitted instead of sputum; a superficial skin swab is taken instead of a swab of pus (a specimen of pus in a sterile bottle is always preferable to a swab when possible).
- Inadequate specimen: the specimen may be too small (especially fluids for culture for tubercle bacilli). Rectal swabs are not an adequate substitute for faeces. It is almost impossible to interpret the significance of microbes cultured in tracheal aspirate in a patient who is ventilated,

because of the likely presence of colonizing upper respiratory tract flora. Deep respiratory specimens such as bronchoalveolar lavage fluid are highly preferable to make an accurate diagnosis of pneumonia in such critically ill patients.

◆ Wrong timing: specimens taken after the start of chemotherapy, when the causative organism may no longer be demonstrable, or after the patient has recovered. It is not uncommon for the laboratory to receive rock-hard faeces from patients with 'diarrhoea'. Many laboratories will not process non-diarrhoeal faecal samples.

◆ Wrong container: blood for culture put in a plain (sometimes non-sterile) bottle instead of the correct culture fluid; biopsies put into bactericidal fixatives such as formalin.

◆ Clerical errors: incorrect labelling; incomplete or misleading information on request forms.

## Specimen transport

Prompt specimen transport to the laboratory is essential. Material submitted for culture may contain living cells; any delay in reaching the optimal cultural conditions will result in loss of viability. With fastidious organisms such as gonococci or viruses, this may result in failure to isolate the organism. Conversely, overgrowth of pathogens by fast-growing commensals also commonly occurs during the period between collection of the specimen and processing in the laboratory, potentially obscuring true pathogens or resulting in a false-positive result. For example, urine that is left at room temperature will act as a culture medium; bacteria that may be present in only low numbers may multiply to levels above the quantitative threshold that is used to define a positive result.

Specimens from potential medical emergencies such as bacterial meningitis or malaria should be delivered to the laboratory as soon as possible after collection for immediate processing. For swabs, most laboratories recommend a form of suspended animation in which the specimen is placed in a special transport medium comprising soft, buffered agar containing charcoal to inactivate any toxic substances. The effect of transport delays on microbe survival can be minimized by inoculating culture media next to the patient and incubating them immediately. This may be achieved in special units with laboratories attached (for example, in some genito-urinary medicine clinics) but is not practicable in most situations. An exception is blood culture, where the counsel of perfection should apply.

## Near patient tests

These are becoming more widely available, for example, the detection of group A streptococcal infection in patients presenting with pharyngitis, or the identification of infants infected with respiratory syncytial virus and presenting with bronchiolitis. Unfortunately, however, such rapid detection methods are sometimes less accurate or complete than the laboratory 'equivalent' tests, meaning that backup testing is required, thus increasing costs. Such methods often do not permit the assessment of the antimicrobial susceptibility of the pathogen, meaning that conventional culture may be required as a supplementary test.

There is likely to be an expansion in the number of molecular tests that can be performed close to the patient, as opposed to requiring transport to a diagnostic laboratory. It is possible to detect an increasing number of potential pathogens, including MRSA and *Clostridium difficile* in nasal swabs and faecal specimens, respectively, using a simple to perform PCR-based, near patient tests. Such tests offer an opportunity for rapid diagnosis of colonization or infection but demonstration of the cost-effectiveness of these types of tests, which are often considerably more expensive, hinders their uptake.

## Specimen processing

The flow diagram (Fig. 12.1) outlines the main steps that occur when a specimen is submitted for bacteriological investigation: microscopy (especially for specimens from normally sterile sites), culture, identification, and antimicrobial susceptibility testing. Even with the most rapidly growing bacteria and with improved methods, results of culture and sensitivity often take 48 hours.

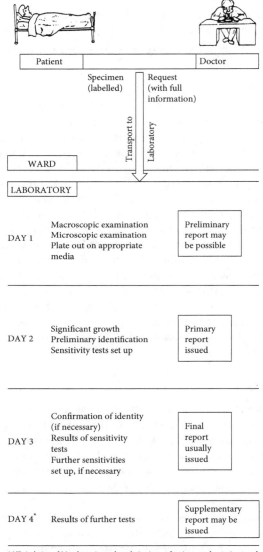

**Fig. 12.1** The various steps between obtaining a specimen from a patient and the issue of the final report. Note the importance of the period before the specimen arrives in the laboratory: unless the specimen is properly taken and transported, it may be useless and, unless the request card is properly completed, the wrong tests may be done and/or incorrect interpretations of the results made.

This may be further delayed if there is a mixture of organisms or if slow-growing pathogens, such as *M. tuberculosis*, obligate intracellular pathogens (e.g. chlamydiae), or viruses, are involved. Not all microorganisms are readily cultivable, and a report of 'sterile' or 'no growth' does not definitively mean that the specimen contained no organisms but rather that the laboratory was unable to isolate a pathogen from the specimen. Conversely, many diagnostic specimens will grow microbes that would normally be expected to be found in particular anatomical sites, and it is important to distinguish these from pathogens; in practice this may be hard or impossible to achieve with certainty. A prime role of the medical microbiologist is to interpret such results and advise on further testing and treatment as appropriate.

Because of the inevitable delay in obtaining culture results, there is a need to inform clinicians of important preliminary findings before the complete results are known. Microscopy results are usually available on the same day as the specimen is received and in urgent cases can be reported within 1 hour or less. For example, a Gram-film of cerebrospinal fluid can be done very quickly and may give the physician a reliable guide to primary therapy (which may be life-saving) while waiting for cultural confirmation of the result. Similarly, positive blood cultures and other findings serious to the individual patient or his immediate contacts are usually telephoned directly to the doctor. When the antibiotic sensitivity is predictable (e.g. *Str. pyogenes* is always susceptible to penicillin), this advice may be given with the initial report. With many bacteria, the report 'susceptibility to follow' is all that can be imparted before antimicrobial testing, although a 'best guess' based on known patterns of resistance in the hospital or community may be suggested.

## Non-culture methods

Rapid advances in immunological and molecular techniques continue to provide new antigen and nucleic acid detection methods. These were initially used to make a diagnosis of infection where viruses or other difficult-to-culture pathogens were suspected. However, the diagnosis of some infections has been transformed by the availability of nucleic acid amplification tests. For example, detection of meningococcal-specific DNA in blood or cerebrospinal fluid makes specific diagnosis of a potentially life-threatening infection possible within hours. This approach can also identify the *Neisseria meningitidis* group and so detect early clusters of cases. One drawback of this approach is that without a viable pathogen it is not be possible to perform standard antimicrobial susceptibility tests (see 'Antimicrobial susceptibility testing' ). However, newer technologies, including specific gene detection and whole genome sequencing, offer the potential to detect mutations or genes associated with antimicrobial resistance; such approaches have been in place for several years to determine the susceptibility of HIV and *M. tuberculosis*, for example, making earlier treatment decisions possible.

## Detection of difficult-to-culture microorganisms

Some microorganisms are notoriously difficult, or indeed impossible, to culture in vitro. This applies to many viruses, *Chlamydia trachomatis*, a common sexually transmitted pathogen, and some very slow-growing bacteria (e.g. *M. tuberculosis*). For these pathogens, culture techniques are being (e.g. for *M. tuberculosis*) or have been (e.g. for many virus and *Chl. trachomatis*) replaced by other methods. For example, tests based on virus culture shifted to the detection of antiviral antibodies, usually using an enzyme immunoassay (EIA), and now increasingly to direct detection of viral nucleic acid with or without quantification or typing.

Viral load measurements of the human immunodeficiency virus (HIV) are now routinely performed by a quantitative (sometimes referred to as real-time) polymerase chain reaction

(PCR) method as part of HIV disease management. The results are used to assess patient prognosis and the effectiveness of antiretroviral therapy. Periodic monitoring of viral load can promptly identify treatment failure potentially due to the emergence of resistance to antiviral drugs. Hepatitis C virus (HCV) infection is detected initially by demonstration of anti-HCV antibodies (using an EIA). Also called 'western blots', recombinant immunoblot assays are frequently used to confirm HCV antibody tests. Positive results are followed up by more specific tests that provided evidence of whether virus is circulating ('active') in the blood or quiescent. This is usually performed by a quantitative PCR test for HCV RNA. The next question in active HCV infection is which virus type is present, as some 'genotypes' are associated with poor response to antiviral treatment. This is answered using a PCR test. Patients with genotypes 2 and 3, for example, are two to three times more likely to respond to interferon therapy than patients with genotype 1. New therapeutic options for genotype 1 infections are discussed in Chapter 34.

## Other molecular and mass spectroscopy tests

Micro-array technology is a method of DNA analysis that involves fixing potentially thousands of DNA probes on to a glass slide. After exposing the slide to a specimen containing pathogens, the DNA fragments that have bound to the probes are detected by chemiluminescence or fluorescence systems, the sensitivity of which may be increased using PCR. This approach has been successfully applied for the detection of rifampicin-resistant strains of *M. tuberculosis*, thus allowing informed choices to be made at the start of therapy. Such approaches offer an alternative source of antimicrobial susceptibility information. However, when many different mechanisms of resistance are possible, some of which may not be characterized by the presence of specific genes, then susceptibility testing by these approaches may not be possible. It is also possible that some genes although present may not be expressed in vivo.

Techniques based on microorganism genotype (e.g. DNA fingerprint) rather than phenotype (e.g. whole cell protein and lipopolysaccharide profiles, antibiotic susceptibility profile, biochemical tests) are now used preferentially to determine the relatedness of clinical isolates. These techniques are useful in the investigation of outbreaks of infection, and in determining routes and sources of infection, including clusters of cases caused by antibiotic-resistant pathogens. The most powerful of these is next generation sequencing (often referred to as whole generation sequencing), and this technique is likely to be used more commonly in coming years, particularly as costs fall to those of older, less discriminatory typing methods.

Other techniques for microorganism detection and identification are used in some larger microbiology laboratories. Broad-range PCR is an alternative, cultivation-independent approach for identifying pathogens that recognizes conserved sequences of bacterial chromosomal genes encoding ribosomal RNA (rDNA). The resulting amplified DNA fragments are sequenced and compared with database results for known microorganisms. Broad-range bacterial PCR has also been used to identify previously uncharacterized pathogens directly in clinical specimens.

Matrix-assisted laser desorption/ionization time of flight (MALDI-TOF) is a form of mass spectrometry that allows the analysis of biomolecules (including proteins, peptides, and sugars). MALDI/TOF is now commonly used for the identification of microorganisms such as bacteria or fungi. A colony of the microorganism is smeared directly on the sample target and overlaid with matrix. The mass spectra generated are analysed and compared with stored profiles. Microorganism identification by this procedure is much faster, more accurate, and cheaper than other procedures based on biochemical tests, which have hitherto dominated in clinical microbiology laboratories. There is increasing interest in the potential use of such methods to identify microorganisms directly in samples such as blood cultures. The advantage here is that delays in waiting for colonies of bacteria to grow, for example on plates inoculated from blood cultures that have signalled positive, could be circumvented.

## Tests of inflammatory markers

Tests of inflammatory markers such as C-reactive protein (CRP) and procalcitonin can be used to aid decision making to initiate or discontinue antibacterial treatment. The strongest evidence for these tests is in respiratory tract infection (see Chapter 21).

## Antimicrobial susceptibility testing

### Purpose of susceptibility testing

Since therapy of infection normally begins, quite properly, before laboratory results are available, antibiotic susceptibility testing primarily plays a supplementary role in confirming that the organism is susceptible to the agent that is being used. Sometimes it may enable the prescriber to change from a toxic to a less toxic agent, from a broad-spectrum to a more targeted (narrow-spectrum) agent, or from an expensive to a cheaper one.

If the patient is failing to respond to the empirical antimicrobial agent(s), by this time the laboratory should have succeeded in establishing the susceptibility pattern of the offending organism (if it is bacterial) and can advise the clinician as to how treatment might be modified. Susceptibility testing of non-bacterial pathogens is not usually possible, although limited antifungal testing is carried out in some centres. Antiviral susceptibility testing (or genotyping that infers susceptibility) is available for certain viruses, for example, HIV, HCV, cytomegalovirus, and herpes simplex.

Many laboratories record and disseminate data on the susceptibility patterns of common pathogens in the hospital and in the community to aid the choice of effective therapy. Patterns of bacterial susceptibility and resistance vary considerably from place to place, and hospitals, or even wards, often have their own particular resistance problems, so the results need to be tailored to the individual circumstance. Regional, national, and international resistance trends are monitored by laboratory networks reporting to a central point.

### Test methods

Most diagnostic microbiology laboratories test antibiotic susceptibility of bacteria by some form of agar diffusion test in which the organism under investigation is exposed to a diffusion gradient of antibiotic provided by an impregnated disc of filter paper (Fig. 12.2). The disc diffusion method is flexible, simple, and cheap and a result can usually be obtained within a day with rapidly growing pathogens such as *Staphylococcus aureus*, *Pseudomonas aeruginosa*, and various enterobacteria; it is less suitable for fastidious or slow-growing bacteria such as anaerobes, streptococci, *Haemophilus* spp., and *Neisseria* spp., for which alternative procedures are preferable. *M. tuberculosis* is very slow growing and needs special media for cultivation and susceptibility testing. These approaches are being replaced by semi-automated commercial devices, primarily when high-throughput susceptibility testing is needed. Molecular methods that are able to detect DNA sequences associated with resistance traits (see 'Non-culture methods' ) are gradually becoming more common.

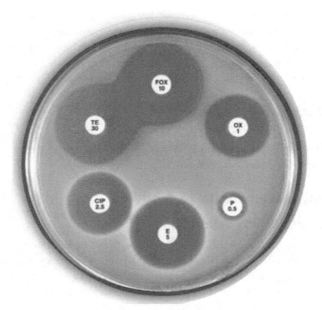

**Fig. 12.2** Example of a disc susceptibility test. The lawn of *Staph. aureus*, present after incubation for 18 hours, shows zones of inhibition (indicating susceptibility) around discs containing cefoxitin (FOX), ciprofloxacin (CIP), erythromycin (E),oxacillin (OX), and tetracycline (TE) but not (indicating resistance) around a penicillin (P) disc.

Reproduced from My Scientific Blog: Research and Articles, *Antibiotic Susceptibility test and Minimum Inhibitory Concentration tests*, available from http://upendrats.blogspot.co.uk/2012/06/antibiotic-susceptibility-test-and. html, Copyright © 2012, with permission from Upendra Thapa Shrestha.

## Minimum inhibitory and bactericidal concentrations

A more accurate estimate of the susceptibility of a bacterial isolate to antimicrobial agents can be obtained by titration in broth or on agar plates containing graded dilutions of antibiotics. The concentration that completely inhibits growth after a defined incubation period (usually overnight) is known as the minimum inhibitory concentration. The minimum inhibitory concentration can also be more easily (but more expensively) estimated by use of a commercial variant of the disc diffusion test, the 'Etest'.

If broth dilution procedures are used, the minimum bactericidal concentration of antibiotic for the test strain may additionally be determined if so desired. The criterion for bactericidal activity is generally taken to be a 1,000-fold reduction in the original inoculum after overnight incubation. This end point is entirely arbitrary and takes no account of the rate of killing, which may be more important.

Estimation of bactericidal concentrations achieved in the patient's serum during therapy is sometimes used in infections (notably bacterial endocarditis) in which bactericidal activity is essential to a cure. The patient's serum, obtained 1 hour after a dose, is titrated against the organism responsible for the infection (so-called back titration). The results are susceptible to methodological variation, and their interpretation has been widely questioned; indeed recent guidelines do not recommend the use of these tests.

**Table 12.1** Some aspects of infection that may cause the results of in vitro tests not to be reflected during treatment.*

| Microorganism | Phenotype different in vivo |
|---|---|
| | Growth rate different in vivo |
| | May be adherent (e.g. device related) |
| Location of infection | Intracellular vs extracellular |
| | Body compartment (CSF, lung, urine, etc.) |
| | May be associated with large collection of pus |
| | May be associated with foreign body |
| | May be within biofilm |
| Host immune response (and other defence mechanisms) | Contributes to recovery |
| | May be influenced by disease |
| | May be influenced by drugs (including antibiotics) |
| Pharmacology of drug | Pharmacokinetic behaviour |
| | Distribution (intracellular or extracellular) |
| | Metabolism in vivo |
| | Penetration to the site of infection (CSF, pus, sputum, etc.) |

* CSF, cerebrospinal fluid.

## Clinical relevance of antibiotic sensitivity tests

A laboratory report of susceptibility or resistance by no means guarantees that the results will translate into clinical success or failure if the agent is used in therapy. Patients may fail to respond to antibiotics judged to be fully active against the offending microbe, or may recover despite the use of agents to which the organism is resistant. These situations arise because laboratory tests offer relatively crude estimates of susceptibility that fail to take into account many crucial features of the infection in the patient (Table 12.1). None the less, antibiotic sensitivity testing offers a generally reliable guide to therapy, particularly in the seriously ill patient in whom laboratory tests may provide an indispensable guide to patient care. The caveat here is that the timing of the start of antibiotic administration likely determines outcome in the very ill patient. Even delays of a few hours may reduce the clinical efficacy of antimicrobial treatment, despite the microorganism being susceptible.

## What the laboratory reports

The final report reaching the clinician must be self-explanatory, even dogmatic. It is not practicable, or desirable, to test each organism isolated against all antibiotics. A restricted range of antimicrobial agents is usually tested against isolates considered significant, with a different selection for Gram-positive and Gram-negative bacteria. Usually, only two or three of the susceptibilities tested are reported even if more are performed. Such restricted reporting has the important function of reinforcing local antibiotic policies and of discouraging clinicians from using inappropriate (or more expensive) agents.

**Table 12.2** Examples of a restricted range of antimicrobial agents selected for primary susceptibility testing of some common pathogens.

| Organism | Antimicrobial agents tested[a] |
|---|---|
| *Staphylococcus aureus* | Benzylpenicillin |
| | Flucloxacillin (methicillin) |
| | Erythromycin |
| | Vancomycin |
| *Streptococcus pyogenes* (and other streptococci) | Benzylpenicillin |
| | Erythromycin |
| Anaerobes | Benzylpenicillin |
| | Clindamycin |
| | Metronidazole |
| *Escherichia coli* (and other enterobacteria) | Ampicillin (amoxicillin) |
| | Cephalosporins[b] |
| | Trimethoprim |
| | Ciprofloxacin |
| | Gentamicin |
| *Pseudomonas aeruginosa* | Piperacillin–tazobactam (ticarcillin–clavulanate) |
| | Gentamicin (tobramycin) |
| | Ciprofloxacin (ofloxacin) |
| | Meropenem (imipenem) |
| Urinary isolates | Ampicillin (amoxicillin) |
| | Cephradine or an alternative oral cephalosporin |
| | Trimethoprim |
| | Nalidixic acid (ciprofloxacin) |
| | Nitrofurantoin |

[a] Agents shown in brackets are examples of acceptable alternatives.

[b] A representative of the earlier (e.g. cefradine, cefalexin) and later (e.g. cefuroxime, cefotaxime) cephalosporins; is usually chosen for primary testing.

Primary testing is ordinarily restricted to a few old and well-tried agents that are perfectly adequate for most common infections (Table 12.2). More extensive (second-line) testing, particularly of expensive, broad-spectrum agents, is reserved for resistant isolates or bacteria from patients with serious infections that are presenting problems of management. Extended testing may also provide useful epidemiological information of trends of antimicrobial susceptibility and of clusters of multiply resistant bacteria, evidence of cross-infection or spread from a common source.

Most infections are caused by a single organism, often a well-known pathogen. In these cases, there is usually no problem in deciding what to test and report. However, some specimens (e.g. those from abdominal wounds) are often infected with mixtures of organisms, and each must be individually identified and tested against appropriate antimicrobial agents. Laboratories usually restrict the reporting of such results to discourage a blanket therapy approach covering each and every microorganism that is recovered from specimens taken from normally non-sterile sites.

The choice of antibiotic tested varies with the site of infection and the pharmacological properties of the drug. Some agents, such as nitrofurantoin and nalidixic acid, achieve therapeutic concentrations only in urine and are of no value in other infections. Information about the individual patient may alter drug testing as follows:

* if the patient is allergic to penicillins, alternatives will be sought in pregnancy, and sulphonamides and trimethoprim should be avoided if possible because of the risk of folate deficiency;

* in a patient with worsening renal failure, it may be preferable to avoid aminoglycoside therapy; and

* tetracyclines should not be used in late pregnancy or in young children owing to deposition in teeth.

These limitations of susceptibility testing or reporting can be taken into account by the laboratory only if the appropriate information is given on the request card.

In some cases there may be many alternative possible antimicrobial agents for an identified infection. Some groups of agents, such as aminopenicillins (ampicillin, amoxicillin) or tetracyclines, are so similar in terms of their antibacterial spectrum that only one representative of each needs to be tested. With other drugs, where there is differential susceptibility of bacteria to different members of the group, such a decision is less easy. An organism susceptible to cefalexin, one of the earliest cephalosporins, is also usually susceptible to all subsequent members of that group and this is often used as a screen for cephalosporin-susceptible bacteria. However, the converse is not true; an organism resistant to cefalexin may be susceptible to later cephalosporins, and a definitive statement in this regard can be made only by testing the appropriate compound. The same principle applies to nalidixic acid and newer, more active quinolones.

## Interpreting antimicrobial susceptibility reports

Consider a report on pus from an abscess that grew *Staph. aureus* which was resistant to penicillin but susceptible to erythromycin and cloxacillin. The statement 'this organism is resistant to penicillin' means that penicillin would not influence the outcome. The infection may well improve due to host defences or to adequate drainage of pus but, since penicillin-resistant staphylococci are invariably β-lactamase producers, any penicillin that reached the abscess would be rapidly destroyed. Such a statement is based on sound laboratory and clinical evidence. If the *Staph. aureus* isolate was found to have relatively low-level resistance (i.e. where inhibition of growth is incomplete but less than that produced using a susceptible control organism), the likelihood of clinical resistance to penicillin is more difficult to determine; factors such as site of infection and drug penetration may be important in this respect. The laboratory will try to weigh up the evidence and score the result as 'susceptible' or 'resistant'; the term 'reduced (or intermediate) susceptibility' is sometimes used but this is a less satisfactory alternative and leaves the clinician uncertain how to interpret the result.

The statement 'this organism is susceptible to cloxacillin' implies that use of this antibiotic (or a related β-lactamase-stable penicillin) would influence the outcome. This is more difficult to support than a statement about resistance. Treatment with the antibiotic may elicit little response in the patient because insufficient drug may have penetrated into a large collection of pus; the dosage prescribed and route of administration may be important here. More importantly (although unlikely in the present example, since *Staph. aureus* is commonly incriminated in infected wounds), the wrong organism (an innocent bystander) may have been tested. Host factors that may also influence therapeutic outcome are described in Chapter 13.

## Conclusion: when in doubt, consult the laboratory

When in doubt, whether about the optimal specimen to submit, the interpretation of a test result, or the most appropriate treatment, the laboratory should be consulted. For unusual diseases and problem cases, it is often possible to seek help from specialized units such as tropical hospitals and institutes. In some countries, reference laboratories are available that provide expertise in particular areas. In the United Kingdom many of these operate under the aegis of Public Health England (formerly, the Health Protection Agency). Worldwide, the Centers for Disease Control and Prevention, Atlanta, Georgia, United States, offer a service for the diagnosis and therapy of unusual infectious diseases.

### Key points

- Supplying appropriate clinical details on request forms is crucial so that the correct tests and interpretations of results are made.
- An antibiotic susceptibility test result is relevant for a given pathogen recovered from a specific site and is not necessarily valid for the same pathogen in a different site; this is because antibiotics generally penetrate some sites better than others.
- A report that a pathogen is antibiotic susceptible does not assure of treatment success; a pathogen that is reported as resistant to an antibiotic is very unlikely to respond to treatment with this agent.
- PCR-based tests are becoming the methods of choice for increasing numbers of infections, as they often offer increased sensitivity and more rapid results than other tests.
- PCR-based tests usually do not permit the assessment of antibiotic resistance, other than the detection of specific genes/mutations associated with a resistant phenotype.

### Further reading

Fawley, W. N. and Wilcox, M. H. (2005) Molecular diagnostic techniques. *Medicine*, **33**(3): 26–32.

Mancini, N., Carletti, S., Ghidoli, N., Cichero, P., Burioni, R., and Clementi, M. (2010) The era of molecular and other non-culture-based methods in diagnosis of sepsis. *Clinical Microbiology Review*, **23**(1): 235–51.

Maurin, M. (2012) Real-time PCR as a diagnostic tool for bacterial diseases. *Expert Review of Molecular Diagnostics*, **12**(7): 731–54.

# Chapter 13

# General principles of the treatment of infection

## Introduction to general principles of treating infection

Antimicrobial agents are among the most commonly prescribed drugs. Their use has had a major impact on the prevention and control of infections in man. More recently, effective antiviral drugs against HIV, hepatitis B, and hepatitis C have revolutionized the treatment of these infections. Likewise, new antifungal agents have had a substantial impact on the outcome from severe invasive fungal diseases. At the same time, however, resistance to all antimicrobial agents has been steadily increasing and now poses one of the most serious threats to global health. In this context, the principles governing the appropriate and safe use of antimicrobial agents are increasingly important and are the subject of this chapter.

## General issues

The appropriate use of antimicrobial therapy requires an initial clinical assessment of the nature and severity of the infection and the likely causative agent. This assessment should be supported, whenever practicable, by laboratory investigation aimed at establishing the microbial cause and its susceptibility to antimicrobial agents appropriate for the treatment of the infection. The choice of drug, its dose, route, and frequency of administration are also dependent upon an appreciation of its pharmacokinetic and pharmacodynamic properties (see Chapter 14), together with evidence from clinical trials and treatment guidelines.

## Clinical assessment

The practice of infectious disease practice differs from all other medical specialties in the need to consider the biology of two organisms: the patient and the infectious agent. A helpful approach in the assessment of an infected patient, and the determination of the likely cause of the illness, is to ask the following question: why did this person, from this place, get this disease, at this time? The question summarizes the key considerations required to begin the diagnostic and treatment process and is an elegant reminder that an infectious disease depends on the complex interaction between the virulence of the infectious agent, the susceptibility of the host, and the nature of their shared environment.

These questions can only be satisfactorily answered by a well-directed history (Box 13.1), but answers to the following questions are essential:

- Is the patient particularly susceptible to some or all infectious agents?
- What is the duration of illness?

To answer the first requires an enquiry spanning vaccination history, travel, illicit and immune-suppressive drugs, and risk factors for HIV. Without answers to both questions, it is almost impossible to construct a sensible differential diagnosis and antimicrobial treatment plan.

## Box 13.1 Key elements in the history: why did this person, from this place, develop this disease at this time?

### Person

- age
- occupation
- immune-suppressed or immune-competent (e.g. pregnancy, drugs, splenectomy, cancer, HIV/AIDS)
- high risk sexual behaviour or intravenous drug use
- vaccination/prophylaxis

### Place

- contact with infected individuals (e.g. tuberculosis, or chickenpox in family member)
- duration of potential exposure to infection
- travel (e.g. to malarial or arbovirus-endemic area)
- season of exposure (e.g. enterovirus infections commoner in summer/autumn
- animals (e.g. cat scratches; tick, animal, or mosquito bites)
- food and water (e.g. eating unpasteurized dairy products or swimming in fresh water)

### Time

- time from potential exposure to disease (e.g. chickenpox, mumps, malaria)
- duration of symptoms before presentation
- duration and nature of any prior treatment (e.g. antibiotics given prior to assessment)

The physical examination should be directed by the history, focusing on defining the organs affected by the infection and its severity. Definition of the focus of infection is essential: it will help refine the likely cause, suggest possible diagnostic sampling of tissue, and determine both antimicrobial and non-drug (e.g. drainage of pus) management.

## Laboratory assessment

Few infective conditions present such a typical picture that a definitive clinical and microbiological diagnosis can be made without recourse to the laboratory. Therefore, whenever possible, a clinical diagnosis should be supported by appropriate laboratory investigations to confirm the cause of the infection. A summary of the key diagnostic tests for a range of common infections is given in Box 13.2. Many doctors (including infectious diseases physicians) consider the microbiology laboratory a black box to which specimens are sent and from which answers mysteriously appear. Like clinical medicine, there is art as well as science to traditional diagnostic microbiology. Its value depends on the quality of the specimens submitted and the human attributes of those who practise it. There are several ways to get the most out of your diagnostic laboratory but good communication between ward and laboratory is essential.

## Box 13.2 The application of key diagnostic tests for infectious diseases

### 1. Microscopy (blood/cerebrospinal fluid/urine/tissue)

◆ bacteria (categorized as Gram-stain positive or negative)

◆ mycobacteria (acid-fast bacilli demonstrated by Zhiel–Neelsen stain; e.g. tuberculosis)

◆ fungi (e.g. invasive hyphae in tissue or yeast forms in cerebrospinal fluid (CSF))

◆ parasites (e.g. malarial parasites in blood)

◆ electron microscopy for viruses (superseded by nucleic acid amplification tests)

### 2. Microbial culture (blood/CSF/urine/tissue)

◆ most bacteria, including mycobacteria

◆ most fungi

◆ viral culture now rarely available in routine diagnostic labs

◆ parasite culture rarely available

### 3. Nucleic acid amplification tests (blood/CSF/tissue)

◆ mainstay of viral diagnostics; includes quantitative counts (e.g. HIV viral load)

◆ increasingly common diagnostic method for non-culturable or hard-to-culture bacteria (e.g. *Mycobacteria tuberculosis*)

◆ occasional use in parasitic diagnosis (e.g. *Toxoplasma gondii*)

◆ rarely used for fungal diagnosis

### 4. Antigen detection tests

◆ most commonly used for fungal infections (e.g. *Cryptococcus neoformans*)

◆ parasitic infections (e.g. cysticercosis)

◆ occasional, hard-to-culture bacteria (e.g. *Legionella* urinary antigen)

### 5. Serology (detection of pathogen-specific antibodies)

◆ diseases with hard-to-culture bacteria (e.g. syphilis (blood and CSF), Lyme disease, brucellosis)

◆ common viral diagnostic tests (e.g. Epstein–Barr virus, mumps, flaviviruses such as Japanese encephalitis virus, West Nile virus)

◆ common parasitic diagnostic tests (e.g. *Toxocara canis*, *Toxop. gondii*, schistosomiasis, strongyloidiasis)

## Assessment of sepsis and the systemic inflammatory response

Sepsis is defined as the combination of symptoms or signs of a localized primary site of infection plus evidence of a systemic inflammatory response. This systemic inflammatory response syndrome (SIRS) is often the first sign that infection is spreading from the primary site and that the patient may, for example, be bacteraemic (see Chapter 26).

Infection is not the only cause of SIRS. Other causes include accidental or elective trauma (it is a normal reaction to elective surgery); chronic inflammatory conditions (e.g. arteritis, systemic lupus erythematosus); and malignancy (especially lymphoma but also solid tumours). In addition, the syndrome can be a response to infection by any type of pathogen: bacterial, fungal, protozoal, or viral.

Severe sepsis is characterized by hypotension, organ/tissue hypoperfusion leading to acute confusion, hypotension, oliguria, and hypoxia or lactic acidosis.

The greater the severity of infection and organ/tissue dysfunction, the higher is the mortality, which increases from 10–20 per cent with sepsis to 25–50 per cent with severe sepsis and 55–80 per cent with septic shock.

## Selection of antimicrobial chemotherapy

### Initial empirical therapy

Acute and potentially life-threatening infections require immediate treatment, usually well before any information is available regarding the causative agent or its likely antimicrobial susceptibility. In these circumstances, initial 'empirical' antimicrobial therapy is chosen based on the likely infectious causes of the presenting clinical syndrome, taking into consideration the possibility of antimicrobial drug resistance. For example, it is common practice in the United Kingdom to combine a β-lactam (penicillin or cephalosporin) with an aminoglycoside, such as gentamicin, in the initial treatment of serious infections. However, if methicillin-resistant *Staphylococcus aureus* (MRSA) infection is possible, or infection with Gram-negative bacteria expressing extended spectrum β-lactamases is suspected, the physician may add vancomycin or use a carbapenem to mitigate these respective risks. Likewise, if there is evidence that the infection has arisen in association with mucosal surfaces, such as the gut or the female genital tract, then metronidazole is frequently added to meet the possibility of a mixed anaerobic and aerobic bacterial infection. Once a definitive diagnosis is established, it is important to adjust the therapeutic regimen to one that is most appropriate.

### Definitive therapy

Once a causative agent has been identified, antimicrobial therapy should be adjusted to ensure the most effective treatment is given. The choice of antimicrobial, its dose, route of administration, and duration is dependent on the type of organism, its known or tested drug susceptibility, the pharmacological properties of the antimicrobials available, and evidence from relevant clinical trials.

### Antimicrobial susceptibility testing

Infectious agents may be inherently resistant to some antimicrobials or acquire resistance through genetic mutation. Acquired resistance can be detected either by demonstrating the specific mutation causing the resistance (genotypic susceptibility testing), or by seeing whether known concentrations of the antimicrobial kill the organism in the laboratory (in vitro phenotypic susceptibility testing). In general, genotypic methods are used for viruses and hard-to-culture bacteria. Their main limitations are that they require prior knowledge of the genetic mechanism of resistance and that the target mutation(s) must be reliably associated with phenotypic resistance. Phenotypic in vitro susceptibility testing is widely used for common bacterial and fungal species and has the advantage of not requiring knowledge of the resistance mechanism. However, both genotypic and phenotypic methods only provide indirect evidence of the likely clinical response of a particular pathogen to a specific drug or drugs. Confirmation of clinical efficacy can be determined only in vivo, hence the importance of clinical evaluation of all new antimicrobial agents.

## Antimicrobial pharmacokinetic and pharmacodynamics

The aim of chemotherapy is to eliminate an infection as rapidly as possible. To achieve this, a sufficient concentration of the drug or drugs selected must reach the site of infection to kill the responsible organisms. Antimicrobial pharmacokinetics describes the relationship between the dose of the drug given and its concentration over time in blood and other relevant tissues. It encompasses drug absorption, distribution, metabolism, and excretion. Pharmacodynamics describes the relationship between drug concentrations and organism killing and clinical effect. These aspects are discussed in more detail in Chapter 14.

Antibacterial agents are sometimes separated into either bactericidal or bacteriostatic agents according to their ability to kill or inhibit bacterial growth in vitro. The clinical relevance of this distinction is controversial. Examples of bactericidal drugs include the β-lactam and glycopeptide antibiotics; bacteriostatic agents include the tetracyclines, sulphonamides, and chloramphenicol. In the treatment of most infections, however, the choice between a bactericidal and a bacteriostatic agent is not critical. Historically, bactericidal agents have generally been preferred for the treatment of infective endocarditis and for infections associated with severely impaired host immune responses, for example, neutropenic sepsis.

## Route, dose, and duration of therapy

The optimal route of administration, dose, and duration of therapy for most infections is not well defined. However, there are some guiding principles which can help select the best treatment regimen. Choosing the right dose and route of administration requires knowledge of the drug's pharmacokinetic, pharmacodynamic, and toxicity profiles. The ideal antimicrobial regimen is well tolerated, kills the organism effectively, limits the emergence of resistant organisms, and does not allow the infection to recur.

In general, antimicrobial agents are administered topically, by mouth, or by intravenous or intramuscular injection. The oral bioavailability of antimicrobial agents is highly variable; some are very well absorbed orally (e.g. fluoroquinolones, linezolid), others are variably absorbed (e.g. many beta-lactams), and some are not absorbed at all (e.g. aminoglycosides and glycopeptides). If the infection is severe, and oral absorption uncertain, intravenous administration is preferred. Intramuscular administration requires absorption through the tissue capillaries and is generally rapid except in conditions of cardiovascular collapse and shock, when tissue perfusion is impaired. Relatively avascular sites such as the vitreous humour of the eye are difficult sites in which to achieve adequate drug concentrations following systemic administration, and direct injection is often preferred in such cases.

The choice of antimicrobial dose depends upon the relationship between the blood and tissue concentrations achieved over time and the killing effect on the responsible organism. This relationship varies for different classes of antibiotics. For example, as β-lactam antibiotics kill susceptible bacteria more effectively the longer their concentration is maintained, maintained administration, or continuous infusion, may be preferable. The killing effects of other drugs (e.g. aminoglycosides) are dependent on the peak concentrations achieved in relation to the minimum inhibitory concentration and necessitate less frequent but higher doses. Drug toxicity may limit the dose given. For example, β-lactams are generally very well tolerated and can be given in frequent high doses, whereas aminoglycosides and glycopeptides have significant nephrotoxicity at high dose.

Treatment should continue until all microorganisms are eliminated from the tissues or until the infection has been sufficiently controlled for the normal host defences to eradicate it. This end point is hard to determine and varies according to the infection. Clinical observation and evidence of the resolution of the inflammatory process, such as the return of body temperature and white cell count to normal, can help the decision to stop antimicrobial therapy. However, for more serious infections, physicians should be guided by evidence from clinical trials. This is especially true for hard-to-treat, recalcitrant infectious, such as those caused by *Staphylococcus aureus* and *Mycobacterium tuberculosis*, where failure to treat for long enough exposes the patient to a high risk of disease recurrence.

## Combination antimicrobial therapy

The possible advantages of using more than one antimicrobial agent in combination include synergistic killing, overcoming prior but unknown antimicrobial resistance, and reducing the risk of de novo resistance developing. Aside from a few notable exceptions—the treatment of tuberculosis, cryptococcal meningitis, and falciparum malaria for example—the clinical benefits of combination therapy remain uncertain. Some drug combinations may even be antagonistic. For example, there is some clinical evidence that the combination of penicillin and tetracycline in the treatment of pneumococcal meningitis may worsen outcome compared to single-drug treatment. Furthermore, using more than one antibiotic increases the risk of associated adverse reactions.

Some drugs—rifampicin and fusidic acid, for example—should always be used in combination with other antimicrobials, as resistance to these agents develops rapidly if used alone.

## Adverse reactions

Antimicrobial agents, like all other therapeutic substances, have the potential to produce adverse reactions. These vary widely in their nature, frequency, and severity. Many reactions, such as gastrointestinal intolerance, are minor and short lived but others may be serious, life-threatening, and occasionally fatal. Drug reactions are unfortunately a common cause of prolonged stay in hospital or may precipitate hospital admission. Drug reactions may be predictable and dose dependent, for example, nephrotoxicity associated with the use of aminoglycosides, glycopeptides, and the antifungal agent amphotericin. However, many adverse reactions are unpredictable. The subject is discussed more fully in Chapter 17.

## Cost

Antimicrobial drugs vary widely in their cost. In general, generic off-patent drugs cost less than proprietary preparations, and well-established, widely used agents tend to be less expensive. Injectable preparations are usually more expensive than oral preparations, and syrups and drops can be more expensive than tablets and capsules. The *British National Formulary* provides a useful guide to the cost of individual drugs for prescribers in the United Kingdom.

# Failure of antimicrobial chemotherapy

Patients with established infection may fail to respond to antimicrobial therapy for a variety of reasons. Chief among these are

- the patient does not have an infection;
- the infection is caused by an organism which is resistant to the antimicrobial treatment prescribed;
- the patient has a deep focus of infection associated with pus and/or prosthetic material; or
- the patient is not receiving or taking the medication.

A common error in the face of possible treatment failure is to conclude that the infection must be resistant to the antimicrobial used and change quickly to another (often more expensive) agent without properly considering other possible causes of failure. In practice, misdiagnoses and undrained/unremoved deep foci of infection are the commonest reasons for antimicrobial failure. The latter is especially important, especially for health-care-associated infections. It is generally impossible to treat infected intravenous catheters or other prosthetic devices with antimicrobial agents alone; their removal is usually essential. The only exceptions are when the infecting organism is of low virulence (e.g. coagulase negative staphylococci) and the infected device is essential to the ongoing medical care of the patient (e.g. central venous catheter in a severely unwell patient with difficult intravenous access). Otherwise, always seek to define the focus of infection and, if it is associated with pus or prosthetic material, drain or remove it before contemplating changes to the antimicrobial regimen.

## Key points

- Antimicrobial agents are some of humankind's most valuable medicines and must be used with great care and responsibility.
- The appropriate use of antimicrobial therapy requires an initial clinical assessment of the nature and severity of the infection and the likely causative agent.
- Acute and potentially life-threatening infections require immediate treatment, usually well before any information is available regarding the causative agent or its likely antimicrobial susceptibility.
- The choice of antimicrobial, its dose, route of administration, and duration is dependent on the type of organism, its known or tested drug susceptibility, the pharmacological properties of the antimicrobials available, and evidence from relevant clinical trials.

## Further reading

Finch, R. G. (2009) Antimicrobial therapy: principles of use. *Medicine*, **37**(10): 545–50.

Lorian, V. (2005) *Antibiotics in Laboratory Medicine: Making a Difference* (5th edn). London: Lippincott, Williams & Wilkins.

# Chapter 14

# Pharmacokinetic and pharmacodynamic principles

## Introduction to pharmacokinetic and pharmacodynamic principles

All those who prescribe antibiotics for the treatment of infections must understand something of how their concentrations rise and fall after administration (pharmacokinetics) and how these concentrations relate to the killing of microorganisms and clinical outcome (pharmacodynamics). Antibiotics target infecting microorganisms which may cause disease at either single or multiple body sites. Therefore, the ability to achieve sufficient concentrations at the site of infection determines an antibiotic's therapeutic application. A number of pharmacokinetic factors are important in relation to determining infection-site drug concentrations but also influence the safety profile of the agent. These factors are

◆ absorption;

◆ distribution;

◆ metabolism; and

◆ elimination.

The majority of information about the antibiotic pharmacokinetics comes from studies in healthy volunteers. Patients with infections, especially if the infections are severe and life threatening, are likely to have altered antibiotic pharmacokinetics. Drug absorption, distribution, and drug elimination may be very different from that observed in healthy volunteers and may therefore have profound effects on plasma concentrations. The potential importance of these differences is well demonstrated in Fig. 14.1.

Organism killing and clinical outcomes are generally dependent on the antibiotic concentrations achieved at the sites of infection and may differ widely according to the type of organism and antibiotic administered. Pharmacodynamics is the study of this relationship and is of enormous clinical relevance. Most organisms have a threshold above which the concentration of an antibiotic will reliably kill the majority of organisms. For bacteria, this is commonly called the minimum inhibitory concentration (or MIC) and it is usually defined in the laboratory (by an e-test, for example). Understanding the relationship between in vivo antibiotic concentrations (or 'drug exposure'), the MIC of the infecting organism, and the killing of the organism is critical to the optimal use of antibiotics, both for curing the diseases caused and preventing the emergence of antibiotic resistant bacteria.

## Pharmacokinetic principles

### Absorption

Antibiotics can be administered by a variety of different routes. Other than by direct intravenous injection, the concentrations achieved in the blood and the site of infection are dependent

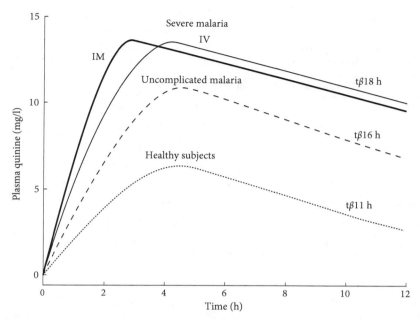

**Fig. 14.1** Plasma concentrations of quinine in healthy subjects compared with patients with uncomplicated and severe malaria following administration of a loading dose of 20 mg (salt)/kg; tβ is the elimination half-life.

Reproduced from White J, 'Antimalarial pharmacokinetics and treatment regimens', *British Journal of Clinical Pharmacology*, Volume 34, Issue 1, pp. 1–10, Copyright © 1992 with permission from John Wiley and Sons.

upon the antibiotic's absorption from that route (e.g. mouth/intestinal tract, muscle). Serial measurements of the concentration of the agent in the serum following administration can be used to calculate both the rates of an antibiotic's absorption/elimination and the volume in which the drug is distributed. The volume of distribution indicates whether the drug is largely confined within the vascular compartment or extends into the extracellular fluid—the site of most infections—or penetrates into cells where some organisms (e.g. mycobacteria and *Salmonella* spp.) multiply.

Many antibiotics do not produce adequate plasma concentrations when given by mouth and are available only as injectable preparations. The fraction of a dose of an oral drug that is absorbed unchanged and available to interact with the target is known as its bioavailability. The degree to which antimicrobial compounds are absorbed when given orally differs greatly (Table 14.1).

Some antibiotics given orally are irregularly absorbed and often produce low plasma concentrations. Sometimes absorption can be improved by chemical modification of the drug (e.g. esterification) to create a 'prodrug' which is converted to its active form following absorption. Examples include erythromycin estolate, pivampicillin, and in the case of antivirals, valaciclovir.

The most direct way of ensuring adequate concentrations of antibiotic in the blood is by intravenous injection. The highest instantaneous concentrations are, of course, achieved by a single rapid intravenous injection but any benefit of this may be offset by rapid excretion, and many agents are given by infusion over 15–20 minutes. Sometimes slow infusion is necessary in order to minimize side effects (as with vancomycin) or local reaction at the injection site.

**Table 14.1** Bioavailability and intestinal elimination of some commonly prescribed antibacterial drugs after oral administration. Note that drugs that are well absorbed may still achieve high concentrations in the faeces because of secretion into bile or other enteral secretions. Similarly, some drugs are eliminated in the intestine after parenteral administration (e.g. ceftriaxone).

| Drug | Bioavailability (%) | Intestinal elimination |
|------|---------------------|------------------------|
| Amoxicillin | 80–90 | Concentrated up to 10-fold in bile |
| Cefalexin | 80–100 | Concentrated up to threefold in bile |
| Cefuroxime axetil | 30–40 | Bile concentrations up to 80% of serum |
| Ciprofloxacin | 70–85 | Concentrated up to 10-fold in bile; additional enteral secretion |
| Erythromycin | 18–45 | Concentrated up to 300-fold in bile |
| Metronidazole | 80–95 | Concentrations in bile similar to serum |
| Rifampicin | 90–100 | Concentrated up to 1000-fold in bile |
| Trimethoprim | 80–90 | Concentrated up to twofold in bile |

Absorption from intramuscular sites is usually rapid but can be modified to suit the clinical need. For example, to maintain prolonged inhibitory levels of penicillin (e.g. to treat syphilis), special depot preparations such as procaine penicillin have been developed (see 'Prolongation of plasma levels' in Chapter 2). These allow slow release from the injection site so that the plasma concentrations are maintained for long periods.

# Distribution

## Protein binding

Antibiotics can bind to plasma proteins, mostly albumin, and this can influence their distribution to tissues and their biological activity. Some antibiotics, such as flucloxacillin, ceftriaxone, fusidic acid, and teicoplanin, are more than 90 per cent protein bound and, in this form, are inactive against bacteria. Only the unbound diffusible fraction of the drug reaches the tissues, and only this fraction exerts antimicrobial effect. As the unbound fraction diffuses away, more of the protein-bound drug dissociates and the equilibrium between the bound and the free compound is maintained. However, the clinical relevance of this property is usually minimal. Inflammatory exudates occurring in response to infection contain high protein concentrations; therefore, protein-bound drug will tend to be delivered to the sites of infection. In this way, protein-bound drug may be looked upon as a prodrug with the valuable property of 'homing in' on to sites of inflammation. Once in the site, as far as is known, the concentration of free and active drug is still defined by the equilibrium between free and bound drug.

## Tissue distribution

Infections can affect any tissue in the body, and the microorganisms may be extracellular, intracellular, or a combination of the two. Antibiotics have variable tissue and cellular penetration and it is important to consider these properties when selecting the likely best therapy (see Table 14.2). For example, aminoglycosides and glycopeptides do not penetrate the blood–brain barrier well, unless it is grossly disrupted by inflammation, and thus are generally not used as first-line treatments for

**Table 14.2** Kinetic requirements for treatment of bacterial infections at different anatomical sites.

| Anatomical site of infection | Natural barrier from blood to interstitial fluid? | Intracellular penetration desirable? | Penetration into luminal secretions required? |
|---|---|---|---|
| Biliary tract | No | None proven; most of the causative organisms are extracellular | No conclusive evidence that antibiotics with high biliary concentrations are any more effective for treating cholecystitis |
| Central nervous system | Yes, the blood–brain barrier | Yes, for tuberculous and listerial meningitis | Yes; effective cerebrospinal fluid concentrations crucial |
| Respiratory tract | No | Essential against agents of atypical pneumonia and tuberculosis but unnecessary for most common pathogens (*Streptococcus pneumoniae* and *Haemophilus influenzae*) | High concentrations in bronchial secretions may be desirable when part of the aim of treatment is reduction of bacterial load in sputum (e.g. in cystic fibrosis). Not essential in most pulmonary infections, including community-acquired pneumonia |
| Skin and soft tissue | No | Not essential, although some evidence that *Staphylococcus aureus* can survive within leucocytes | Not essential; most organisms are extracellular |
| Urinary tract | Prostate only | Only for *Chlamydia trachomatis* (prostatitis/epididymo-orchitis); unnecessary for common causes of urinary tract infection | Effective urinary concentrations essential; drugs that achieve low concentrations in interstitial fluid (nitrofurantoin) are relatively ineffective in pyelonephritis |

bacterial meningitis. Some antibiotics are selectively concentrated in cells and are particularly useful for intracellular infections. For example, rifampicin and azithromycin concentrate within leucocytes and are very effective in the treatment of tuberculosis and salmonella infections, respectively. In general, β-lactam antibiotics do not penetrate cells well and are less useful against intracellular infections.

## Plasma half-life

The time required for the plasma drug concentration to fall by half is called the plasma half-life. Antibiotic half-lives vary considerably; that of benzylpenicillin, for example, is only 30 minutes, whereas the half-life of the antimalarial mefloquine is about three weeks.

The concentration achieved in plasma while the drug is resident in the body can be measured relatively simply from serial blood samples but the calculation of the true half-life must take into account the distribution phase (sometimes called the α phase) during which the compound is migrating from the plasma to the tissues. This is clearly influenced by the route of administration, since absorption from intestinal or intramuscular sites is not instantaneous (Fig. 14.2).

The half-life of a drug that is usually cited is that which follows distribution to the tissues and is designated as the β phase. Any metabolism of the drug, binding to plasma proteins, or alteration

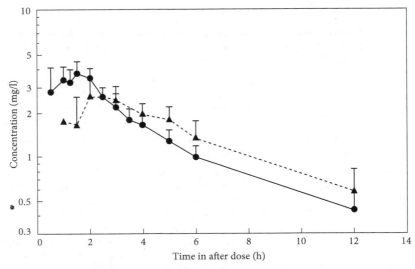

**Fig. 14.2** Mean plasma (●) and inflammatory fluid (▲) concentrations following a single 750 mg oral dose of ciprofloxacin. The distribution (or α) phase lasts for two hours and is followed by the elimination (or β) phase. There is an even longer distribution phase in the inflammatory fluid, where concentrations do not peak until about three hours after administration. There is a lag in diffusion of drug back into the plasma so that, from three hours after administration, tissue fluid concentrations are higher than plasma concentrations.

Reproduced from Catchpole C et al., 'The comparative pharmacokinetics and tissue penetration of single-dose ciprofloxacin 400 mg iv and 750 mg po', *Journal of Antimicrobial Chemotherapy*, Volume 33, Issue 1, pp. 103–110, Copyright © 1994, by permission of Oxford University Press.

in the functional integrity of the organs of excretion (usually the kidney, the liver, or both) will affect the elimination of the drug and hence the plasma half-life.

## Drug accumulation

If large doses are given, or the half-life of the drug is such that complete elimination has not occurred before the next dose is administered, the concentration of drug in the plasma will progressively rise. The excretion phase being logarithmic, the rate of elimination rises as the concentration of drug rises; eventually excretion proceeds as fast as the accumulation, and the drug reaches a steady state (Fig. 14.3). In this example, the first dose results in plasma concentration that exceeds the minimum inhibitory concentration for the organism being treated but not throughout the dosing interval. If it is essential to reach higher concentrations immediately, then a loading dose should be given, which is usually two to three times the maintenance dose.

The possibility of accumulation and its consequences must be considered when an agent with a long half-life is administered or the patient's capacity to eliminate the agent is known or thought likely to be impaired and the agent has dose-related side effects (e.g. vancomycin and gentamicin).

## Metabolism

Many antibiotics are metabolized. Some antibiotics are completely inactivated but the metabolites of others may have their own spectrum of antimicrobial activity. In addition, metabolites may be

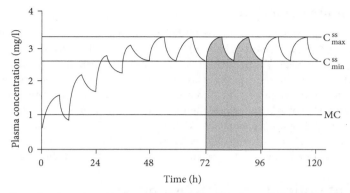

**Fig. 14.3** Illustration of a drug dosed twice daily that takes five doses to reach steady state. The shaded area shows the area under the concentration–time curve at steady state over 24 hours. $C^{ss}_{max}$ is the maximum (or peak) concentration at steady state, and $C^{ss}_{min}$ is the minimum (or trough) concentration at steady state. MIC is the minimum inhibitory concentration for a target pathogen.

Reproduced from *Clinical Pharmacokinetics*, Volume 37, Issue 4, pp. 289–304, Sanchez-Navarro A and Sanchez Recio M, 'Basis of Anti-Infective Therapy: Pharmacokinetic - Pharmacodynamic Criteria and Methodology for Dual Dosage Individualisation', Copyright © 1999, with kind permission from Springer Science and Business Media.

toxic. Furthermore, metabolites may display altered pharmacokinetic characteristics, so that the period for which they are present in the body and able to achieve an antibacterial (or toxic) effect may be longer or shorter than that of the parent compound.

Occasionally, it is necessary to prevent metabolism from occurring. For example, the carbapenem antibiotic imipenem is susceptible to a renal dehydropeptidase that opens the β-lactam ring. Consequently, imipenem is formulated with a dehydropeptidase inhibitor, cilastatin, which protects it from inactivation.

Antibiotics which are metabolized are particularly liable to interact with other drugs. For example, some of the macrolides, fluoroquinolones, and antifungal azoles can inhibit the hepatic metabolism of other drugs in the liver. Conversely, rifampicin is a potent non-specific inducer of hepatic metabolism and may therefore cause therapeutic failure of a very wide range of co-administered drugs by increasing their clearance, for example, immunosuppressive agents (cyclosporin, tacrolimus), anti-asthmatic agents (theophylline), opioid analgesics (alfentanil), anticonvulsants (phenytoin, carbamazepine), calcium antagonists (verapamil, nifedipine, felodipine), and anticoagulants (warfarin).

# Elimination

Most antibiotics are eliminated by the kidneys, so that very high concentrations may be achieved in urine. Excretion is by glomerular filtration or tubular secretion, and sometimes both. The principal compounds excreted in the urine by active tubular secretion are the penicillins and cephalosporins. This process is so effective as to clear the blood of most of the drug during its passage through the kidney, and these compounds generally have a very short half-life of two hours or less. Increasing the frequency of administration can increase the period for which inhibitory levels of rapidly excreted agents are present in the blood. Alternatively, an agent that competes for the active transport mechanism may be used. The oral uricosuric agent probenecid shares the tubular route of excretion of penicillins and can be used to prolong the plasma half-life of these antibiotics.

## Pharmacodynamic principles

The important link between an antibiotic's pharmacokinetics and its clinical effect—or the pharmacokinetic–pharmacodynamic (PK-PD) relationship—was initially identified in the 1940s and 1950s by Dr Harry Eagle. Eagle identified that continuous penicillin concentrations killed bacteria more effectively than short peaks of concentrations, whereas the converse was true of the aminoglycoside antibiotic streptomycin. Moreover, Eagle realized the implications of these observations for patients. He noted that, for penicillin, continuous infusion was the best way to achieve the most rapid cure while sparing patients excess drug-related toxicities and that, for antibiotics like streptomycin, intermittent bolus dose regimens that resulted in high peak concentrations were likely to be the most rapidly effective. These principles remain at the heart of effective antibiotic usage.

## Predictors of optimal antimicrobial activity

Antimicrobial agents can be categorized on the basis of the PK-PD measure that is most predictive of efficacy (see Table 14.3). The three most common PK-PD measures are the duration of time a drug concentration remains above the MIC (T > MIC), the ratio of the maximal drug concentration to the MIC ($C_{max}$:MIC), and the ratio of the area under the concentration–time curve at 24 hours to the MIC ($AUC_{0-24}$:MIC).

## Postantibiotic effects

Some antibiotics continue to suppress microorganism replication even after their concentrations have fallen well below the expected MIC. These postantibiotic effects are defined as the time period beginning after organisms are exposed to an antibiotic until the survivors begin to multiply to a significant degree. This phenomenon was first recognized in the 1940s for penicillin against staphylococci, and moderate-to-long postantibiotic effects are the rule rather than the exception when using β-lactams for Gram-positive bacteria like staphylococci. However, for Gram-negative bacteria, a significant postantibiotic effect is primarily observed with agents that inhibit protein or nucleic acid synthesis, such as aminoglycosides, macrolides, and quinolones. β-Lactams have little postantibiotic effect against Gram-negative bacteria.

**Table 14.3** Pharmacokinetic-pharmacodynamic measures of optimal effectiveness for the common classes of antibiotics.[a]

| Antibiotic class | Best PK-PD measure of activity | Summary of optimal killing activity |
|---|---|---|
| Aminoglycosides | $AUC_{0-24}$: MIC and $C_{max}$:MIC | Concentration dependent |
| β-Lactam antibiotics | T > MIC | Time dependent |
| Glycopeptides | $AUC_{0-24}$: MIC | Concentration dependent |
| Macrolides | $AUC_{0-24}$: MIC | Time dependent |
| Quinolones | $AUC_{0-24}$: MIC and $C_{max}$:MIC | Concentration dependent |
| Tetracyclines | $AUC_{0-24}$: MIC | Mixed time and concentration dependent |
| Metronidazole | $AUC_{0-24}$: MIC and $C_{max}$:MIC | Concentration dependent |

[a] $AUC_{0-24}$:MIC, ratio of the area under the concentration–time curve at 24 hours to the minimum inhibitory concentration; $C_{max}$:MIC, ratio of the maximal drug concentration to the minimum inhibitory concentration; PK-PD, pharmacokinetic-pharmacodynamic; T > MIC, duration of time a drug concentration remains above the minimum inhibitory concentration.

## Relevance of animal models

Much of antibiotic PK-PD data comes from animal models of infection. These experiments typically identify the magnitude of the PK-PD measure necessary for bactericidal efficacy but the data can also be used to guide the optimal dose and dosing interval selection for human clinical trials. When available, patient population exposure–response analyses serve as the ultimate arbiter of dose regimen justification. However, there is much to be learned by comparing predictions made by animal models to PK-PD analyses of human data, because the knowledge gained allows us to improve our ability to make the best translations from animal models to man.

## PK-PD and antibiotic resistance

Antibiotic resistance poses an ever-increasing threat to public health. Animal PK-PD infection models can be used to study the relationship between antibiotic concentrations and the selection of resistant organisms. Measures of antibiotic exposure can be identified that prevent the amplification of resistant subpopulations of bacteria; these thresholds are larger than those associated with clinical efficacy, and bacterial load at the primary effect site is usually critical. The larger the numbers of bacteria, the more likely it is that a resistant mutant will occur. These studies can therefore be used to identify the conditions where resistance emergence is minimized and help clinicians select dosing regimens which are least likely to result in resistance and treatment failure.

## Key points

- ◆ Pharmacokinetics is the study of an antibiotic's concentration within the body over time and is dependent upon its absorption, distribution, metabolism, and elimination. These parameters can change in sick patients, complicating antibiotic administration and making the safe and efficacious use of antibiotics a considerable clinical challenge.

- ◆ Pharmacodynamics is the study of the relationship between antibiotic concentrations (pharmacokinetics) and microorganism killing and clinical effect. It varies by antibiotic and the type and site of infection.

- ◆ A report that a pathogen is susceptible to an antibiotic in a laboratory does not assure treatment success. Predicting treatment success requires knowledge of the likely antibiotic concentrations at the site of infection, and the dosing regimen most likely to achieve the required concentrations to eliminate the infection.

- ◆ Study of the antibiotic dose–concentration response relationship can also be used to predict and prevent the emergence of drug resistant organisms.

## Further reading

Ambrose, P. G., Bhavnani, S. M., Rubino, C. M., Louie, A., Gumbo, T., Forrest, A., and Drusano, G. L. (2007) Pharmacokinetics–pharmacodynamics of antimicrobial therapy: it's not just for mice anymore. *Clinical Infectious Diseases*, **44**(1): 79–86.

Craig, W. A. (1998) Pharmacokinetic/pharmacodynamic parameters: rationale for antibacterial dosing of mice and men. *Clinical Infectious Diseases*, **26**(1): 1–10.

# Chapter 15

# Prescribing in special groups: effects of age, pregnancy, body weight, and hepatic and renal impairment

## Effects of age

The evaluation of new drugs in children and elderly people presents particular problems and is extremely important, since the pharmacological handling of the drugs and their unwanted effects may differ considerably in infants, young children, old people, and normal adults.

## Paediatric prescribing

When selecting antimicrobial therapy, knowledge of age-related infections is important in the initial management, before laboratory information is available. Many infections, although not entirely peculiar to infancy and childhood, are none the less much more frequently encountered in this age group, reflecting the susceptibility of a relatively non-immune population. Neonatal meningitis is primarily caused by group B streptococci and *Escherichia coli*. Meningococcal infection is a disease of early childhood and young adulthood.

Upper respiratory tract infections are extremely common in childhood. Many are caused by viruses but infection is often complicated by secondary bacterial invasion with *Streptococcus pneumoniae* or *Haemophilus influenzae*.

Cystic fibrosis is a disease that generally first becomes manifest in children and, through careful management, many sufferers survive into adult life. A major complication of this disease is recurrent lower respiratory tract infection in which *Staphylococcus aureus* and *Pseudomonas* spp. predominate. Such infections are difficult to control and it is often impossible to eliminate *Pseudomonas* completely from the sputum.

## Pharmacokinetics in children

In childhood, pharmacokinetic and pharmacodynamic factors often differ markedly from those in the adult (see Table 15.1). To arrive at a safe yet effective concentration of a drug is not without difficulties. In fact, for many drugs the dosage regimens have not been accurately determined for every indication. In the case of new antimicrobial agents, until recently pharmacological and toxicological investigations were more commonly carried out in an adult population, so that information in children and particularly in infants and neonates is often extremely limited. To derive the necessary information in childhood requires painstaking and careful observations in sick children, since pharmacokinetic information is not available from healthy children for ethical reasons. Lack of such information may preclude the widespread use of a potentially useful agent in childhood. Recent regulatory changes now actively encourage evaluation in childhood during drug development.

**Table 15.1** Pharmacokinetic differences between paediatric patients and adults.

| | Preterm | Neonate (0–4 weeks) | Infant (<1 year) | Early childhood (1–6 years) |
|---|---|---|---|---|
| Absorption | Slightly reduced | No difference | No difference | No difference |
| **Distribution** | | | | |
| Body water | Greatly increased | Moderately increased | Slightly increased | Slightly increased |
| Body fat | Moderately reduced | Slightly reduced | Slightly reduced | No difference |
| Plasma albumin | Reduced | Reduced | Slightly reduced | No difference |
| **Excretion (renal)** | | | | |
| Glomerular filtration | Moderately reduced | Slightly reduced | Slightly reduced[a] | No difference |
| Tubular secretion | Moderately reduced | Slightly reduced | Slightly reduced[a] | No difference |

[a] First 6 months of life.

Paediatric prescribing recognizes the fact that growth and development, including organ function and metabolism, change in childhood. This is particularly so for the neonatal period, in which chronological age, gestational age, and body weight are all important considerations.

In the neonate and especially the preterm newborn, renal function is less efficient than in the older child, since glomerular and tubular functions continue to mature. The creatinine clearance rate in the neonate is approximately one-third that of the older child. However, most infants achieve an adult glomerular filtration rate between 6 to 12 months of age. Hence, drugs excreted by the kidneys may require dose modification if toxicity is to be avoided.

Kidney function is not the only consideration. The volume of distribution of antibiotics is important in determining the dose that is necessary to achieve a therapeutic concentration at the site of infection. Agents such as the aminoglycosides, which are essentially confined to the extracellular fluid compartment, are affected by the proportionally larger extracellular fluid volume in the preterm and full term neonate compared with the older child and adult. The extracellular fluid volume is approximately 45 per cent of the body weight in the newborn. Parenteral antimicrobial dosing regimens in the *BNF for Children* recommend longer dosing intervals for neonates versus older children.

## Compliance in children

Of particular importance in paediatric prescribing is the acceptability of the medication to the patient. The need to make preparations palatable with syrup and flavourings is important if compliance is to be observed. Children generally find tablet and capsule preparations difficult to swallow—hence the popularity of flavoured syrup suspensions. In addition to palatability, compliance is increased by making the prescribing instructions clear and least disruptive to the normal daily routine. Unnecessary disturbance of sleep patterns is a sure way to reduce compliance.

An important aspect of all prescribing, particularly with paediatric formulations, which may be attractively coloured and sweet-tasting, is the need to warn parents that any residual medication should be discarded. Drugs should not be stored in anticipation of using them for a future infection. The shelf-life of antibiotics is limited, and prolonged storage is associated with loss of potency.

## Prescribing in older people

As with most therapeutic agents, use of antibiotics is greatest in old age. Infection is an important cause of morbidity and mortality in elderly people. Infections of the respiratory tract, urinary tract, and skin structures all become more common with increasing age. This increase in risk of common infections is largely due to an increase in the number of co-morbidities: more than 10 per cent of people aged 85 or more have 6 or more long-term conditions (Fig. 15.1).

## Pharmacokinetic and pharmacodynamic changes in older people

Elderly people are the least homogeneous population in relation to drug prescribing. Multiple long-term conditions (Fig. 15.1) are accompanied by an age-related decline in renal function. Consequently, while the average half-life of drugs increases with age, there is also increasing variability between individuals.

## Adverse drug reactions in older people

Unwanted effects of drugs are more common in older people. While some are idiosyncratic, most are dose related. However, the risk of some idiosyncratic reactions does increase with age. An example is the increased frequency and severity in older people of serious adverse reactions to co-trimoxazole (e.g. Stevens–Johnson syndrome, with extensive skin and mucous membrane ulceration and major blood dyscrasias).

Although age-related reduction in elimination of drugs plays a part, polypharmacy is an important cause of adverse drug reactions in older people. The relationship between risk of

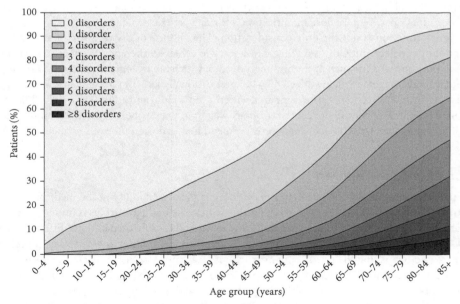

**Fig. 15.1** Number of chronic disorders by age in 2007 in Scotland.

Reprinted from *The Lancet*, Volume 380, Issue 9836, Barnett K et al., Epidemiology of multimorbidity and implications for health care, research, and medical education: a cross-sectional study, pp. 37–43, Copyright © 2012, with permission from Elsevier, http://www.sciencedirect.com/science/journal/01406736

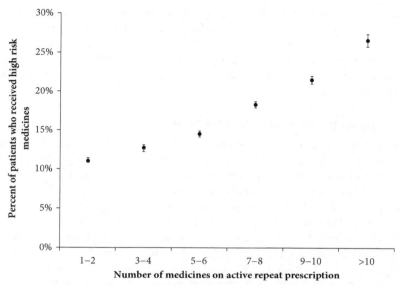

**Fig. 15.2** Percent of patients (with 95% confidence interval) who received high-risk medicines in Scotland in 2007, by the number of medicines on active repeat prescription at the end of the study period. Indicators of high-risk prescribing were required to be ones where the prescribing being measured was clearly stated to be contraindicated or to be avoided in routine practice, either in the *British National Formulary*, 15 national clinical guidelines, prescribing advice, or safety alerts. For every indicator examined, there was explicit guidance at the time of prescription that it carried significant risk of harm and should be routinely avoided, usually on the basis of clear evidence that such prescribing carried a significantly increased risk to patients.

Source: data from Guthrie B et al., High risk prescribing in primary care patients particularly vulnerable to adverse drug events: cross sectional population database analysis in Scottish general practice, *British Medical Journal*, Volume 342, Copyright © 2011, DOI: http://dx.doi.org/10.1136/bmj.d3514

adverse drug reactions and the number of medicines taken is non-linear because the risk of taking high-risk medicines also increases exponentially with the number of medicines taken (Fig. 15.2). The prevalence of patients taking more than five medicines doubled in the United Kingdom between 1995 and 2010 and is now more than 20 per cent, with most of this increase being in people aged 65 or more. At the same time, the number of older people is rising in most countries. In the United Kingdom the number of people aged 85 or more is likely to double to about 3.5 million by 2035.

Poor compliance with medication may be the result of cognitive or visual impairment. Compliance with complex regimens can be assisted by daily 'dosette' containers and supported by written instructions for the patient or carer. Much can be done to mitigate the present high rate of adverse effects of medication.

# Prescribing in pregnancy

Drugs, including antibiotics, are frequently prescribed to pregnant women. Antimicrobial agents are most commonly prescribed in pregnancy for maternal urinary and respiratory tract infections. They may also be prescribed to treat intrauterine infections such as amnionitis.

Pregnancy frequently alters the pharmacokinetic handling of drugs, including anti-infective agents. Plasma concentrations of ampicillin are 50 per cent of those observed in the non-pregnant state, as a result of increased plasma clearance. The same applies to many cephalosporins.

Any decision to prescribe drugs during pregnancy, including antibiotics, should only be taken after careful assessment of the risks and benefits, in order to avoid unnecessary exposure of the developing foetus.

## Placental passage of antimicrobial agents

The placenta is not only an important defence against foetal infection but also largely determines the concentration of a drug in foetal tissues. The transplacental passage of drugs may be by simple diffusion or by an active transport system. As in other membrane situations, molecular weight, protein binding, ionizability, lipid solubility, and blood flow are all important considerations. In addition, the placenta is able to metabolize drugs through oxidation, conjugation, reduction, and hydrolysis. Drugs of low molecular weight (<1 kDa) tend to cross readily.

Antimicrobial agents that achieve good concentrations in foetal tissues include ampicillin, penicillin G, sulphonamides, metronidazole, and nitrofurantoin. The aminoglycosides cross moderately well and have occasionally been associated with foetal ototoxicity. The cephalosporins and clindamycin cross less readily, and erythromycin is particularly poor in this respect.

The general caution restricting all unnecessary prescribing in pregnancy, in particular during the first three months, when organogenesis is maximal, also applies to antimicrobial drugs. For example, the antifolate properties of trimethoprim and the sulphonamides carry a theoretical risk of inducing foetal abnormalities. However, of more importance is the complication of hyperbilirubinaemia that can result should sulphonamides be prescribed in the latter few weeks of pregnancy or during the neonatal period. Displacement of protein-bound bilirubin by sulphonamide may result in toxic concentrations of bilirubin in the basal ganglia of the brain, with the resultant risk of kernicterus.

## Excretion of antimicrobial agents into breast milk

In common with other drugs, antimicrobial agents can enter human breast milk and therefore may potentially affect the suckling infant.

The secretory process may either be active or passive, and the final concentration is determined by factors such as molecular weight, lipid or water solubility, the degree of protein binding, and, of course, maternal serum concentrations. Breast milk has a neutral pH, which will affect the ionization of drugs.

Few antimicrobial drugs pass readily into breast milk to achieve concentrations similar to those in maternal blood. However, isoniazid and some sulphonamides do so. Tetracyclines achieve moderate concentrations and could possibly cause discoloration of primary dentition and enamel hypoplasia; hence, they are contraindicated in early childhood. Erythromycin is found in concentrations approximately half those present in maternal blood. Metronidazole achieves concentrations comparable with maternal serum levels. The penicillins and cephalosporins are generally poorly excreted into human breast milk.

In general, such concentrations are of more theoretical than of practical significance. There have been occasional reports of dapsone- and nalidixic-acid-associated drug toxicity in children with glucose-6-phosphate dehydrogenase deficiency. Disturbance of the bowel flora has been reported with ampicillin; use of clindamycin has resulted in bloody diarrhoea. Before prescribing, the benefit-to-risk ratio must be considered for both mother and infant. Infants who are exposed to antibacterials via drug monitoring should be monitored for unusual signs or symptoms. However, under most circumstances, the short-term administration of antimicrobial agents to lactating mothers need not interfere with breast feeding.

## Prescribing in obesity

The prevalence of obesity in the western world is increasing, particularly in the United Kingdom and United States, where the prevalence in 2009 was 25 per cent and 30 per cent, respectively. Obesity is associated with impaired vascular supply to soft tissues and diminished respiratory reserve function, which predispose to soft-tissue and lower respiratory tract infections, respectively. Despite the growing prevalence of obesity, there is little general guidance about whether or how doses of antimicrobials should be adjusted in clinical practice. Regulatory rules for new antimicrobial drug development require special pharmacokinetic studies in children, elderly people, and patients with renal or hepatic impairment but not for individuals with obesity. As a result, this group is generally under-represented in drug development studies, and few antimicrobial product information sheets provide advice about obesity. Nonetheless, in recent years there have been an increasing number of studies of pharmacokinetics of specific antibacterials in obese adults, so a literature search may be appropriate if there is a clinical problem with a particular drug and no guidance is found in standard textbooks.

The size descriptors that are most commonly used for drug dose adjustment are total body weight, lean body weight, and ideal body weight. Drugs are either hydrophilic or lipophilic (Table 15.2). Hydrophilic drugs distribute mainly in extracellular fluid and do not distribute into fat, whereas lipophilic drugs cross lipid membranes into cells and do distribute into fat. However, about 30 per cent of adipose tissue is water, and hydrophilic drugs vary in their ability to distribute into adipose tissue.

Clearance ($CL$) and volume of distribution ($V$) are the two pharmacokinetic parameters that are most influenced by body size. The available studies do have some consistent findings:

1  Total body weight is the best descriptor of $V$ for most lipophilic drugs. However, not all lipophilic drugs distribute throughout adipose tissue, and some hydrophilic ones do distribute into the water within adipose tissue.

**Table 15.2** Classification of antibacterial drugs as hydrophilic or lipophilic.

| Hydrophilic | Lipophilic |
| --- | --- |
| β-lactams: | Fluoroquinolones |
| • penicillins | Macrolides |
| • cephalosporins | Lincosamides (e.g. clindamycin) |
| • monobactams | Tetracyclines |
| • carbapenem | Tigecycline |
| Glycopeptides | Co-trimoxazole |
| Aminoglycosides | Rifampicin |
| Polymyxins | Chloramphenicol |
| Fosfomycin | |

2 In contrast, *CL* is better correlated to lean body weight than to total body weight. Total body weight greatly overestimates renal function in obese patients. However, since obese patients have slightly increased renal function, ideal body weight underestimates *CL* for most drugs.

3 For drugs that are dosed chronically, *CL* is of primary concern, because failure to estimate *CL* accurately can lead to underdosing or to accumulation. However, for the initial therapy of acute infections, it is important to fill *V* quickly.

The combination of these three factors means that there are no simple dosing rules that fit all hydrophilic or all lipophilic drugs. Moreover the recommended method for calculating lean body weight (LBW 2005) uses a formula that is based on the non-linear relationship between height and total body weight. The available evidence only provides guidance about some drugs (Table 15.3). There are major gaps in information, such as for co-trimoxazole, which is increasingly administered intravenously for the empirical treatment of acute infections in hospital. Drug dosing in the obese patient population remains an inexact science, and more data are needed in this patient population to effectively treat infections. Clinicians managing patients with severe sepsis must be aware of the importance of obesity. Initial doses should be based on total body weight in order to minimize the risk of underdosing. However, advice on maintenance dosing should be sought on calculation of maintenance doses based on lean body weight.

**Table 15.3** Recommendations for dosing in obesity.

| Agent | Suggested dosing weight[a] | Additional dosing recommendations |
|---|---|---|
| **Antibacterial agents** | | |
| Aminoglycosides | IBW | Consider capping dose e.g. at 640 mg for 7 mg/kg; use therapeutic drug monitoring[b] |
| β-Lactam drugs | TBW | Consider using maximum unit dose and dosing more frequently or via continuous infusion |
| Ciprofloxacin | Adjusted body weight (IBW+0.45)×(TBW−IBW) | No data for levofloxacin |
| Clindamycin | Unknown | No data but up to 1200 mg 6 hourly has been used |
| Daptomycin | TBW | Consider reducing final dose by 25% |
| Doxycycline | Unknown | No data |
| Erythromycin | Unknown | No data but up to 6 g/day has been used |
| Glycopeptides | | |
| Vancomycin | TBW | A more frequent dosing interval may be required; use therapeutic drug monitoring |
| Teicoplanin | Unknown | No data[c] |
| Linezolid | Standard dosing | No dose adjustment recommended |

**Table 15.3** (continued).

| Agent | Suggested dosing weight[a] | Additional dosing recommendations |
|---|---|---|
| Metronidazole | Unknown | No data but up to 1 g 6 hourly has been used |
| Sulphamethoxazole–trimethoprim | Unknown | No data but high doses are used routinely for treatment of pneumocystis pneumonia |
| **Antifungal agents** | | |
| Amphotericin B, conventional | TBW | |
| Amphotericin B, lipid preps | IBW | |
| Echinocandins | Unknown | No data |
| Fluconazole | Unknown | Consider higher doses |
| **Antiviral agents** | | |
| Aciclovir | IBW | |
| Cidofovir | Unknown | No data |
| Ganciclovir | Unknown | No data |
| **Calculation of IBW** | | |
| IBW (in kg) | Women: 45.5 kg + 2.3 × (inches over 5 feet)<br><br>Men: 50 kg + 2.3 × (inches over 5 feet) | |

[a] IBW, ideal body weight; TBW, total body weight.

[b] Pai MP et al., Simplified estimation of aminoglycoside pharmacokinetics in underweight and obese adult patients, *Antimicrobial Agents and Chemotherapy*, Volume 55, Issue 9, pp. 4006–11, Copyright © 2011 by the American Society for Microbiology.

[c] Grace E, Altered vancomycin pharmacokinetics in obese and morbidly obese patients: what we have learned over the past 30 years, Journal of Antimicrobial Chemotherapy, Volume 67, Issue 6, pp. 1305–10, Copyright © 2012 by the American Society for Microbiology.

Adapted with permission from Dodds Ashley E., Optimal antibiotic dosing for obese patients a challenge for clinicians, *Infectious Diseases News*, June 2007, Copyright © Healio 2007, available from http://www.healio.com/infectious-disease/news/print/infectious-disease-news/%7Ba0b8d0cb-6d3c-4c3d-b2ce-3d45dcd0bb58%7D/optimal-antibiotic-dosing-for-obese-patients-a-challenge-for-clinicians. Source: data from Janson B, and Thursky K, Dosing of antibiotics in obesity, *Current Opinion in Infectious Disease*, Volume 25, Issue 6, pp. 634–49, Copyright © 2012.

# Prescribing in renal impairment

The use of drugs in patients with reduced renal function can give rise to problems for several reasons:

- reduced renal excretion of a drug or its metabolites may cause toxicity;
- sensitivity to some drugs is increased even if elimination is unimpaired;
- many side effects are tolerated poorly by patients with renal impairment; and
- some drugs are not effective when renal function is reduced.

For many drugs with only minor or no dose-related side effects, very precise modification of the dose regimen is unnecessary, and a simple scheme for dose reduction is sufficient. However, when both efficacy and toxicity are closely related to plasma drug concentration (e.g. for gentamicin treatment of sepsis), recommended regimens should be regarded only as a guide to initial treatment; subsequent doses must be adjusted according to clinical response and serum drug concentration.

The total daily maintenance dose of a drug can be reduced either by reducing the size of the individual doses or by increasing the interval between doses. For some drugs, although the size of the maintenance dose is reduced, it is important to give a loading dose if an immediate effect is required. This is because it takes regular dosing about five times the elimination half-life of the drug to achieve steady-state plasma concentrations. Because the plasma half-life of drugs excreted by the kidney is prolonged in renal impairment, it can take many doses for the reduced dosage to achieve therapeutic plasma concentrations. The loading dose should usually be the same size as the initial dose for a patient with normal renal function.

Many clinical chemistry laboratories now report estimated glomerular filtration rate (eGFR), which is calculated from a formula that uses serum creatinine, age, sex, and race (for Afro-Caribbean patients) and is standardized for a body surface area of 1.73 m². Consequently, eGFR can be inaccurate at both extremes of weight (total body weight <40 kg or >90 kg). In these patients and in patients who are receiving drugs with narrow therapeutic index to treat severe infections, it is preferable to calculate creatinine clearance with the Cockcroft–Gault formula (Table 15.4)

Note that ideal body weight is often used in the Cockcroft–Gault formula because of concerns that using the total body weight of an obese patient in this formula would substantially overestimate glomerular filtration rate. However, the glomerular filtration rate is often increased in obese patients, so the Cockcroft–Gault formula may underestimate renal function in these patients. Conversely, frail elderly patients and some patients with cancer produce very little creatinine, so the Cockcroft–Gault formula overestimates renal function in these patients. This emphasizes the need to use therapeutic drug monitoring to check drug dosing in critically ill obese patients.

## Prescribing in liver disease

There is genetic variability in enzyme function, and neonates or infants have immature enzyme systems, both of which factors can be clinically important (see Chapter 17). Liver disease can influence the clearance of drugs that are metabolized and, in severe liver disease, hypoprotenaemia

**Table 15.4** Cockcroft–Gault formula for estimation of creatinine clearance from serum creatinine.

$$\text{Estimated creatinine clearance in ml/minute} = \frac{(140 - \text{Age}) \times \text{Weight} \times \text{Constant}}{\text{Serum creatinine}}$$

Age in years

Weight in kilograms; **NB use ideal body weight**

Serum creatinine in micromoles/litre

Constant = 1.23 for men; 1.04 for women

can also change clearance and distribution. However, unlike with renal impairment, there is no practical method for assessing hepatic function for dose adjustment. More importantly, all drugs should be used with extreme caution in patients with liver disease because of the dangers of fluid overload, impairment of cerebral function in patients with borderline hepatic encephalopathy, and haemorrhage in patients with reduced clotting.

## Conclusion

The principles of antimicrobial prescribing are common to all patients but greater attention to issues of drug distribution, excretion, and potential for adverse reactions is necessary in patients at the extremes of age and weight, during pregnancy, or with impaired renal or hepatic function. The burden of infection falls most heavily on the very young, the very old, and those with co-morbidities, so antibiotic prescribing is correspondingly more common in these patient groups. In the treatment of infection in these special groups, it is essential to choose the safest and most effective agent and to use it in appropriate dosage for the shortest time necessary.

## Key points

- Immaturity, ageing, and renal or hepatic impairment alter the pharmacokinetics of drug handling and increase the risks of drug toxicity.
- Dosing of antimicrobials in obesity is complex. Initial doses for severe infections should be based on total body weight, to avoid underdosing. However, maintenance doses should be recalculated based on lean body weight to minimize risk of accumulation.
- Collectively, patients in these special groups are the target of most antibiotic prescribing. Obesity is increasingly common and increases the risk of bacterial infections. In some populations, obese patients already account for up to 40 per cent of all patients treated with antibacterial drugs.
- For most drugs, dose adjustment is necessary in these special groups, and advice should be sought about therapeutic drug monitoring for critically ill patients and for patients who require long-term treatment with drugs that have a low therapeutic index.

## Further reading

### Children

Paediatric Formulary Committee. (2014) *BNF for Children*. London: Pharmaceutical Press.

Remington, J. S., Klein, J. O., Wilson, C. B., Nizet, V., and Maldonado, Y. (2011) *Infectious Diseases of the Fetus and Newborn Infant* (7th edn). Philadelphia, PA: Saunders.

### Older people

Barnett, K., Mercer, S. W., Norbury, M., Watt, G., Wyke, S., and Guthrie, B. (2012) Epidemiology of multimorbidity and implications for health care, research, and medical education: a cross-sectional study. *Lancet*, **380**(9836): 37–43.

Duerden, M., Avery, T., and Payne, R. (2013) *Polypharmacy and medicines optimisation. Making it safe and sound*. London, The King's Fund.

Guthrie, B., McCowan, C., Davey, P., Simpson, C. R., Dreischulte, T., and Barnett, K. (2011) High risk prescribing in primary care patients particularly vulnerable to adverse drug events: cross sectional population database analysis in Scottish general practice. *BMJ*, **342**: d3514.

Scottish Antimicrobial Prescribing Group. (2013) *Good Practice Recommendations for Antimicrobial Use in Frail Elderly Patients in NHS Scotland.* <http://www.scottishmedicines.org.uk/files/sapg/SAPG_Recommendations_for_antibiotic_use_in_frail_elderly_-_February_2013.pdf>, accessed 26 November 2014.

## Obesity

Dodds Ashley, E. (2007) *Optimal Antibiotic Dosing for Obese Patients: A Challenge for Clinicians.* <http://www.healio.com/infectious-disease/news/print/infectious-disease-news/%7Ba0b8d0cb-6d3c-4c3d-b2ce-3d45dcd0bb58%7D/optimal-antibiotic-dosing-for-obese-patients-a-challenge-for-clinicians>, accessed 26 November 2014.

Falagas, M. E. and Karageorgopoulos, D. E. (2010) Adjustment of dosing of antimicrobial agents for body-weight in adults. *Lancet*, **375**(9710):248–51.

Green, B. and Duffull, S. B. (2004) What is the best size descriptor to use for pharmacokinetic studies in the obese? *British Journal of Clinical Pharmacology*, **58**(2): 119–33.

## Formula for calculating LBW 2005

Han, P.Y., Duffull, S.B., Kirkpatrick, C.M., and Green, B. (2007) Dosing in obesity: a simple solution to a big problem. *Clinical Pharmacology and Therapeutics*, **82**(5):505–8.

Janson, B. and Thursky, K. (2012) Dosing of antibiotics in obesity. *Current Opinion in Infectious Diseases*, **25**(6):634–49.

Pai, M. P. and Bearden, D.T. (2007) Antimicrobial dosing considerations in obese adult patients. *Pharmacotherapy: The Journal of Human Pharmacology and Drug Therapy*, **27**(8):1081–91.

## Renal and hepatic impairment

Joint Formulary Committee. (2014) *British National Formulary* (68th edn). London: Pharmaceutical Press.

# Chapter 16

# OPAT: outpatient parenteral antimicrobial therapy

## Introduction to OPAT

Outside hospitals antibiotics are generally administered by the oral route. However, over the past 20 years there has been increasing development of services for the administration of intravenous (IV) antibiotics to patients in the community. Various terms have been used to describe this, including community-based parenteral anti-infective therapy, hospital in the home therapy and non-inpatient parenteral antimicrobial therapy. However, OPAT is the term most commonly used (see <http://www.e-opat.com/>).

In the United States over 250,000 patients receive OPAT annually. Establishment of OPAT has been slower in other countries, probably because of differences in health-care financing. In the United States hospitals are reimbursed for each patient treated, so there is a clear financial incentive to treat as many patients as possible and to minimize the duration of hospitalization. In contrast, in most other countries hospitals are reimbursed for delivering treatment to populations and geographic regions. However, OPAT is becoming increasingly common in Australia and Europe.

## Indications for OPAT and patient selection

OPAT was first developed for children with cystic fibrosis, and who consequently had recurrent pulmonary infections, and subsequently for adult patients with osteomyelitis. Initially, carers or patients were trained to administer parenteral antibiotics at home but increasingly services were developed for parenteral administration by health professionals, either in patients' homes or in outpatient clinics. Bone and joint infection, which requires prolonged parenteral therapy, is still the commonest indication for OPAT in the United Kingdom (Fig. 16.1). However, short-term OPAT treatment for skin and soft-tissue, urinary tract, or respiratory infections is increasingly common (Fig. 16.1).

The most important determinants of suitability for OPAT therapy are the patient and their carers (Box 16.1). Patients must be clinically stable and have home circumstances that support OPAT, including effective communication with health-care professionals. Consequently, although pneumonia is the commonest indication for parenteral antibiotics in hospital, it is not among the commonest indications for OPAT (Fig. 16.1), because most patients with pneumonia require other support from hospitals during the time that they need parenteral therapy. In contrast, many patients with skin and soft-tissue infection are suitable for OPAT (Fig. 16.1).

## OPAT team and service structure

The first requirement for OPAT is a multidisciplinary team capable of delivering the treatment and all the necessary support services (Table 16.1). In addition to a clinical database, the development

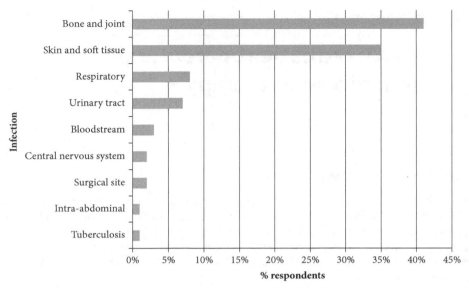

**Fig. 16.1** Most common indication for OPAT from a survey of 193 NHS Trusts and Health Boards in England, Northern Ireland, Scotland, and Wales, in 2013.

Source: data reproduced with kind permission of British Society for Antimicrobial Chemotherapy UK, Outpatient Parenteral Antimicrobial Therapy Initiative Landscape Survey 2013.

---

## Box 16.1 Components of good clinical practice for OPAT

1 Patient selection

   1.1 No clinical contraindications to discharge from hospital.

   1.2 Appropriate home environment with adequate support.

   1.3 Patients and carers are fully aware of the benefits and risks of OPAT.

   1.4 Patients and carers are clearly given the opportunity to decline OPAT.

   1.5 Patients and carers are willing and able to comply with the follow-up plan.

2 OPAT team structure

   2.1 The OPAT team should have clear managerial and clinical governance lines of responsibility.

   2.2 The OPAT team should have an identifiable, medically qualified lead clinician who has identified time for OPAT in his/her job plan.

   2.3 Selection of patients for OPAT should be made by a medically qualified infection specialist.

   2.4 There should be a written, multidisciplinary care plan with clear lines of responsibility between the referring team, the OPAT team, and the community care teams. This care plan should be available and accessible to all relevant members of the clinical team at all times, including out of hours.

**Box 16.1 Components of good clinical practice for OPAT** *(continued)*

3 Antimicrobial management and drug delivery

3.1 The OPAT team must ensure correct and continued prescription of antimicrobials throughout OPAT, although prescriptions may be written by the referring team under the direction of the OPAT team.

3.2 Storage, reconstitution, and administration of antimicrobials must comply with published standards.

3.3 Insertion and care of intravascular devices must comply with local and national standards.

3.4 Training of patients or carers should comply with national standards, and evidence of competence should be documented.

3.5 All administered doses of IV antimicrobial therapy should be documented.

3.6 The first dose of a new antimicrobial should be administered in a supervised setting.

4 Monitoring of the patient during OPAT

4.1 Patients with skin and soft-tissue infection should be monitored daily by the OPAT team to ensure timely switch to oral therapy.

4.2 Weekly multidisciplinary meetings should be held to review progress of all patients on OPAT.

4.3 Patients receiving in excess of one week of OPAT should have a plan for regular review and blood tests (weekly for the first month, and at least every two weeks thereafter).

4.4 The OPAT team is responsible for monitoring clinical response and results of blood tests.

4.5 The OPAT team is responsible for providing a mechanism for 24 hour immediate access to advice and urgent review of OPAT patients.

5 Outcome measurement

5.1 Patient satisfaction and patient experience surveys

5.2 Drug-related and vascular-access adverse events (Fig. 16.2)

5.3 Readmissions to hospital

5.4 Audit with evidence of the impact of programme improvements

Adapted from Chapman AL et al., Good practice recommendations for outpatient parenteral antimicrobial therapy (OPAT) in adults in the UK: a consensus statement, *Journal of Antimicrobial Chemotherapy*, Volume 67, Issue 5, pp. 1053–1062, Copyright © 2013. Source: data from Muldoon EG et al, Are we ready for an outpatient parenteral antimicrobial therapy bundle? A critical appraisal of the evidence, *Clinical Infectious Disease*, Volume 57, Issue 3, pp. 419–424, Copyright © 2013.

of OPAT services requires a strong business case to ensure the necessary support services (see <http://www.e-opat.com/>). This is particularly important for hospitals that are not reimbursed on a per-patient basis. In these systems, reducing length of hospital stay does not necessarily increase hospital income or reduce operational costs. It is more important to emphasize the benefits to patients, which include reduction in risk of health-care associated infections, particularly

**Table 16.1** Information about OPAT services from a survey of 193 NHS Trusts and Health Boards in England, Northern Ireland, Scotland, and Wales, in 2013.

|  | Respondents (%) |
|---|---|
| **OPAT delivered by a multidisciplinary team** | 72 |
| **Specialty of deliverers of OPAT** | |
| Specialist nurse | 22 |
| Clinical microbiologist | 20 |
| Antimicrobial pharmacist | 19 |
| Infectious disease physician | 11 |
| Physician not specializing in infectious disease or acute medicine | 10 |
| Acute medicine physician | 9 |
| Business manager/project lead | 4 |
| Emergency medicine consultant | 3 |
| Surgeon | 2 |
| **Model of care** | |
| Ambulatory care centre | 29 (NHS: 23; private: 6) |
| At home by a health-care professional | 42 (NHS: 34; private homecare: 8) |
| At home by the patient or carer | 16 |
| Multiple models used | 13 |
| **Number of patients treated per year** | |
| <50 | 10 |
| 50–99 | 23 |
| 100–199 | 43 |
| 200–299 | 16 |
| ≥300 | 8 |

Data reproduced with kind permission of British Society for Antimicrobial Chemotherapy UK, Outpatient Parenteral Antimicrobial Therapy Initiative Landscape Survey 2013.

*Clostridium difficile* infection. OPAT should be seen as the best standard of care and not simply a method for cost containment.

Although best practice recommendations in the United Kingdom and the United States emphasize the importance of a multidisciplinary OPAT team, a recent survey of UK hospitals showed that only 72 per cent could sustain a multidisciplinary OPAT team (Table 16.1). The survey also shows the increasing range of medical specialties that are involved with OPAT (Table 16.1)

There are three basic models of care: an ambulatory care centre, a nurse attending the patient's home, or self-administration by the patient or a carer. In the United Kingdom the majority of OPAT is delivered in the patient's home but 13 per cent of OPAT services use multiple models of care (Box 16.1). The private sector accounted for 14 per cent of care delivery in the United Kingdom in 2013 (Box 16.1).

## Antimicrobial management and drug delivery

The most suitable antibiotics are those that can be administered once daily or less frequently; consequently, teicoplanin, ceftriaxone, daptomycin, ertapenem, and teicoplanin are the commonest OPAT antibiotics in the United Kingdom (Fig. 16.2). Daptomycin is a lipopeptide antibacterial with a spectrum of activity similar to vancomycin. Ertapenem is a carbapenem with a spectrum of activity similar to imipenem (Chapter 2). Amikacin and gentamicin are also used by >10 per cent of OPAT centres, despite the need for therapeutic drug monitoring (Fig. 16.2). OPAT is rarely used to deliver antiviral drugs because most of them are available in oral formulations, and patients who require parenteral therapy usually have other clinical problems that require hospitalization. The antifungal drug caspofungin has been used for OPAT in patients with endocarditis. Piperacillin–tazobactam was the only penicillin used by >10 per cent of OPAT centres but a wide range of other β-lactams was used by 47 per cent of OPAT centres, despite the fact that these drugs require continuous infusion or administration at least three times daily (Fig. 16.2).

Standard peripheral IV cannulas are not suitable for most patients with OPAT because the cannulas must be changed every two to three days. Peripherally inserted central catheters (PICC) provide a more durable alternative that can be inserted or removed in the outpatient setting, and have a low infection rate. Because of their central positioning, such catheters are suitable for the administration of concentrated antibiotic solutions.

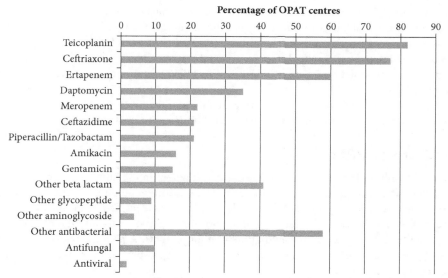

**Fig. 16.2** Drugs most commonly used for OPAT from a survey of 193 NHS Trusts and Health Boards in England, Northern Ireland, Scotland, and Wales, in 2013. Centres were asked to identify all drugs that they used. Nine drugs from three classes (β-lactams, glycopeptides, and aminoglycosides) were used by at least 10 per cent of centres. However, antibacterials from other classes were used by over 50 per cent of centres.

Source: data reproduced with kind permission of British Society for Antimicrobial Chemotherapy UK, Outpatient Parenteral Antimicrobial Therapy Initiative Landscape Survey 2013.

IV injection over 5–10 minutes is the most convenient method for administration of OPAT for patients and staff. IV infusion at home is technically possible through compact, battery-operated, computerized infusion pumps. However, these generally are expensive to purchase and can be difficult for patients to manage.

## Monitoring of the patient during OPAT

It is essential that there is clear communication with definition of responsibility for delivery of OPAT, and review of progress with treatment between the OPAT team, the referring clinical team, and teams in the community (Box 16.1). Although the home environment has many advantages for the patient, the careful regular monitoring that occurs in hospitals is not possible at home. Patients receiving OPAT need to be seen at least weekly for the first month, either in their home or in an outpatient setting (Box 16.1). Patients treated for skin/soft-tissue or other acute infections require daily review (Box 16.1). Specific factors to assess on review include response to therapy, evidence of drug adverse effects, and other complications such as infection related to the venous cannula. It is important that there are clear policies for monitoring of specific drugs. In addition to prevention of side effects, measurement of serum drug concentrations is used to ensure effective therapy. This is particularly important for achieving optimum dosing frequency. For example, with teicoplanin, most patients can maintain effective concentrations for treatment of bone and joint infections via three times' weekly administration. This is much more convenient than daily administration for patients and does not require weekend services for OPAT. However, it is critical to ensure that effective serum concentrations can be maintained.

Comparison of OPAT delivered by health-care professionals versus by the patient or a carer has not revealed significant differences in adverse effects (Fig. 16.3). Line-related complications were more common with self-administered OPAT but overall these were rare events (0.6% of 2,009 infections), so the difference was not statistically significant. Further evidence is required about the safety of patient-administered OPAT, including assessment of retention of competencies.

Serious adverse effects of OPAT are rare (Fig. 16.3); consequently, a register is required to provide aggregate safety data from multiple hospitals (<http://www.e-opat.com/>).

## The future of OPAT

There is currently wide variation across the United Kingdom in the number of patients treated with OPAT each year (Box 16.2), and the hospitals treating >300 patients annually include general hospitals as well as university hospitals. Funding was identified as the major barrier to extending OPAT services, and agreement of national or regional tariffs for OPAT would likely be required to facilitate realizing the full potential for patients. A national register of patients would also increase understanding of the reasons for current practice variation (see <http://www.e-opat.com/>).

OPAT needs to be seen as one example of a range of options for transferring patients from acute care into the community, and providers of OPAT should be aware of gaps in the evidence about cost-effectiveness of transferring care from hospitals into the community (Box 16.1). In particular, the need to develop a standardized approach towards documenting details of service provision and outcomes should inform the development of a register for OPAT patients (see <http://www.e-opat.com/>).

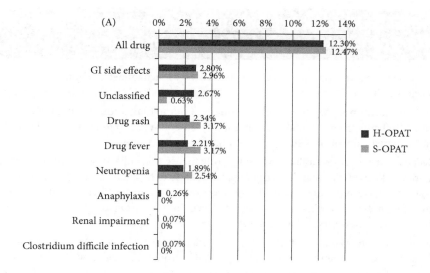

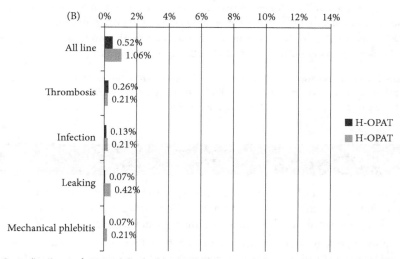

**Fig. 16.3** Complications of OPAT delivered by health-care professionals (H-OPAT; *n* = 1,536) versus self-administered by the patient (S-OPAT; *n* = 473). (A) Drug-associated complications. (B) Line-associated complications.

Data reproduced with kind permission of British Society for Antimicrobial Chemotherapy UK, Outpatient Parenteral Antimicrobial Therapy Initiative Landscape Survey 2013.

**Box 16.2 Selected key points from a review of evidence about shifting care from hospitals into the community.**

1  The effectiveness of community care solutions is very much influenced by the quality of those services rather than simply the setting (primary or secondary) in which they are provided.

2  Patients seem more satisfied with treatment at home than with hospital inpatient care. Early discharge from hospital into community-based care settings is associated with better patient satisfaction scores and equivalent quality-of-life scores.

3  Because existing research has not consistently focused on collecting robust financial data, there is little evidence that discharging patients early to hospital-at-home care delivers cost savings to the health-care system. The delivery of significant cost savings is likely to depend on inpatient services being decommissioned; yet, there is little evidence that commissioners do this once a new service has been set up.

4  Studies evaluating community-based care are often highly selective in terms of who is offered the service. Consequently, it is difficult to generalize from the available evidence as to whether community-based care would be as effective when used across a broader range of patients.

5  Developing a consistent framework for research and analysis, identifying key factors that can be monitored and evaluated across interventions and settings, would help to inform commissioning decisions. A consistent analytical framework for summarizing information would support the collection of comparable information that could show how to successfully implement systemic and strategic changes to service provision.

Reproduced with permission from Munton T et al, Getting out of hospital? The evidence for shifting acute inpatient and day case services from hospitals into the community, *Health Foundation*, Copyright © 2011, available from http://www.health.org.uk/publications/getting-out-of-hospital/

## Key points

♦ Over the past 20 years, there has been increasing development of services for administering IV antibiotics to patients in the community. This practice is most common in the United States but is now increasingly common in Australia and Europe.

♦ The most important determinants of suitability for OPAT are the patient and their carers. Patients must be capable of self-management and clinically stable. The commonest indications for OPAT are infections that require long or repeated courses of IV treatment and skin and soft-tissue infections.

♦ Patients must be supported by a multidisciplinary team capable of delivering the treatment and all the necessary support services.

♦ Standard peripheral IV cannulas are not suitable for most patients with OPAT, who usually require PICC. The most convenient antibiotics for OPAT are given once daily by short IV injection.

♦ Patients receiving OPAT need to have written care plans that include contacts for urgent advice or review that must be accessible at all times by all health professionals who are involved with the patient's care.

## Further reading

Chapman, A. L. (2013) Outpatient parenteral antimicrobial therapy. *BMJ*, **346**: f1585.

Chapman, A. L., Seaton, R.A., Cooper, M. A., Hedderwick, S., Goodall, V., Reed, C., Sanderson, F., and Nathwani, D. (2012) Good practice recommendations for outpatient parenteral antimicrobial therapy (OPAT) in adults in the UK: a consensus statement. *Journal of Antimicrobial Chemotherapy*, **67**(5):1053–62.

Eaves, K., Thornton, J., and Chapman, A. L. (2013) Patient retention of training in self-administration of intravenous antibiotic therapy in an outpatient parenteral antibiotic therapy service. *Journal of Clinical Nursing*, **23**(9–10), 1318–22.

Matthews, P. C., Conlon, C. P., Berendt, A. R., Kayley, J., Jefferies, L., Atkins, B. L., and Byren, I. (2007) Outpatient parenteral antimicrobial therapy (OPAT): is it safe for selected patients to self-administer at home? A retrospective analysis of a large cohort over 13 years. *Journal of Antimicrobial Chemotherapy*, **60**(2): 356–62.

Muldoon, E. G., Snydman, D. R., Penland, E. C., and Allison, G. M. (2013) Are we ready for an outpatient parenteral antimicrobial therapy bundle? A critical appraisal of the evidence. *Clinical Infectious Diseases*, **57**(3):419–24.

Munton, T., Martin, A., Marrero, I., Llewellyn, A., Gibson, K., and Gomersall, A. (2011) *Getting out of Hospital? The Evidence for Shifting Acute Inpatient and Day Case Services from Hospitals into the Community*. <http://www.health.org.uk/publications/getting-out-of-hospital/?utm_medium=email&utm_source=The+Health+Foundation&utm_campaign=Getting+out+of+hospital+-+list+2&dm_i=4Y2,GZ4V,36GS4C,1DV4I,1>, accessed 27 November 2014.

Nathwani, D. (2010) 'Non-inpatient parenteral antimicrobial therapy (NIPAT)', in J. Cohen, W. G. Powderly, and S. M. Opal (eds) *Infectious Diseases*. London: Mosby/Elsevier, pp. 1333–9.

PAUSE. (2007) 'Vignette 21: outpatient parenteral antibiotic therapy', *PAUSE: Prudent Antibiotic User Website*. <http://www.pause-online.org.uk>, accessed 27 November 2014.

The British Society for Antimicrobial Chemotherapy. (2014) *OPAT: Outpatient Parenteral Antimicrobial Therapy*. <http://www.e-opat.com/>, accessed 27 November 2014.

Chapter 17

# Adverse drug reactions, and patient safety

## Introduction to adverse drug reactions

The World Health Organization (WHO) defines an adverse drug reaction as 'a drug related event that is noxious and unintended and occurs at doses used in humans for prophylaxis, diagnosis or therapy of disease or for the modification of physiological function'(WHO 2014). This definition of adverse drug reactions (ADRs) excludes overdose (including prescribing or administration errors), therapeutic failure, and reactions occurring because of drug withdrawal. Nonetheless, ADRs are common: they occur in 25 per cent of all patients taking prescription medicines in primary care, cause 7 per cent of all acute admissions to hospital, and affect at least 15 per cent of hospital inpatients (Fig. 17.1). Importantly, between 33 per cent and 72 per cent of ADRs are preventable (Table 17.1). Consequently, improving medication safety ranks alongside reducing wrong-site surgery and health-care-associated infection in the WHO's top three priorities for improving patient safety.

## Classification of ADRs

### Type A reactions

Type A ADRs are due to the pharmacological effect of the drug. They are predictable and dose related; hence, they are usually readily reversible on removing the drug or reducing the dose. The pharmacological mechanism underlying type A ADRs is often different from that responsible for the drug's intended therapeutic effect. For example, macrolide antibiotics cause a dose-related increase in gastric and intestinal motility, which results in abdominal pain, vomiting, and diarrhoea. This is independent of their effect on bacterial protein synthesis, and macrolides have been modified to retain their effect on intestinal motility but lose their antibacterial activity. In contrast, both *Clostridium difficile* infection and colonization with antibiotic-resistant bacteria are examples of type A ADRs that arise from antibacterial effects.

### Type B reactions

Type B reactions are idiosyncratic, cannot be predicted from the known pharmacology of the drug, and are not dose related. The most common mechanism for type B reactions is immunologically mediated hypersensitivity but other important mechanisms include receptor abnormality, abnormal biological system unmarked by the drug, abnormalities in drug metabolism, drug–drug interactions, and drug–disease interactions (Table 17.2).

## Epidemiology of ADRs caused by antimicrobials

In primary care, antibiotics feature in the top five classes of drugs associated with ADRs (Table 17.1). However, antimicrobial ADRs caused in primary care are usually not serious, so they

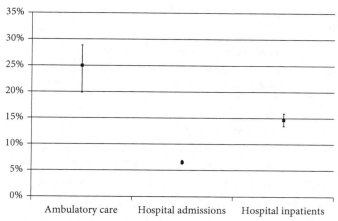

**Fig. 17.1** Prevalence of ADRs in ambulatory care, as a cause of hospital admission and in hospital inpatients.

Source: data from: Ambulatory care: Gandhi TK et al., Adverse drug events in ambulatory care, *New England Journal of Medicine*, Volume 348, Number 16, pp. 1556–64, Copyright © 2003 Massachusetts Medical Society; Hospital admissions: Pirmohamed M et al., Adverse drug reactions as cause of admission to hospital: prospective analysis of 18 820 patients, *British Medical Journal*, Volume 329, Issue 7463, pp. 15–9; Copyright © 2004; Hospital inpatients: Davies EC et al., Adverse drug reactions in hospital in-patients: a prospective analysis of 3695 patient-episodes, *PLoS One*, Volume 4, Issue 2, e4439, Copyright © 2009 Davies et al.

**Table 17.1** Characteristics of adverse drug reactions in ambulatory care, causing hospital admissions, or in hospital inpatients.[a]

|  | **Ambulatory care** | **Hospital admissions** | **Hospital inpatients** |
| --- | --- | --- | --- |
| Type A (predictable; %) | Not stated | 95 | 94 |
| Preventable (%) | 39 | 72 | 53 |
| Top five drug classes | 1. Cardiovascular | 1. Cardiovascular | 1. Antibacterials |
|  | 2. SSRIs | 2. NSAIDs | 2. Analgesics |
|  | 3. NSAIDs | 3. Anticoagulants | 3. Cardiovascular |
|  | 4. Antibacterials | 4. Antidepressants | 4. Anticoagulants |
|  | 5. Corticosteroids | 5. Opioid analgesics | 5. Corticosteroids |
| Risk factors | Number of medicines | Increasing age | Number of medicines |

[a] Note that, while antibacterials comprise the fourth most common drug class involved in adverse drug reactions in ambulatory care, they comprise the most common drug class for adverse drug reactions in hospital inpatients; NSAIDs, non-steroidal anti-inflammatory drugs; SSRIs, selective serotonin reuptake inhibitors.

Source: data from: Ambulatory care: Gandhi TK et al., Adverse drug events in ambulatory care, *New England Journal of Medicine*, Volume 348, Number 16, pp. 1556–64, Copyright © 2003 Massachusetts Medical Society; Hospital admissions: Pirmohamed M et al., Adverse drug reactions as cause of admission to hospital: prospective analysis of 18 820 patients, *British Medical Journal*, Volume 329, Issue 7463, pp. 15–9; Copyright © 2004; Hospital inpatients: Davies EC et al., Adverse drug reactions in hospital in-patients: a prospective analysis of 3695 patient-episodes, *PLoS One*, Volume 4, Issue 2, e4439, Copyright © 2009 Davies et al.

**Table 17.2** Mechanisms of type B, idiosyncratic adverse drug reactions, with examples from antimicrobial chemotherapy.

| Mechanism | Example from antimicrobial chemotherapy |
|---|---|
| Receptor abnormality | Seizures associated with relatively low doses of beta-lactams and quinolones. Both classes of drugs inhibit the GABA-A receptor but normally this only occurs with very high doses or accumulation due to severe renal impairment. |
| Abnormal biological system unmarked by the drug | Primaquine induced haemolysis in patients deficient in glucose 6-phosphate dehydrogenase. |
| Abnormalities in drug metabolism | Isoniazid induced peripheral neuropathy in people who are slow acetylators because they are deficient in the enzyme N-acetyl transferase. |
| Immunological | Anaphylaxis due to Type 1 hypersensitivity to beta-lactams. |
| | Acute interstitial nephritis due to flucloxacillin. |
| | Eosinophilic pneumonia due to nitrofurantoin. |
| Drug-drug interactions | Increased incidence of hepatitis when isoniazid is prescribed with rifampicin. |
| Drug-disease interactions | Rash that occurs in 90% of patients with infectious mononucleosis when given aminopenicillins but does not recur on re-challenge after recovery. Similarly rashes due to co-trimoxazole are much more common in patients with HIV infection. |

Reproduced from *British Medical Journal*, Pirmohamed M et al., 'Adverse drug reactions', Volume 316, Issue 7140, pp. 1295–8, Copyright © 1998, with permission from BMJ Publishing Group Ltd.

do not feature in the top five classes of drugs causing admission to hospital (Table 17.1). The commonest severe ADRs that cause hospital admission are postural hypotension, acute kidney injury, and bleeding. Antimicrobials could contribute to these serious ADRs through dehydration caused by diarrhoea or vomiting or through interaction with anticoagulants; however, they are rarely solely responsible for hospital admission. In contrast, antibacterial drugs are the commonest class causing ADRs in hospital inpatients and are implicated in half of fatal ADRs. Renal failure and *C. difficile* infection are the two principal mechanisms for fatal antibacterial ADRs.

Over 90 per cent of ADRs that cause hospital admission or affect hospital inpatients are type A, which are predictable from the pharmacological effects of the drug, and >50 per cent are preventable (Table 17.1). In hospital the ADRs associated with cephalosporins, macrolides, and penicillins are virtually identical (Table 17.3).

## Improving medication safety

The WHO (2011) multiprofessional edition of the *Curriculum Guide for Patient Safety* uses cases to illustrate threats to medication safety, and it is striking that three of the seven cases involve antimicrobials and that they are all both predictable and preventable:

1 fatal acute kidney injury caused by a patient receiving 240 mg of gentamicin, three times daily for a week—the intended dose was 80 mg, three times daily (240 mg per day) but the instruction was misinterpreted as 240 mg per dose;

2 retroperitoneal haemorrhage caused by interaction between warfarin and a course of antibacterials; and

3 severe oral and oesophageal candidiasis caused by prescription of antibacterials to a patient with severe immunodeficiency.

**Table 17.3** Adverse drug reactions associated with antibacterial use in hospital inpatients. Note that the reactions for penicillins, cephalosporins, and macrolides are almost identical.

| | |
|---|---|
| **Penicillins** | *Clostridium difficile* infection |
| | Candidal infection |
| | Bleeding and increased international normalized ratio |
| | Diarrhoea and vomiting |
| | Rash |
| **Cephalosporins** | *Clostridium difficile* infection |
| | Candidal infection |
| | Bleeding and increased international normalized ratio |
| | Diarrhoea and vomiting |
| | Neutropenia |
| | Rash |
| | Renal failure |
| **Macrolides** | *Clostridium difficile* infection |
| | Candidal infection |
| | Bleeding and increased international normalized ratio |
| | Diarrhoea and vomiting |
| | Rash |
| | Renal failure |
| **Aminoglycosides** | Acute kidney injury |

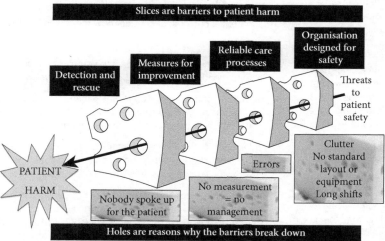

**Fig. 17.2** Swiss cheese model of patient safety.

Adapted from *British Medical Journal*, Reason J, 'Human error: models and management', Volume 320, Issue 7237, pp. 768–70, Copyright © 2000, with permission from BMJ Publishing Group Ltd.

Prescribing errors that lead to patient harm almost always have multiple causes. Moreover, lack of knowledge or skills is almost never the sole cause of prescribing errors and rarely even a contributory factor. Rather, prescribing errors are caused by a combination of latent threats in the healthcare environment (poor design or cluttered, untidy workplaces), factors that impact on individuals (fatigue, stress) or teams (short staffing), and most importantly failure to detect and mitigate errors before they cause harm or to learn from them after the event (Fig. 17.2). When a prescribing error does cause patient harm, it is never the first link in the chain of events (Table 17.4). This is because there were already latent threats in the environment that made it easy to make the error

**Table 17.4** Identification of contributory factors to an incident from the World Health Organization (2011) *Patient Safety Curriculum Guide*. Even though the description of the incident gives no details about the societal, regulatory, or organizational influences on the hospital, there are at least eight different contributory factors.

| Description of incident | Contributory factors |
|---|---|
| Sarah, a 42-year-old woman, was admitted for the resection of a small, localized, non-metastatic malignant duodenal tumour. Sarah was otherwise healthy, without any family history of malignancy. Upon her return to the ward, the patient quickly developed a high fever, which remained unchanged for a week. A prescription for antibiotics was written: IV. Gentamicin 80 MGR X 3 P/D. The nurse copied the following order: IV. Gentamicin 80 MGR X 3 P/DOSE. The nurse who copied the order mistook the letter 'D' to mean 'dose', while the physician who wrote the order actually meant 'day'. Over the next 10 days, the patient received 240 mg of gentamicin, three times daily. During that time, the patient began showing signs of renal failure and hearing impairment. On the tenth day of treatment, as the nurse manager was taking stock of the drugs administered, the error was discovered. The treatment was stopped but the patient's general status deteriorated due to acute renal failure. Ten days later, the patient died of generalized organ failure. | Work environment and equipment (latent threats) 1. The prescription for gentamicin was ambiguous. Most hospitals have inpatient prescription records that clearly specify the unit dose and the times at which this should be administered. However, there is still considerable variation between hospitals and a need for clearer, standardized documentation. Individual behaviour 2. Communication: the nurse did not check that her interpretation was correct. For a dangerous drug like gentamicin it is essential to use closed loop communication, which means that the receiver checks for shared understanding with the deliverer. 3. Decision making: review should be part of every clinical decision. How will the outcome be monitored and who is responsible? 4. Situation awareness: both the doctor and the nurse lacked situation awareness; they did not predict gentamicin toxicity as a potential outcome or consider how they could minimize the risk. Team behaviour 5. Coordination: nobody checked the prescription for 10 days. There is no mention of monitoring of gentamicin levels. 6. Culture: nobody spoke up for the patient. It is hard to believe that other nurses who administered the 240 mg doses of gentamicin did not think that this was unusual enough to question. 7. Leadership: the error was identified by the nurse manager because of stock checking rather than monitoring a patient who was receiving a dangerous drug for a life-threatening infection. 8. Group processes and cooperation: once gentamicin is prescribed, then the tasks required for monitoring need to be clearly assigned to team members. This includes responsibility for daily clinical review, sampling gentamicin levels, checking results, and acting on them. |

Adapted from the WHO Patient Safety Curriculum Guide, Multiprofessional Edition, 2011 with permission from the World Health Organization.

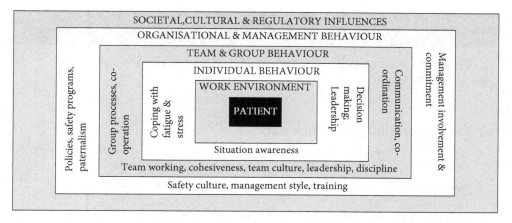

**Fig. 17.3** Human factors approach to patient safety.
Adapted from Moray N., 'Culture, politics and ergonomics', *Ergonomics*, Volume 43, Issue 7, pp. 858–868, Copyright © 2000, with permission from the Taylor and Francis Group,www.tandfonline.com.

(Table 17.4). In contrast, a safe health-care environment would make it easy to do the right thing and very hard to do the wrong thing. In addition, patient harm is not an inevitable consequence of the prescribing error. A safe health-care system would encourage staff to speak up when things go wrong so that harm can be avoided. Addressing these problems requires the application of human factors science or ergonomics to clinical practice (Fig. 17.3).

## Clinical Human Factors

Clinical human factors has been defined as 'enhancing clinical performance through an understanding of the effects of teamwork, tasks, equipment, workspace, culture, organization on human behaviour and abilities, and application of that knowledge in clinical settings' (Clinical Human Factors Group 2014).

The human factors approach to patient safety (Fig. 17.3) sets the patient at the centre of a set of interactions with the health-care environment, the individual health-care professional, the health-care professional's team, the organization in which they work, and the societal, cultural, and regulatory influences under which they operate (Fig. 17.3). Applying the human factors approach to one of the case studies in the WHO (2011) *Patient Safety Curriculum Guide* identifies at least eight contributory factors that lay behind the incident, even though the description of the incident does not include details of the regulatory system (Table 17.4) Having identified the contributory factors, the team should then use these as targets for improvement and undertake tests of change (see Box 17.1)

## Box 17.1 Ten performance requirements for health-care professionals to improve medication safety

### 1 Know which medications are high risk

♦ In hospitals at least 50 per cent of prescriptions are written by doctors in their first 2 years after qualification. The high-risk medicines that they will prescribe regularly are antimicrobials, anticoagulants, insulin, opiate analgesics, and sedatives.

**Ten performance requirements for health-care professionals to improve medication safety** *(continued)*

## 2 Be very familiar with the medications prescribed and/or dispensed

- It is better for prescribers to know a few drugs well than many superficially.

## 3 Tailor prescribing for each patient

- Factors to consider include allergies, pregnancy, breastfeeding, co-morbidities, other medications the patient may be taking, and the size and weight of the patient.
- Remember that every additional medicine multiplies the risk of ADR by 1.14.

## 4 Practise taking thorough medication histories

- Include the name, dose, route, frequency, and duration of every drug the patient is taking.
- Ask about
  - recently ceased medications;
  - over-the-counter medications, dietary supplements, and complementary medicines; and
  - any medications they have been advised to take but do not actually take.
- Look up any medications you are unfamiliar with.
- Identify medications that can be ceased and medications that may be causing side effects.
- Always include a thorough allergy history. When collecting an allergy history, remember that, if a patient has both a potentially serious allergy and a condition for which staff may want to prescribe that medication, this is a high-risk situation. Alert the patient and alert other staff.

## 5 Use memory aids

- Have a low threshold for looking things up. Prescribers should view relying on memory aids as a marker of safe practice rather than a sign that their knowledge is inadequate.
- Examples of memory aids include pocket-sized guidelines, and information technology such as computer software (decision/dispensing support) packages and personal digital assistants.

## 6 Communicate clearly

- The safe use of medication is a team activity and the patient is also a member of the team. Clear, unambiguous communication will help to minimize assumptions that can lead to error.
- Bad handwriting can lead to dispensing errors. Health professionals should write clearly and legibly, including their name and contact details.
- Pharmacists or nurses who cannot read the writing should contact the person who signed the prescription to check the details.
- In an emergency, use SBAR:

**Ten performance requirements for health-care professionals to improve medication safety** *(continued)*

- Situation: Mrs Smith in Bed 2 has severe community-acquired pneumonia.
- Background: she was admitted direct to the ward and has not had any antibiotics; she is allergic to penicillin.
- Assessment: she is hypotensive and needs intravenous (IV) antibiotics immediately.
- Recommendation: 'Please give IV levofloxacin, 200 mg, immediately. Will you be able to do that?'

♦ Close the loop: the nurse would close the loop by saying 'OK, I will give the patient 200 mg IV levofloxacin as soon as possible'.

## 7 Encourage patients to be actively involved in the medication process

♦ Educate your patients about their medication(s) and any associated hazards.

♦ Remember that patients and their families are highly motivated to avoid problems. If they are made aware of the important role they play in the medication process, they can contribute significantly to improving the safety of medication use.

♦ Information should be both verbal and written and should cover the following aspects:
  1 name of the generic drug;
  2 purpose and activity of the medication;
  3 dose, route, and administration schedule;
  4 special instructions, directions, and precautions;
  5 common side effects and interactions; and
  6 how the effects of the medication (e.g. efficacy, side effects, etc.) will be monitored.

♦ Encourage patients to keep a written record of the medications that they take and details of any allergies or problems they have had with medications in the past. This list should be presented whenever they interact with the health-care system.

## 8 Develop checking habits

♦ If checking becomes a habit, then it is more likely to occur even if the clinician is not actively thinking about being vigilant.

♦ Always read the label on the ampoule before drawing up a medication.

♦ Check the five Rs:
  1 right patient;
  2 right drug;
  3 right dose;
  4 right route; and
  5 right time.

♦ Check for allergies.

♦ High-risk medications and situations require extra vigilance. Develop situation awareness: gather and interpret information, then predict what is likely to happen next. Always ask

**Ten performance requirements for health-care professionals to improve medication safety** *(continued)*

'What is the worst that could happen?' and 'How would I detect this to prevent harm occurring to the patient?'

◆ Remember that computerized prescribing does not remove the need for checking. Computerized systems solve some problems (e.g. illegible handwriting, confusion around generic and trade names, recognizing drug interactions) but also present a new set of challenges.

## 9 Understand and practise drug calculations, including adjustments based on clinical parameters (e.g. renal clearance)

◆ Be familiar with how to manipulate units and adjust volumes, concentrations, and doses. Practice the calculations you will need to make to prescribe aminoglycosides and glycopeptides and to adjust doses in response to serum levels.

◆ Practise calculating adjustments based on clinical parameters.

◆ In high-stress and/or high-risk situations, consider ways to decrease the chance of a calculation error, for example, by using a calculator. Avoid doing arithmetic in your head (use a pen and paper instead).

◆ Ask a colleague to perform the same calculation to see if you concur. Note: asking them to check your calculation is very unlikely to identify an error; instead, ask them to perform the same calculation from scratch.

## 10 Report and learn from errors

◆ If you think something is wrong, speak up, however junior a member of the team you are.

◆ Learn from errors through investigation, discussion, and problem-solving.

◆ If an error can occur once, it can occur again. Consider strategies to prevent the recurrence of errors at both an individual practitioner level and an organizational level.

◆ Be familiar with how to report errors, adverse reactions, and adverse events involving medication.

◆ Reporting errors is just the first step. Improvement will only come through applying the model for improvement (see Chapter 20):

  • What are we trying to accomplish? Set a measurable aim (e.g. >95% reliability in 3 months).

  • How will we know that change is an improvement? Use regular measurement to feedback progress to the team, with action planning if the goal has not been reached.

  • What changes can we make to bring about improvement? Use small tests of change on one patient or professional and then scale up successful tests.

Adapted with permission from WHO Multi-professional Patient Safety Curriculum Guide, http://www.who.int/patientsafety/education/curriculum/en/index.html, Copyright © World Health Organization, 2011. All rights reserved.

## Key points

♦ ADRs are common, and antimicrobial drugs are among the commonest causes of ADRs in both primary and secondary care.

♦ More than 90 per cent of ADRs are predictable, and more than 50 per cent are avoidable.

♦ ADRs have multiple contributory factors and are rarely due to simple lack of knowledge or skills.

♦ Preventing ADRs requires teamwork, with involvement of the patient as part of the team.

## Further reading

Clinical Human Factors Group. (2014) *What is Human Factors?* <http://chfg.org/what-is-human-factors>, accessed 27 November 2014.

Coombes, I. D., Stowasser, D. A., Coombes, J. A., and Mitchell, C. (2008) Why do interns make prescribing errors? A qualitative study. *Medical Journal of Australia*, **188**(2): 89–94.

Davies, E. C., Green, C. F., Taylor, S., Williamson, P. R., Mottram, D.R., and Pirmohamed, M. (2009) Adverse drug reactions in hospital in-patients: a prospective analysis of 3695 patient-episodes. *PLoS ONE*, **4**(**2**): e4439.

Flin, R., O'Connor, P., and Crichton, M. (2008) *Safety at the Sharp End: A Guide to Non-Technical Skills*. Aldershot: Ashgate.

Flin, R., Winter, J., Sarac, C., and Raduma, M. (2009) *Human Factors in Patient Safety: Review of Topics and Tools*. <http://www.who.int/patientsafety/research/methods_measures/human_factors/human_factors_review.pdf>, accessed 27 November 2014.

Gandhi, T. K., Weingart, S. N., Borus, J., et al. (2003) Adverse drug events in ambulatory care. *New England Journal of Medicine*, **348** (16): 1556–64.

Pirmohamed, M., Breckenridge, A. M., Kitteringham, N. R., and Park, B. K. (1998) Adverse drug reactions. *BMJ*, **316**(7140): 1295–8.

Pirmohamed, M., James , S., Meakin, S., Green, C., Scott, A. K., Walley, T. J., Farrar, K., Park, B. K., and Breckenridge, A. M. (2004) Adverse drug reactions as cause of admission to hospital: prospective analysis of 18 820 patients. *BMJ*, **329**(7456): 15–19.

World Health Organization. (2011) *Patient Safety Curriculum Guide: Multi-Professional Edition*. <http://whqlibdoc.who.int/publications/2011/9789241501958_eng.pdf>, accessed 27 November 2014.

World Health Organization. (2014) *Annex: Glossary of Terms*. <http://www.who.int/medicines/areas/quality_safety/safety_efficacy/Annex1Glossaryof Terms.pdf>, accessed 27 November 2014.

# Chapter 18

# Chemoprophylaxis and immunization

## Chemoprophylaxis

Chemoprophylaxis is the prevention of infection by the administration of antimicrobial agents, as distinct from prevention by immunization. Individuals who require prophylaxis differ from the normal population in that they are known to be exposed to a particular infectious hazard or their ability to respond to infection is impaired.

Prophylaxis should be confined to those periods for which the risk is greatest, so that the problems of disturbance of the normal flora, superinfection with resistant organisms, untoward reactions, and cost will be minimized. The benefits and risks of chemoprophylaxis depend on

- the likelihood of infection in the absence of prophylaxis;
- the potential severity of the consequences of infection;
- the effectiveness of prophylaxis in reducing the likelihood of infection and the severity of the consequences; and
- the likelihood and consequences of adverse effects from prophylaxis.

Prevention strategies for infectious disease can be characterized by the traditional concepts of primary, secondary, and tertiary prevention. *Primary prevention* can be defined as the prevention of infection. *Secondary prevention* includes measures for the detection of early infection, and effective intervention before symptoms occur. *Tertiary prevention* consists of measures to reduce or eliminate the long-term impairment and disabilities caused by established infection.

Failure to consider fully the risks of prophylaxis or to be realistic about the benefits has made unnecessary chemoprophylaxis one of the commonest forms of antibiotic misuse. Nonetheless, it is important to recognize that the judgement about what is and is not necessary chemoprophylaxis may require complex decisions about the balance of benefits and risks to individual patients and to the population. The example of prevention of neonatal infection by group B streptococci (see 'Neonatal infection with group B streptococci') shows how national guidelines committees can produce different recommendations based on their risk assessment of the same evidence.

## Primary chemoprophylaxis

Most indications for primary chemoprophylaxis involve starting prophylaxis before a period of defined risk (e.g. elective surgery, travel to regions with endemic malaria, or intrapartum exposure of neonates to maternal infections) or following exposure to a patient who is known to have a contagious, dangerous infection (e.g. meningococcal meningitis).

### Prophylaxis in surgery

Reducing the risk of surgical infection is probably the commonest indication for chemoprophylaxis and accounts for up to a third of total antibiotic use in an acute hospital. There is no doubt

**Table 18.1** American Society of Anesthesiologists (ASA) classification of physical status.

| ASA score | Physical status |
|---|---|
| 1 | Normal healthy patient |
| 2 | Patient with a mild systemic disease |
| 3 | Patient with a severe systemic disease that limits activity, but is not incapacitating |
| 4 | Patient with an incapacitating systemic disease that is a constant threat to life |
| 5 | Moribund patient not expected to survive 24 hours with or without operation |

Adapted from Dripps RD, 'New classification of physical status', *Anesthesiology*, Volume 24, Copyright © 1963, with permission from the American Society of Anesthesiologists.

that prophylaxis can reduce the risk of surgical infection but at best it is only one component of effective infection control. Unnecessary use or duration of prophylaxis puts patients at risk of infection by *Clostridium difficile* or antimicrobial resistant bacteria with no compensating benefit.

## Classification of operations by risk of infection

The aim of chemoprophylaxis is to reduce the risk of surgical site infection, meaning infection in any part of the operative field from the superficial wound down to the deepest tissues involved in the operation. Postoperative infections can occur at other sites, for example, the respiratory or urinary tract, but chemoprophylaxis is targeted at surgical site infection.

The US Centers for Disease Control's (CDC) National Nosocomial Infections Surveillance (NNIS) risk index is an internationally recognized method for infection risk adjustment. Risk adjustment is based on three major risk factors:

♦ the American Society of Anesthesiologists (ASA) score, reflecting the patient's state of health before surgery (Table 18.1);

♦ wound class, reflecting the state of contamination of the wound (Table 18.2); and

♦ duration of operation, reflecting technical aspects of the surgery.

Primary prevention by chemoprophylaxis is only achievable for clean, clean-contaminated, or contaminated wounds, because the process of infection has started pre-operatively in dirty wounds. The risk of infection rises progressively according to the NNIS score (Fig. 18.1). The relative weightings of the elements in this score mean, for example, that a prolonged operation with a clean wound in a patient with co-morbidities carries approximately a 5 per cent risk of wound infection, which is markedly higher than the 3.5 per cent risk for a contaminated wound in a patient with no co-morbidities and a short operation. Such data underscore the risk associated with the underlying fitness of the patient at the time of surgery.

In addition to the probability that an infection will occur, it is important to consider the consequences of infection for the patient and the health service. Surgical site infection following colon surgery is associated with substantially increased risk of mortality, and prophylaxis significantly reduces death within 30 days of surgery. An increasing proportion of surgical procedures involve the implantation of devices such as prostheses (e.g. artificial joints) or cardiac pacemakers. Postoperative infection can rarely be controlled without removal of these devices, resulting in long-term morbidity, which can be reduced through surgical prophylaxis. Because of these dire consequences, even small reductions in the risk of surgical site infection by prophylaxis may be justifiable.

**Table 18.2** Classification of surgical operations according to risk of contamination of the wound by bacteria.

| Class | Conditions of operation |
|---|---|
| Clean | No inflammation is encountered and the respiratory, alimentary or genito-urinary tracts are not entered. There is no break in aseptic operating theatre technique |
| Clean-contaminated | The respiratory, alimentary or genito-urinary tracts are entered but without significant spillage |
| Contaminated | Acute inflammation (without pus) is encountered, or there is visible contamination of the wound. Examples include: gross spillage from a hollow viscus during the operation; compound injuries operated on within 4 h |
| Dirty | Presence of pus, a previously perforated hollow viscus, or compound injuries more than 4 h old |

Reprinted from *American Journal of Medicine*, Volume 91, Issue 3B, Culver DH et al, 'Surgical wound infection rates by wound class, operative procedure, and patient risk index: National Nosocomial Infections Surveillance System', pp. 152S–157S, Copyright © 1991, with permission from Elsevier, http://www.sciencedirect.com/science/journal/00029343

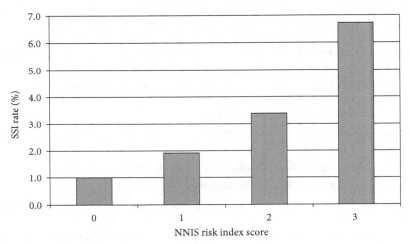

**Fig. 18.1** Surgical site infection rate according to National Nosocomial Infections Surveillance risk index score; NNIS, National Nosocomial Infections Surveillance; SSI, surgical site infection.

Reprinted from *American Journal of Medicine*, Volume 91, Issue 3B, Culver DH et al, 'Surgical wound infection rates by wound class, operative procedure, and patient risk index: National Nosocomial Infections Surveillance System', pp. 152S–157S, Copyright © 1991, with permission from Elsevier, http://www.sciencedirect.com/science/journal/00029343.

## Principles of surgical prophylaxis

The key to successful surgical prophylaxis is to achieve effective antimicrobial concentrations in the wound before bacterial contamination occurs (Fig. 18.2). Prophylaxis can still be effective if it is administered within 2 hours after the start of the operation but later administration is much less effective. However, prophylaxis should not be administered too early before the start of the operation, or antibiotic concentrations in the surgical site will have declined below effective levels

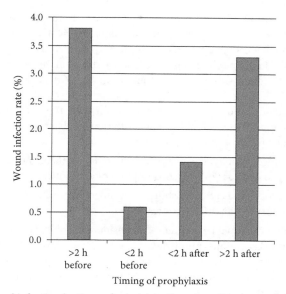

**Fig. 18.2** Risk of wound infection by time of administration of antibiotic prophylaxis. Data from a prospective study of 2,847 patients undergoing elective clean or clean–contaminated surgery and who received prophylactic antibiotics. The timing of prophylaxis refers to the time of administration of the first dose in relation to the start of the operation.
Source: data from Classen DC et al., The timing of prophylactic administration of antibiotics and the risk of surgical-wound infection, *New England Journal of Medicine*, Volume 326, Number 5, pp. 281–286, Copyright © 1992 Massachusetts Medical Society. All rights reserved.

before bacterial contamination occurs. The ideal time to administer intravenous prophylaxis is in the anaesthetic room no more than 30 minutes before the start of surgery and before any tourniquet is applied to reduce blood supply to the surgical site. For drugs with a short half-life (2 hours or less) additional doses may be required during the operation if it is prolonged or if there is substantial blood loss (1,500 ml or more) or haemodilution by 15 ml/kg or more.

It follows that there is no value in administering additional doses of prophylaxis once the wound has been closed. For most operations, a single dose of prophylaxis is all that is required. There is still some controversy about the benefits and risks of extending prophylaxis for up to 24 hours postoperatively, the argument in favour being that wounds are insufficiently sealed to prevent bacterial contamination. However, there is absolutely no doubt that prophylaxis should not continue for more than 24 hours after surgery. Extended antibiotic 'prophylaxis' risks selecting for antibiotic resistant bacteria or causing complications such as *Clo. difficile* infection and other drug-related adverse events.

## Guidelines for surgical prophylaxis

Unequivocal evidence for the effectiveness of antibiotic prophylaxis comes from controlled clinical trials with a 'no treatment' or placebo arm. Once effectiveness has been established for a specific operation, it may be considered unethical to do placebo-controlled trials in similar operations. For example, the recommendation to give prophylaxis before total knee replacement is based on expert opinion that the strong evidence supporting prophylaxis for total hip replacement supports prophylaxis for all total joint replacements. Guidelines should be explicit about the expected standard of care by distinguishing between operations for which prophylaxis should be the rule, those for which local policy makers or surgeons may identify exceptions, and operations for which prophylaxis should not be given at all. These judgements are based on a combination of the evidence about effectiveness of prophylaxis and estimates of the consequences of surgical site infection for the patient.

For example, evidence graded recommendations for each type of surgery, are available at <http://www.sign.ac.uk/pdf/sign104.pdf>. Four different levels of recommendations are made regarding the case for surgical antibiotic prophylaxis:

◆ Highly recommended: prophylaxis unequivocally reduces major morbidity, reduces hospital costs, and is likely to decrease overall consumption of antibiotics.

◆ Recommended: prophylaxis reduces short-term morbidity, reduces hospital costs, and may decrease overall consumption of antibiotics.

◆ Should be considered: prophylaxis should be considered for all patients. Local policy makers may wish to identify exceptions (prophylaxis may not reduce hospital costs and could increase antibiotic use). Notably, for clean-contaminated procedures or procedures involving insertion of a prosthetic device, good-quality evidence for the clinical effectiveness of surgical antibiotic prophylaxis is lacking.

◆ Not recommended: prophylaxis has not been proven to be clinically effective and, as the consequences of infection are short-term morbidity, it is likely to increase hospital antibiotic consumption for little clinical benefit.

However effective prophylaxis is at reducing the risk of surgical site infection, there must be a point when the risk of infection is so low without prophylaxis that the benefits are questionable.

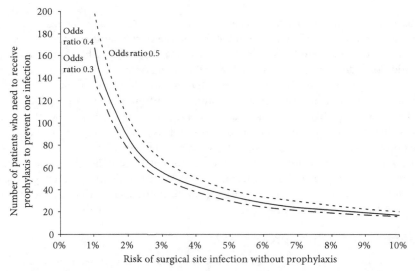

**Fig. 18.3** The relationship between the number of patients who must receive surgical prophylaxis to prevent one surgical site infection and the risk of infection without prophylaxis. The three lines show results for operations in which the odds ratio of infection with prophylaxis versus no prophylaxis is 0.3 (—·—), 0.4 (—), and 0.5 (....).

The number of patients that must receive prophylaxis to prevent one surgical site infection rises exponentially as the risk of infection diminishes (Fig. 18.3). For clean wound surgery in a patient with no other risk factors, the probability of surgical site infection is only 1 per cent. If prophylaxis halves the risk of infection, that means that 200 patients must receive prophylaxis in order to prevent one surgical site infection. The balance between benefits and risks of prophylaxis therefore depends on how a surgical site infection will be managed if it occurs. An infected hip prosthesis may require 2 months or more of antibiotic treatment (over 200 doses of flucloxacillin); consequently, administration of single doses of prophylaxis to 200 patients is still likely to reduce total antibiotic use in the hospital if it prevents one infection.

The choice of agents for chemoprophylaxis should be guided by local susceptibilities of prevalent surgical site infection pathogens and antibiotic policies (Table 18.3). The single dose for prophylactic use is in most circumstances the same as would be used therapeutically. In most instances, prophylactic antibiotics are given intravenously but there are some exceptions (Table 18.3).

**Table 18.3** Perioperative surgical antibiotic prophylaxis administration.

| Strength of evidence | Recommendation |
| --- | --- |
| **Choice of antibiotics** | |
| C | The antibiotics selected for prophylaxis must cover the expected pathogens for that operative site. |
| ☑ | The choice of antibiotic should take into account local resistance patterns. |
| ☑ | Narrow spectrum, less expensive antibiotics should be the first choice for prophylaxis during surgery. |
| **Route of administration—general** | |
| ☑ | Prophylactic antibiotics for surgical procedures should be administered intravenously. |
| **Route of administration—surgery specific** | |
| B | Intranasal mupirocin should be used prophylactically for patients undergoing high risk surgery who are identified with *S. aureus* or MRSA. |
| B | A single dose of topical antibiotic is recommended for insertion of grommets. |
| B | In addition to intravenous antibiotics, impregnated cement is recommended for cemented joint replacements. |
| A | Intracameral antibiotic prophylaxis is recommended for cataract surgery. |
| B | Intracameral of intravitreal intraocular antibiotic prophylaxis is recommended at completion of surgery for penetrating eye injuries *(dependent on extent of injury and the presence or absence of an intraocular foreign body).* |
| **Duration of prophylaxis—general** | |
| B | A single dose of antibiotic with a long enough half-life to achieve activity throughout the operation is recommended. |

*(continued)*

**Table 18.3** (continued).

| Strength of evidence | Recommendation |
| --- | --- |
| Duration of prophylaxis—surgery specific | |
| C | An additional intraoperative dosage of antibiotic is recommended for cardiac surgery longer than four hours when using an antibiotic with pharmacokinetics equivalent to cefazolin. |
| B | Up to 24 hours of antibiotic prophylaxis should be considered for arthroplasty. |
| ☑ | Additional dosage may be indicated for longer surgery or shorter-acting agents to maintain activity for the duration of the operation. |

A: High quality evidence e.g. meta-analysis, systematic review, or randomised control trial.

B: High quality case control or cohort study evidence.

C: Lower quality case control or cohort study evidence.

☑: Good practice recommendation based on the clinical experience of the guideline development group.

This table is reproduced from SIGN guideline QRG104, *Antibiotic Prophylaxis in Surgery* by kind permission of the Scottish Intercollegiate Guidelines Network, SIGN, Edinburgh, Copyright © 2008 (SIGN publication no. QRG104), available from URL: http://www.sign.ac.uk. These recommendations were produced only for NHS Scotland in 2014 by SIGN, and are due for review in 2017. The current status of SIGN guidelines in Scotland is available at www.sign.ac.uk. The grant of permission to any other person or body outside the UK to reprint or otherwise use the SIGN guidelines in any way is given on the strict understanding that such a person or body is not the intended user of the guidelines and the guidelines are used entirely at the person's or body's own risk. SIGN, Healthcare Improvement Scotland and NHS Scotland accept no responsibility for any adverse outcomes resulting from such use.

# Prophylaxis for travellers

## Malaria

Protecting travellers to areas where malaria is common fulfils all of the criteria for successful chemoprophylaxis. The chances of acquiring the disease are high, the results can be grave, and the period at risk is well defined: from arrival in the area until four weeks after departure—the time taken for any parasites that may have been acquired to be finally eliminated. Although resistance is an increasing problem in malaria, it is still possible to identify a drug that is suitable for prophylaxis for most travellers (see 'Antimalarial prophylaxis' in Chapter 35). Failure to take chemoprophylaxis or to continue chemoprophylaxis for four weeks after leaving a region of endemic malaria are the commonest reasons for malaria presenting in countries where malaria is not endemic.

As in surgery, chemoprophylaxis for malaria should be seen as only one component of risk reduction. They should also do all that they can to avoid contact with malaria vectors: using protective clothing, window netting, and insect repellents, and sleeping under insecticide-impregnated bed netting.

Apart from transient visitors to endemic regions, the only other clear candidates for antimalarial chemoprophylaxis are resident women during pregnancy.

## Other prophylaxis for travellers

Chemoprophylaxis can reduce the risk of traveller's diarrhoea but early treatment of symptomatic cases is highly effective and is preferable.

# Primary prevention of other bacterial infections

## Endocarditis

Prevention of bacterial infective endocarditis (IE) in people with abnormal heart valves or other endocardial disease is a controversial subject. Until relatively recently, it was routine practice to administer antibiotics to achieve effective plasma concentrations of antimicrobial drugs before the start of procedures that carry substantial risk of causing bacteraemia and therefore contamination of the endocardium. However, in 2008, the National Institute for Health and Clinical Excellence (NICE) changed the advice concerning the need for antibiotic prophylaxis against IE: prophylaxis should not be given to adults and children with structural cardiac defects at risk of IE who are undergoing dental (and non-dental) interventional procedures. This change in practice was based on a review of the available evidence that found no consistent association between having a dental (or non-dental) interventional procedure and the development of IE. It was concluded that the clinical and cost-effectiveness of antibiotic prophylaxis is not proven and that its use may actually lead to a greater number of deaths through fatal anaphylactic reactions than not using preventive antibiotics.

## Selective decontamination of the digestive tract

Chemoprophylaxis has a possible role in the prevention of ventilator-associated pneumonia but there is a lack of consensus about whether to use this approach routinely as part of a risk reduction strategy that includes a bundle of other measures. Selective decontamination of the digestive tract, started at the time of intubation and targeted at Gram-negative aerobic bacilli and fungi, reduces the risk of ventilator-associated pneumonia, especially in trauma victims. However, adoption of such prophylaxis is very variable across the world, largely because of ongoing controversy about long-term outcome and specifically whether mortality is affected. Concern about antibiotic resistance selection also remains a concern.

Another example of selective decontamination of the digestive tract is oral administration of co-trimoxazole or quinolones to afebrile neutropenic patients. However, this is no longer recommended practice in most national guidelines because the risks from selection of drug-resistant bacteria are thought to outweigh any clinical benefit. Again, evidence that mortality is reduced by this approach is lacking.

## Neonatal infection with group B streptococci

Colonization of the vagina or rectum with group B streptococci (*Streptococcus agalactiae*) is very common in pregnancy (prevalence 20–30%). It does not usually cause morbidity in mothers but can cause serious neonatal infections (10% overall mortality but 23% mortality in premature infants of less than 35 weeks' gestation). However, routine intrapartum chemoprophylaxis does not significantly reduce neonatal mortality, and most guidelines recommend targeted intrapartum prophylaxis. There are three different approaches, each advocated by at least one set of national guidelines:

◆ Risk-based assessment: intrapartum prophylaxis with penicillin is offered to women with known risk factors (e.g. previous baby with neonatal group B streptococcal disease; group B streptococcal bacteriuria during pregnancy; premature delivery) or intrapartum fever. The UK Royal College of Obstetricians and Gynaecologists (2012 guidelines) currently advocate this approach.

- Bacteriological screening: vaginal and rectal swabs are taken from all women between 35 and 37 weeks of gestation, and intrapartum prophylaxis is offered to those with positive swabs. Prophylaxis is also offered to women who go into labour before swabs have been taken or cultured. This approach is currently advocated by the Centers for Disease Control and Prevention in the United States.

- Bacteriological screening with targeted prophylaxis: the screening process is the same as in the second option but intrapartum prophylaxis is offered only to women who also have one of the risk factors outlined in the first option.

In 2007 the UK Royal College of Obstetricians and Gynaecologists reviewed practice on group B streptococcal intrapartum antibiotic prophylaxis in 13 countries. Seven guidelines recommended universal bacteriological screening, four guidelines promoted a risk-based strategy, one recommended universal bacteriological screening but women would only be offered prophylaxis if they had a positive streptococcal culture and another risk factor, and one gave no strong preference. The arguments for and against are based on estimation of the benefits, costs, and risks of each strategy. The reason that the UK guidelines do not favour routine bacteriological screening is that they estimate that at least 24,000 women would need to be screened and about 700 women receive intrapartum prophylaxis to prevent one neonatal infection, whereas with risk-based assessment the number of women who must be treated to prevent one neonatal infection is about 200. The risk assessments and decisions made by the national guideline groups will have been heavily influenced by the different legal systems in the United Kingdom and North America, and differences in disease epidemiology according to ethnicity and social status.

## Post-exposure prophylaxis of bacterial infections

Examples of primary post-exposure chemoprophylaxis for bacterial infection include

- exposure to *Neisseria meningitidis*;
- exposure of vulnerable, unvaccinated children to *Bordetella pertussis*;
- prevention of ophthalmia neonatorum in babies born to mothers with gonorrhoeal or chlamydial infection; and
- prophylaxis following sexual assault.

For *N. meningitidis*, there are two distinct situations. The first is prophylaxis of contacts of sporadic cases, which is confined to close contacts (e.g. household or mouth-kissing contacts, and health-care workers who have been heavily exposed to respiratory droplets or secretions). The second is in epidemic situations, where chemoprophylaxis may be used to supplement vaccination strategies for group A or C strains and for epidemics caused by group B strains. Sulphonamides are no longer effective for prophylaxis of meningococcal infection because of drug resistance; the current agent of choice is ciprofloxacin (with rifampicin as a second-line choice).

## Primary prevention of recurrent bacterial infections

All of the previous examples involve short-term risk reduction but there are a few situations where risk reduction has to be continued for prolonged periods, for example, for the prevention of bacterial infection following splenectomy or rheumatic carditis or for the prevention of recurrent infections. Patients who have their spleens removed (e.g. following trauma) or who have poorly functioning spleens are at greatly increased risk of infection by certain microorganisms (including capsulated bacteria such as pneumococci and meningococci, and malaria parasites).

Such individuals need to be offered advice (including carrying warning cards/bracelets), appropriate vaccinations, and antibiotic prophylaxis (typically involving penicillin, amoxicillin, or erythromycin).

For recurrent infections, it may be possible to identify repeated short periods of risk. For example, some women with recurrent urinary tract infection may be able to achieve satisfactory control by taking a single dose of antibiotics following sexual intercourse, which is really repeated post-exposure prophylaxis.

## Primary prevention of viral infections by chemotherapy

An example of prophylaxis before exposure is intrapartum treatment of mothers who are known to be human immunodeficiency virus (HIV) positive in order to reduce the risk of perinatal infection. The principles of prophylaxis here are the same as for neonatal group B streptococcal infection.

Examples of post-exposure antiviral chemoprophylaxis include exposure to influenza A virus (amantadine, rimantadine), influenza A or B virus (zanamivir or oseltamivir), and HIV (antiretroviral drugs). There are two common indications for post-exposure prophylaxis against HIV: after occupational or environmental exposure and after sexual exposure.

## Secondary chemoprophylaxis

Secondary prevention strategies involve the identification of early or asymptomatic infection with subsequent treatment so that such infections are eradicated and sequelae are prevented. Although most secondary prevention programmes involve intervention at the individual level through the use of chemoprophylaxis, they may also operate within the context of a population-based or institution-based screening effort. Routine screening programmes for sexually transmitted diseases such as *Chlamydia* infection are examples of secondary prevention strategies. Contact investigations for partners of persons with sexually transmitted diseases are also part of a secondary prevention strategy focused on those with known exposure. Another example of a secondary prevention programme that uses chemoprophylaxis is the screening of high-risk populations for tuberculosis infection and subsequent therapy with an antimicrobial drug such as isoniazid to prevent active disease.

## Tertiary prophylaxis

Tertiary prevention efforts are measures to eliminate long-term impairment and disability that may result from an existing condition. Because most infectious diseases are treatable, tertiary prevention activities are less common than those used with chronic diseases such as hypertension, diabetes, and coronary artery disease. However, this concept is still applicable to the control of infectious diseases; for example, some chronic viral infections cannot be eradicated and there are a number of latent infections that cause symptoms only in immunosuppressed patients.

Treatment of HIV infection now relies on highly active antiretroviral therapy (HAART) with combinations of drugs that reduce viral load to undetectable levels and restore counts of CD4 lymphocytes to $> 200/mm^3$. Provided that the patient can tolerate the treatment and there is no major resistance to antiviral drugs in the infecting strain of HIV, this treatment can maintain normal immunity for many years and prevent recurrence of latent opportunistic infections (see Chapter 31). However, once the CD4 lymphocyte count falls below $200/mm^3$, the cumulative risk for developing an acquired immune deficiency syndrome (AIDS)-defining opportunistic infection is 33 per cent by year 1, and 58 per cent by year 2, so chemoprophylaxis must be considered.

Latent infection means that many patients are already infected with these organisms before they become immunosuppressed. With normal immunity, the infections may have been asymptomatic from the start or may have caused a transient illness but then remain dormant for very long periods. *Pneumocystis jiroveci* (formerly *carinii*) rarely if ever causes symptomatic infection in people with normal immunity, whereas herpes simplex does cause recurrent symptoms even with normal immunity. However, in immunosuppressed people the frequency and consequences of symptomatic infection are greatly increased. Other indications for tertiary prophylaxis of latent infection include

- primary immunodeficiency;
- severe malnutrition;
- after organ transplantation; and
- cytotoxic or immunosuppressive treatment of cancer, connective tissue disorders, and other diseases, including long-term corticosteroids.

The general principles of chemoprophylaxis are the same for long-term suppression of latent infection as for short-term primary or secondary prevention. However, with long-term prophylaxis the issues of inducing resistance, risk of adverse effects, and cost-effectiveness are even more important.

Resistance or cross-resistance has become increasingly common with prophylaxis for the *Mycobacterium avium* complex, fungal infections, and *P. jiroveci*. For example, following prophylaxis with clarithromycin for *M. avium* complex infections, over half of the infections that occur are caused by strains that are resistant to clarithromycin and therefore delay clinical recovery and require treatment with alternative less effective or more toxic agents. Prophylactic regimens may also lead to the development of cross-resistance against more common pathogens. For example, rifabutin used for prophylaxis of infections with opportunistic mycobacteria may result in the emergence of rifampicin-resistant strains of *M. tuberculosis*, and the use of antibiotics such as clarithromycin, azithromycin, or co-trimoxazole may lead to the development of resistance among organisms such as pneumococci that were not the primary targets of prophylaxis.

Patients with HIV infection are particularly vulnerable to adverse reactions to drugs. The reason is probably a combination of immunomodulation or other HIV-related idiosyncrasy, pre-existing organ damage in late-stage disease, and interactions among the large number of potentially toxic drugs that these patients require (see Chapter 31).

The balance of risks and benefits of taking long-term prophylaxis versus treating symptomatic infections when they occur determine cost-effectiveness. The issue is not purely financial: the costs of prophylaxis include the inconvenience to the patient of having to take large numbers of medicines all the time and the negative impact of these medicines on quality of life. In general, long-term prophylaxis is cost-effective for *P. jiroveci* or opportunistic mycobacteria but not for fungal infection or cytomegalovirus.

## Immunization

The contribution of immunization to reducing the morbidity and mortality due to infectious diseases is enormous. For example, the introduction of vaccines (initially separately and then in a combined product) against measles, mumps, and rubella (MMR) was followed by dramatic reductions in the incidences of these diseases. In the 1950s and 1960s, approximately half a million recorded cases of measles occurred each year in England and Wales. Routine measles vaccination was introduced in 1968 and, by the time the combined MMR vaccine followed in 1988, the annual incidence of measles had fallen fivefold to approximately 100,000 cases. A decade later there were 56 confirmed cases of measles in the United Kingdom. After (subsequently unfounded) controversy about the safety of MMR vaccination began, compliance dropped sharply in the United Kingdom from 92 per cent in 1996 to 84 per cent in 2002. In some parts of London, compliance was as low as 61 per cent in 2003, which was far below the rate needed to avoid an epidemic of measles. Depressingly, in 2008 there were 1,370 confirmed cases of measles. The incidence started to fall again, coincident with enhanced population vaccination rates as the safety concerns have been refuted, but further outbreaks in 2013 emphasize the need to achieve and maintain high levels of vaccination.

A full review of immunization is beyond the scope of this text but it should be noted that the complexity of immunization schedules continues to increase markedly as new vaccines are discovered and new age groups are included (for example, the elderly now routinely receive pneumococcal, influenza, and shingles vaccines). This can be seen, for example, by comparing the recommended UK immunization schedules in 1996 and 2014 (Tables 18.4 and 18.5). New recent additions include extended coverage pneumococcal conjugate and human papilloma virus vaccines. It is very likely that further vaccines will be introduced given the substantial health benefits (and profits) achieved to date.

**Table 18.4** UK immunization schedule 2014.

| AGE | Immunisation (Vaccine Given) |
| --- | --- |
| 2 months | **DTaP/IPV(polio)/Hib** (diphtheria, tetanus, pertussis (whooping cough), polio, and *Haemophilus influenzae* type b)—all-in-one injection, plus:**PCV** (pneumococcal conjugate vaccine)—in a separate injection. |
| | Rotavirus. |
| 3 months | **DTaP/IPV(polio)/Hib** (2nd dose), plus:**MenC** (meningitis C)—in a separate injection. |
| | Rotavirus (2nd dose). |
| 4 months | **DTaP/IPV(polio)/Hib** (3rd dose), plus:**MenC** (2nd dose)—in a separate injection, plus:**PCV** (2nd dose)—in a separate injection. |
| Between 12 and 13 months | **Hib/MenC** (combined as one injection—4th dose of Hib and 3rd dose of MenC) plus:**MMR** (measles, mumps and rubella—combined as one injection), plus:**PCV** (3rd dose)—in a separate injection. |
| 2 and 3 years | Influenza (annual). |
| Around 3 years and four months | Pre-school booster of:**DTaP/IPV(polio)** (diphtheria, tetanus, pertussis (whooping cough) and polio), plus:**MMR** (second dose)—in a separate injection. |
| Around 12–13 years (girls) | **HPV** (human papillomavirus)—**three injections** The second injection is given 1–2 months after the first one. The third is given about six months after the first one. |
| Around 13–18 years | **Td/IPV(polio) booster** (a combined injection of tetanus, low-dose diphtheria, and polio). |
| Adults | **Influenza and PCV** if you are aged 65 or over or in a high-risk group.**Td/IPV(polio)**— at any age if you were not fully immunised as a child. |
| | Varicella zoster (shingles) when aged 70 years. |

Reproduced from NHS Choices, 'The NHS Vaccination Schedule', under the Open Government License v. 2.0, available from http://www.nhs.uk/Conditions/vaccinations/Pages/vaccination-schedule-age-checklist.aspx.

**Table 18.5** UK Immunization schedule 1996.

| Age | Vaccine |
| --- | --- |
| 2 months | D/Ta/P, PV and Hib 1st dose |
| 3 months | D/Ta/P, PV and Hib 2nd dose |
| 4 months | D/Ta/P, PV and Hib 3rd dose |
| 12–15 months | MMR |
| 3–5 years | Booster D/Ta and PV, MMR second dose |
| 10–14 years or infancy | BCG |
| 13–18 years | Booster D/Ta and PV |

Reproduced from *Green Book*, 1996 edition, under the Open Government License v. 2.0, available from http://webarchive.
nationalarchives.gov.uk/20080910134953/http:/dh.gov.uk/en/publichealth/healthprotection/immunisation/greenbook/
dh_4097254.

## Key points

- The patient's state of health before surgery, type of wound (clean, contaminated, dirty), and duration of operation are key determinants of infection risk.
- Antibiotic prophylaxis should be preferably be given just before (e.g. in the 30 minutes before) surgery starts.
- Antibiotic prophylaxis is indicated in many but importantly not all surgical operations, as a way of reducing infection risk and overall antibiotic consumption.
- Practice varies considerably concerning intrapartum antibiotic prophylaxis against group B streptococcal infection.
- Immunization coverage (compliance) in the at-risk population is crucial in determining the overall effectiveness of a vaccine.

## Further reading

**Public Health England.** (2013) *Immunisation against Infectious Disease.* <https://www.gov.uk/government/uploads/system/uploads/attachment_data/file/266583/The_Green_book_front_cover_and_contents_page_December_2013.pdf>, accessed 27 November 2014.

**Royal College of Obstetricians and Gynaecologists and London School of Hygiene and Tropical Medicine.** (2007) *The Prevention of Early-Onset Neonatal Group B Streptococcal Disease in UK Obstetric Units: An Audit of Reported Practice in England, Scotland, Wales and Northern Ireland.* <https://www.rcog.org.uk/globalassets/documents/guidelines/research--audit/neonatal_audit_full_250507.pdf >, accessed 5 December 2014.

**Scottish Intercollegiate Guidelines Network.** (2014) *Sign 104: Antibiotic Prophylaxis in Surgery.* <http://www.sign.ac.uk/pdf/sign104.pdf>, accessed 27 November 2014.

# Chapter 19

# Guidelines, formularies, and antimicrobial policies

## Introduction to guidelines, formularies, and antimicrobial policies

The discovery of antibiotics undoubtedly transformed the outcome of severe bacterial infection. However, a less comfortable aspect of the antibiotic revolution was that within 10 years over 80 per cent of patients with acute bronchitis were receiving antibiotics without any evidence of clinical benefit. A link between antimicrobial prescribing and resistance has been clear from the start of the therapeutic use of sulphonamides and penicillin. Collateral damage to the normal bacterial flora also results in infection by other pathogens such as *Clostridium difficile* and fungi. Logic dictates that antimicrobial drugs should only be prescribed when benefit outweighs risk and that unnecessary use should be avoided.

## Definition of terms

The terms guidelines, formularies, and policies are often used interchangeably but they are separate, complementary components of a strategy for prudent antimicrobial use.

- *Guidelines* provide advice about what drug should be prescribed for a specific clinical condition. They may take the form of a care pathway or flow chart outlining processes of care including investigations and therapies other than just antimicrobial compounds (e.g. use of fluid replacement and oxygenation in a pneumonia guideline).

- A *formulary* is a limited list of drugs available for prescription. It may include information about available formulations (by route of administration), dosing instructions, and advice about drug safety or interactions but it does not include detailed guidance for use.

- An *antimicrobial policy* is a set of statements about an organization's strategy for promoting prudent antimicrobial prescribing. This can include a limited list of antimicrobial agents that are generally available to all prescribers—in other words, an antimicrobial formulary. However, an antimicrobial policy should also contain guidelines about treatment of specific conditions.

  - *Restrictive policies*. In addition to guidance, antimicrobial policies may include enforcement strategies such as requiring authorization of initial prescription or automatic stop orders (e.g. orders for intravenous vancomycin will be stopped after three days unless authorization for continued use is obtained from a consultant microbiologist).

  - *Persuasive policies*. This term is used to distinguish policies that do not include enforcement strategies and rely on persuading professionals to follow the policy. This term is preferred to educational because most restrictive policies have an educational component.

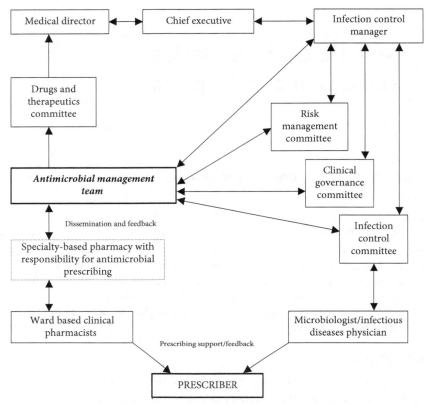

**Fig. 19.1** Model pathway for implementing improvements in antimicrobial prescribing practice in hospitals. The antimicrobial management team has a central coordinating role in feedback of information to individual prescribers, clinical teams, and senior management.

Reproduced from Nathwani D., Antimicrobial prescribing policy and practice in Scotland: recommendations for good antimicrobial practice in acute hospitals, *Journal of Antimicrobial Chemotherapy*, Volume 57, Issue 6, pp. 1189–1196, Copyright © 2006, with permission from Oxford University Press

An antimicrobial management team is a multidisciplinary team in which each member is given specific roles and which collectively takes responsibility for implementation of local policies (Fig. 19.1). To be effective, the team must have full support from organizational leadership and provide regular feedback to individual clinicians and clinical teams about their compliance with policies. This rule applies equally to primary care and to hospital care; the key point is that guidelines, formularies, and policies will not change practice unless they are actively implemented.

## National policies and laws

Self-medication with antimicrobial drugs is the norm in countries where they are freely available over the counter; self-medication is estimated to account for over 90 per cent of all antimicrobial drug use in the Philippines. There are undoubtedly some potential advantages to increasing the availability of antibacterial agents without prescription, such as convenience for the patient, faster initiation of treatment, and a reduction in primary care workload. However, in the European

Union and North America, the risks of increasing access are thought to outweigh these benefits. The degree of control of supply of antimicrobial compounds is highly variable between countries. In the most conservative countries, free sale is banned, professional limits are placed on prescription practices by law, and there is statutory control of advertising. No advertising is allowed to the lay public, and the content of professional advertising is limited by law. To be effective, these comprehensive restrictions need to be backed up by tightly controlled availability of antimicrobial drugs and rigorous enforcement of regulations.

## Benefits of standardization

Antimicrobial formularies and policies should be seen as part of more general efforts to promote rational prescribing. In any therapeutic area, there are likely to be several drugs that have similar effectiveness for specific conditions and there are advantages to standardizing which of the options is chosen for common indications. There are additional benefits to standardizing the range of antimicrobial drugs used (Table 19.1). At the same time, there may be concerns that continuous use of a limited range of antimicrobial compounds will promote the development of resistance by focusing the selection pressure onto a narrow range of drugs. Although this sounds logical, several lines of evidence indicate that use of a restricted range of antimicrobial agents is strongly associated with lower total use. Prudent antimicrobial prescribers are conservative about whom they give these drugs to as well as the range of compounds that they use.

## Prudent antimicrobial prescribing

Prudent antimicrobial prescribing has been defined as: the right drug for the right condition for the right amount of time. Any unnecessary use in human medicine should be minimized to reduce selective pressure in the environment. There are five key questions that need to be addressed for prudent antimicrobial prescribing:

1  Does the patient need antimicrobial therapy?
2  If needed, what are the most appropriate drug, route, dosage, and frequency of administration?
3  When and how should response to treatment be reviewed?
4  When should treatment be stopped?
5  Who is responsible for review of response to treatment and for stopping treatment?

## Content of antimicrobial policies

See Table 19.2. Antimicrobial policies should promote prudent prescribing by ensuring that an effective range of antimicrobial drugs is maintained. They should define effective treatment (including appropriate dosages), avoid unnecessary treatment, reduce the emergence of antimicrobial resistance, promote good practice, and contain costs. Contact details should be given for further advice, for example, about public health and infection control issues or about therapeutic drug monitoring. Policies should be dated and state when the document will be revised. In the UK the National Audit Office recommends at least annual revision of hospital policies. However, now that most antibiotic policies are web based, they can be updated regularly without requiring expensive reprinting and dissemination of printed documents.

Ideally policy recommendations should be linked to evidence. This can be relatively easy to achieve if the local policy is adapted from a national document based on systematic review of

**Table 19.1** General and specific benefits of limiting the range of drugs used for conditions through guidelines, formularies, and policies.

| Category | Benefits |
| --- | --- |
| Knowledge | *General*: |
| | Promotes awareness of benefits, risks and cost of prescribing |
| | Focuses learning about safety and drug interactions on a limited range of drugs |
| | Reduces the impact of aggressive marketing by the pharmaceutical industry |
| | Encourages rational use of drugs based on analysis of pharmacology, clinical effectiveness, safety, and cost |
| | *Specific to antimicrobial agents*: |
| | Targets education about local epidemiology of pathogens towards knowledge of their susceptibility to a limited range of compounds |
| | Promotes awareness of the strengths and weaknesses of specific antimicrobial drugs |
| Attitudes | *General*: |
| | Acceptance by clinicians of the importance of setting standards of care and prescribing |
| | Acceptance of peer review and audit of prescribing |
| | *Specific to antimicrobial agents*: |
| | Recognition of the complex issues underlying antimicrobial chemotherapy |
| | Recognition of the importance of the special expertise required for full evaluation of antimicrobial chemotherapy: |
| | Diagnostic microbiology |
| | Epidemiology and infection control |
| | Clinical diagnosis and recognition of other diseases mimicking infection |
| | Pharmacokinetics and pharmacodynamics of antimicrobial agents |
| Behaviour | *General*: |
| | Increased compliance with guidelines and treatment policies |
| | Reduction of medical practice variation |
| | *Specific to antimicrobial agents*: |
| | Improved liaison between clinicians, pharmacists, microbiologists, and the infection control team |
| Outcome | *General*: |
| | Standardization is a key strategy for improving patient safety. |
| | Improved efficiency of prescribing by increasing sensitivity (patients who can benefit receive treatment) and specificity (treatment is not prescribed to patients who will not benefit: |
| | Improved clinical outcome |
| | Reduces medicolegal liability |
| | *Specific to antimicrobial agents*: |
| | Limits emergence and spread of drug-resistant strains |

**Table 19.2** Recommended template for antimicrobial guidelines.

Antimicrobial guidelines should be evidence-based and prepared in line with best practice recommendations for treatment guidelines. 4 The provision of costing information within the guideline should be discussed locally.

Recommendations for the content and detail of local antimicrobial policies.

1. Title page

    1.1. Name of policy

    1.2. Specify the condition and patient group where appropriate

    1.3. Date

    1.4. Version

    1.5. Review date

    1.6. Authors

    1.7. Contact details for enquiries for normal hours and out of hours

    1.8. Contact details for microbiological and pharmacological information

    1.9. Details of electronic availability

2. Introduction section

    2.1. Statement as to whether the guideline is mandatory or for guidance only

    2.2. Contents

    2.3. Guidance on the local procedure for microbiological samples

    2.4. Abbreviations used in the text

    2.5. Reference should be made to guidance in the British National Formulary under Prescription writing. These notes lay out a standard for expressing strengths and encourage directions in English not Latin abbreviations.

3. Summary list of available antimicrobials

    3.1. The antimicrobials that are recommended in the guidelines should be listed, with clear indications to the route of administration and should state whether they are:

• Unrestricted

• Restricted (approval of a specialist is required)

• Permitted for specific conditions (for example, co-trimoxazole for Pneumocystis)

4. Regimens for treatment and prevention of common infections

| Treatment | Prophylaxis |
|---|---|
| • First-line recommendation | • First-line recommendation for empirical therapy |
| • Second-line recommendation | • Second-line recommendation for empirical therapy |
| • Timing | • Dose |
| • Dose | • Timing of initial dose |
| • Route of administration | • Route of administration |
| • Duration of treatment | • Details of repeat dosing if required |
| • Rules for intravenous to oral switch | |

evidence. However, it is unreasonable to expect individual primary or secondary care organizations to conduct their own systematic reviews of evidence. This would involve massive duplication of effort and it is highly unlikely that all have the necessary skills. National and international organizations should take responsibility for regular review of evidence to support development of antimicrobial policies. National templates are an efficient method for defining the core evidence for antimicrobial policies, while still leaving much decision making to local policy makers, who can select a range of effective antimicrobial agents based on local information about susceptibility patterns and drug costs.

Recommendations about treatment of specific conditions should include advice about withholding therapy (Box 19.1). Antimicrobial treatment should not be prescribed, for example, for patients with asymptomatic bacteriuria (except in pregnancy; see Chapter 23) or for most patients with upper respiratory symptoms (see Chapter 21).

Advice should be given about methods for assessment of severity of infections and criteria for diagnosis of sepsis, severe sepsis, and septic shock (see Chapter 26). Advice about chemoprophylaxis (see Chapter 18) should be included in addition to treatment of infection. Hospital policies should include guidance on criteria for intravenous administration and for switching patients from intravenous to oral formulations.

## Implementation of policies

There is increasing emphasis on the need for antimicrobial management teams, who work closely with infection control teams (Fig. 19.1). The core skills of the team should include diagnosis of infection, assessment of severity, surveillance of prescribing and resistance, pharmacokinetics, and pharmacodynamics. It is critical that the team has the full support of senior management and good communication with risk management and clinical governance teams. There are potential risks to reducing antimicrobial use, and it is unlikely that the antimicrobial management team has all the skills necessary to assess these risks or to devise a balanced set of measures that will reassure everybody that change in prescribing is an improvement.

Antimicrobial management teams are becoming well established in hospitals and the same model can be adapted to primary care. The need to interact with infection control, risk management, and clinical governance is just as necessary, especially in residential care and nursing homes. Multidisciplinary involvement in prescribing is increasingly common in primary care.

## Do antimicrobial policies work?

The first aim should be to change antimicrobial prescribing, which may have a variety of secondary aims (e.g. improving clinical effectiveness, limiting drug resistance, and reducing unnecessary prescribing costs; see Chapter 20).

There is a lot of evidence about the effectiveness of interventions to change antimicrobial prescribing but unfortunately much of it is unreliable. The Cochrane Library contains two reviews on interventions to improve antimicrobial prescribing in primary and hospital care. Over half of the studies in primary care and hospitals were rejected because the articles reported uncontrolled evaluations. It is impossible to assess the impact of an intervention without some information on what would have happened in its absence. This does not mean that randomized controlled trials are the only acceptable method for evaluation; much simpler designs can be used. These include controlled before—and—after studies (Table 19.3) and interrupted time series (Fig. 19.2).

## Box 19.1 Recommended approach for prudent antimicrobial use in primary care through minimizing unnecessary use in respiratory infection

1 Detailed history and examination.

2 Ask directly about patient's expectation for antibiotics.

3 Decision options:

3.1 No antibiotic—reassure patients that antibiotics are not needed because they are likely to make little difference to the symptoms and may have side effects.

3.2 Delayed antibiotics—reassure patients that antibiotics are not needed because they are likely to make little difference to the symptoms and may have side effects. Advise on using delayed antibiotics if symptoms are not settling within a recognized time frame.

3.3 Immediate antibiotics—consider in the following situations:

3.3.1 Children under 2 years with bilateral otitis media.

3.3.2 Acute otitis media in children with otorrhoea.

3.3.3 Acute sore throat with three or more CENTOR criteria (tonsillar exudate, tender anterior cervical lymphadenopathy, lymphadenitis, fever and an absence of cough).

3.3.4 Systemically very unwell.

3.3.5 Pre-existing co-morbidity.

3.3.6 Those who are over 65 with acute cough and at least two of the following, or over 80 with acute cough and at least one of the following: admission to hospital in the past 12 months; diabetes; heart failure; glucocorticoids.

4 Advise patients on the likely timescale for the illness:

4.1 Acute otitis media—four days.

4.2 Acute sore throat —one week.

4.3 Acute rhinosinusitis—two and one-half weeks.

4.4 Acute bronchitis—three weeks.

5 Give symptom management advice and safety-net (delayed) antibiotic prescription.

Adapted with permission from Scottish Antimicrobial Prescribing Group (SAPG), *Prudent Antimicrobial use in Primary Care-Respiratory 2012*, Copyright © SAPG 2012, available from http://www. scottishmedicines.org.uk/files/sapg/Prudent_antimicrobial_use_respiratory.pdf

Note that in Scotland this simple advice has been superseded by the Scottish Reduction in Antimicrobial Prescribing (ScRAP) Programme, Full details and all educational resources are available at http://www.nes.scot.nhs.uk/education-and-training/by-discipline/pharmacy/about-nes-pharmacy/ educational-resources/resources-by-topic/infectious-diseases/antibiotics/scottish-reduction-in-antimicrobial-prescribing-%28scrap%29-programme.aspx

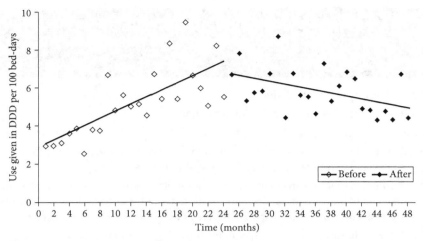

**Fig. 19.2** Example of an interrupted time series that showed significant reduction in use of 'alert antibiotics':

1. Immediate reduction in use on introduction of the policy: −0.7 defined daily dose (DDD), 95 per cent confidence interval (CI), −1.8 to 0.4, $P = 0.2$.

2. Sustained reduction in use in the 24 months after introduction of the policy: −0.3 DDD per month, 95 per cent CI, −03 to −0.2, $P < 0.0001$.

Reproduced from Ansari F et al., Outcomes of an intervention to improve hospital antibiotic prescribing: interrupted time series with segmented regression analysis, *Journal of Antimicrobial Chemotherapy*, Volume 52, Issue 5, pp. 842–48, Copyright © 2003, with permission from Oxford University Press.

**Table 19.3** Example of a controlled before-and-after study that showed a large reduction in primary care antimicrobial drug prescribing for acute bronchitis with no adverse effect on rates of repeat consultation for bronchitis or pneumonia.

|  | Antimicrobial prescribing (%) | | Repeat consultations (%) | |
| --- | --- | --- | --- | --- |
|  | **Before** | **After** | **Before** | **After** |
| Control (no intervention) | 82 | 77 | 6 | 7 |
| Partial intervention[a] | 78 | 76 | 4 | 4 |
| Full intervention[b] | 74 | 48 | 6 | 5 |

[a] Supply of patient information leaflets to doctors' offices.

[b] Supply of leaflets plus information targeted at households at the start of the winter as well as a clinician intervention consisting of group education, practice-profiling, and one-to-one education of individual prescribers.

Source: data from Gonzales R et al., Decreasing antimicrobial use in ambulatory practice: impact of a multidimensional intervention on the treatment of uncomplicated acute bronchitis in adults, *Journal of the American Medical Association*, Volume 281, Number 16, pp. 1512–1519, Copyright © 1999 American Medical Association. All Rights Reserved.

There are striking differences in the methods that have been used to change antimicrobial prescribing in primary and hospital care. Less than 10 per cent of the interventions in primary care were restrictive, whereas nearly half of the hospital interventions included some form of restriction. This difference arises from the very different structures of primary and hospital care. First, practitioners in primary care are more likely to be independent rather than salaried employees of an organization. Second, it is much easier to restrict supply of drugs in a single hospital than in a primary care organization that may include tens or even hundreds of offices in different locations. A further difference is that 31 per cent of the primary care interventions targeted patients, either alone or alongside interventions on professionals. Again, this reflects the very different context, because shared decision making between patients and professionals is the norm in primary care, whereas it is still uncommon in hospitals, especially during inpatient care of acute illness. Taken together, the Cochrane reviews evaluated eight different persuasive and five different restrictive strategies and found that all are supported by at least one successful study. Consequently there is a lot of evidence about the changes that can be made to prescribing. More importantly there is increasing evidence to show that change in prescribing results in improvement to both clinical and microbial outcomes (see Chapter 20).

## Which antimicrobial policies work best?

In hospitals restrictive interventions do have a much greater immediate impact on prescribing than persuasive ones, so restriction is justified when there is a need for rapid change in prescribing (Fig. 19.3). However, restrictions can have unintended consequences. Clinicians may be very resentful about having restrictions imposed on their practice, in which case they will find ways to overcome them, which are considered in more detail in Chapter 20. Comparison of the effectiveness of restrictive versus persuasive interventions suggests that the initially greater impact of restrictive interventions reduces over time (Fig. 19.3). Unless there is a very clear justification for needing an immediate impact on prescribing (e.g. an outbreak of infections caused by multiresistant bacteria), it may be more effective in the long term to use a slower, persuasive strategy.

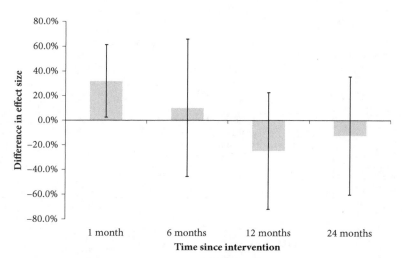

**Fig. 19.3** Difference in the effect on hospital antibacterial prescribing of restrictive versus persuasive interventions. At 1 month there is a 32 per cent difference in effect size (restrictive-persuasive; 95% confidence interval, 2–61%). There is no significant difference at 6, 12, or 24 months. Data are from 40 studies conducted in 46 hospitals.

Adapted from Davey P et al., 'Interventions to improve antibiotic prescribing practices for hospital inpatients', *Cochrane Database of Systematic Reviews* (Online), Volume 4, CD003543, Copyright © 2013 The Cochrane Collaboration, published by John Wiley & Sons Ltd, with permission.

In primary care, multifaceted interventions that aim to influence patients as well as professionals have generally produced much greater changes in prescribing than interventions that are aimed only at patients or professionals. Delayed prescriptions have been consistently successful in reducing prescribing for respiratory tract infections. The doctor says to the patient or parent that in their opinion there is no need to prescribe an antimicrobial drug; they provide an information sheet explaining how the symptoms will resolve without treatment but they also say that they will leave an antimicrobial prescription at reception to be collected if required. Between 50 and 70 per cent of these delayed prescriptions are never collected.

The most successful guidelines and policies involve the professionals who are the targets for change in development, dissemination, and implementation. Involvement in implementation is best accomplished by feedback of information about practice. Evidence about behaviour change interventions from psychology has shown that they are most effective when feedback is linked to a goal and to action planning (Fig. 19.4). The goal should be a clear, measurable target, and action planning should be used to agree specific responses when feedback shows a gap between performance and the target (Fig. 19.4). A meta-analysis of randomized clinical trials showed that control theory independently explained some of the variation in the effectiveness of audit and feedback in medicine (Table 19.4). However, only 3 per cent of interventions included both action planning and target setting, 14 (10%) just included target setting, 41 (29%) just included action planning, and 84 (60%) included neither action planning nor target setting.

Setting a measurable target is relatively straightforward, for example, 95 per cent reliability for recording of indication for antibiotic treatment and compliance with antibiotic policy (Fig. 19.5). The aim will be even more specific if it is timed (e.g. achieve 95% compliance with policy within 6 months). Finally, it is important to link the antimicrobial prescribing target to a higher-order goal, for example, in Scotland the target for compliance with a primary care antibiotic policy (Fig. 19.6)

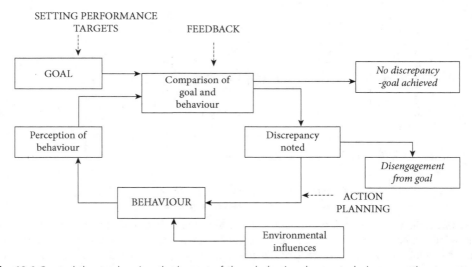

**Fig. 19.4** Control theory showing the impact of three behavior change techniques: setting targets, providing feedback and action planning.

Reprinted from *Social Science & Medicine*, Vol 70, Gardner B et al, 'Using theory to synthesise evidence from behaviour change interventions: the example of audit and feedback', 1618–25, 2010, with permission from Elsevier.

**Table 19.4** Characteristics that influence the effectiveness of audit and feedback based on multivariate meta-regression with data from 80 randomized clinical trials that had low risk of bias.

| Characteristic of the feedback or recipient | Impact on the effectiveness of the intervention | Significance of effect |
| --- | --- | --- |
| Format of feedback | Both verbal and written more effective than either alone | $P = 0.020$ |
| Source of feedback | From a superior or colleague more effective than from the investigators or the employer or a professional standards review organization | $P < 0.001$ |
| Frequency of feedback | Monthly feedback more effective than less frequent feedback | $P < 0.001$ |
| Instructions for improvement | More effective with both explicit, measurable target and action planning versus action planning alone, which was more effective than interventions with no action planning | $P < 0.001$ |
| Direction of change required | More effective if the intervention intended to decrease current behaviour versus increase current behaviour | $P < 0.001$ |
| Baseline performance | More effective if the baseline performance was poor | $P = 0.007$ |
| Profession of recipient | No difference if the recipient was a physician versus non-physician | $P = 0.561$ |

Adapted from Ivers N et al. 'Audit and feedback: effects on professional practice and healthcare outcomes,' *Cochrane Database of Systematic Reviews*, Issue 6, CD000259, Copyright © 2012 The Cochrane Collaboration, with permission from John Wiley & Sons.

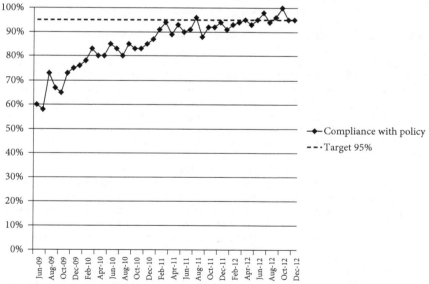

**Fig. 19.5** Improvement in recording of indication in the notes, and in compliance with hospital antibiotic policy in hospitals in Scotland. Hospitals collect data monthly from acute medical and surgical admissions units. By December 2010 all 56 hospital units in 14 health boards were collecting data, and compliance had improved from 60 per cent to 85 per cent. The aim was to achieve 95 per cent compliance with policy, a level which occurred in April 2012.

Source: data reproduced with permission from Scottish Antimicrobial Prescribing Group (SAPG). Quarterly reports on this national indicator are publicly available from http://www.scottishmedicines.org.uk/SAPG/Policies_and_Guidance

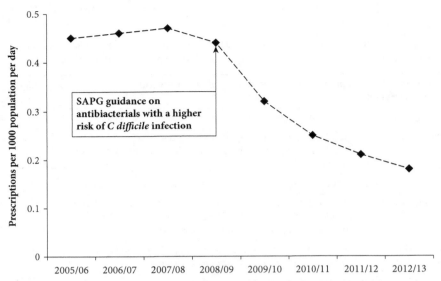

**Fig. 19.6** Reduction in use of antibiotics associated with a higher risk of *C. difficile* infection (ciprofloxacin, cephalosporins, clindamycin, and co-amoxiclav) in primary care in Scotland after introduction of national target for reduction in *C. difficile* in 2009.

Adapted with permission from Scottish Antimicrobial Prescribing Group (SAPG), *Primary Care Prescribing Indicators 2010*, Copyright © 2010 SAPG, available from http://www.isdscotland.org/isd/6463.html; and Scottish Antimicrobial Prescribing Group (SAPG), *Primary Care Prescribing Indicators Annual Report 2012–13*, Copyright © 2013, SAPG, available from http://www.isdscotland.org/Health-Topics/Prescribing-and-Medicines/Publications/2013–10–29/2013–10–29-SAPG-Primary-Care-PI-Report-2012–2013.pdf?4099673033

**Table 19.5** Examples of action planning from hospital and primary care interventions that changed antimicrobial prescribing.

| | |
|---|---|
| Hospital intervention to reduce unnecessary vancomycin use | For patients whose prescribing was deemed not to conform with the agreed guidelines, the prescribing doctor and supervising medical officer were given immediate concurrent feedback on the very same day. This entailed the issue of a memo signed by a consultant physician or microbiologist, detailing the suspected 'errant' prescribing for the specific patient, together with an explanation. Depending on what was appropriate, the memo also included explicit advice to (i) discontinue such treatment entirely, (ii) prescribe an alternative medication/intervention (pending further information if necessary), or (iii) avoid such prescribing in the future under similar circumstances. The memo also provided contact telephone/fax numbers to enable the relevant doctors to seek clarification, justify, or challenge the advice given. Patients for whom prescribing prompted memos with a suggestion to discontinue treatment with either drug were also followed up (repeatedly if necessary) to document whether the advice had been complied with. |
| Primary care intervention to reduce total antibiotic prescribing | Each individual prescriber in this group received audit and feedback plus face-to-face interactive educational meetings with clinical pharmacologists who were experts in prescribing (academic detailing). The interactive discussions normally lasted about two hours. They were reminded through personal visit two weeks later. They also received feedback from audits for one month post-intervention with written specific recommendations for improvement and they were reminded two weeks later. |

Source: data from Kumana CR et al., Curtailing unnecessary vancomycin usage in a hospital with high rates of methicillin resistant *Staphylococcus aureus* infections, *British Journal of Clinical Pharmacology*, Volume 52, Issue 4, pp. 427–32, Copyright © 2001; and Awad AI et al., Changing antibiotics prescribing practices in health centers of Khartoum State, Sudan, *European Journal of Clinical Pharmacology*, Volume 62, Issue 2, pp. 135–43, Copyright © Springer-Verlag 2006.

was explicitly linked to a national goal of reduction in *C. difficile* infections (CDI). Action planning requires discussion or written advice to prescribers about how they can modify their behaviour to improve performance in response to feedback (Table 19.5).

## Antibiotic policy implementation at the population level

The European Surveillance of Antimicrobial Consumption (ESAC) has developed methods for sustainable measurement of prescribing and indicators of prescribing quality. In Scotland the ESAC indicators were adopted in 2009 as national targets to support the higher-order goal of reduction in CDI. In hospitals there has been a steady increase in the number of participating hospital units and in their compliance with local antibiotic policies (Fig. 19.5); in primary care there has been a 49 per cent reduction in use of antibiotics associated with CDI (Fig. 19.6) since 2009, with an associated marked decrease in CDI (Fig. 19.7).

## Implications for research and practice

The most important deficiency to address is in the quality of the research evidence. The criteria for reliable evidence are simple and readily accessible through the ORION guidelines for transparent reporting of *Outbreak Reports* and *Intervention studies Of Nosocomial infection*. All that remains is for sponsors of research and journal editors to refuse to support collection and publication of poor quality evidence.

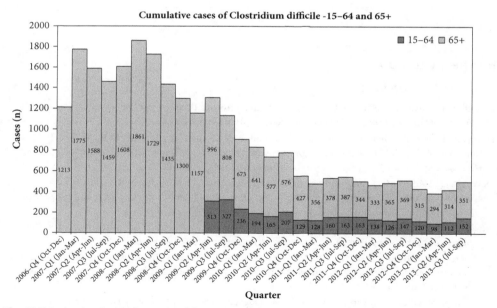

**Fig. 19.7** Reduction in CDI in Scotland from 2009 in association with the reduction in use of antimicrobials with higher risk of CDI in hospitals and primary care.

Source: data from The Quarterly Surveillance Report on the Surveillance of Clostridium difficile infection (CDI) in Scotland, October-December 2013, Copyright © Health Protection Scotland - a division of NHS National Services Scotland, available from http://www.hps.scot.nhs.uk/documents/ewr/pdf2014/1413.pdf

Measurement of antimicrobial prescribing, surveillance of important microbial outcomes, and balancing measures of clinical outcome should be part of routine practice in primary and hospital care. Antimicrobial resistance is a key public health problem so measures of prudent prescribing are important for patient safety.

## Key points

- Antimicrobial policies should include guidelines about management of specific infections, in addition to providing a list of recommended and restricted drugs (a formulary).

- Prudent antimicrobial prescribing means treating the right patient at the right time for the right duration.

- Antimicrobial policies should contain recommendations for treatment and prophylaxis. They should include advice about patients who should not receive antimicrobials.

- Restrictive antimicrobial policies are more effective in the short term but persuasive policies have more sustained effects. Restrictive policies may be justified when the need is urgent (e.g. to control an outbreak of drug-resistant infections).

- Feedback of information about prescribing is an effective method for professional behavioural change. Feedback is most effective when linked to a specific aim (e.g. 50% reduction in unnecessary intravenous antibiotics within six months) and when discrepancy between performance and the aim is addressed through action planning.

## Further reading

### Antimicrobial policies

Arnold, S. R. and Straus, S. E. (2005) Interventions to improve antibiotic prescribing practices in ambulatory care. *Cochrane Database of Systematic Reviews*, **Issue 4**: Art. No. CD003539.

Davey, P., Brown, E., Charani, E., Fenelon, L., Gould, I.M., Holmes, A., Ramsay, C. R., Wiffen, P. J., and Wilcox, M. (2013) Interventions to improve antibiotic prescribing practices for hospital inpatients. *Cochrane Database of Systematic Reviews*, **Issue 4**: Art. No. CD003543.

Davey, P. G., Nathwani, D., and Rubinstein, E. (2010) 'Antimicrobial Policies', in R. G. Finch, D. Greenwood, and S. R. Norrby, eds, *Antibiotic and Chemotherapy. Anti-infective agents and their use in therapy*. London: Churchill Elsevier, pp. 126–43.

European Commission. (2014) *Key Documents on Antimicrobial Resistance*. <http://ec.europa.eu/health/antimicrobial_resistance/key_documents/index_en.htm>, accessed 28 February 2014.

Gardner, B., Whittington, C., McAteer, J., Eccles, M. P., and Michie, S. (2010) Using theory to synthesise evidence from behaviour change interventions: the example of audit and feedback. *Social Science and Medicine*,**70**(10): 1618–25.

Ivers, N., Jamtvedt, G., Flottorp, S., Young, J. M., Odgaard-Jensen, J., French, S. D., O'Brien, M. A, Johansen, M., Grimshaw, J., and Oxman, A. D. (2012) Audit and feedback: effects on professional practice and healthcare outcomes. *Cochrane Database of Systematic Reviews*, **Issue 6**: Art. No. CD000259.

Malcolm, W., Nathwani, D., Davey, P., Cromwell, T., Patton, A., Reilly, J., Cairns, S., and Bennie, M. (2013) From intermittent antibiotic point prevalence surveys to quality improvement: experience in Scottish hospitals. *Antimicrobial Resistance and Infection Control*, 2(1): 3.

Nathwani, D., Sneddon, J., Malcolm, W., et al. (2011) Scottish Antimicrobial Prescribing Group (SAPG): development and impact of the Scottish National Antimicrobial Stewardship Programme. *International Journal of Antimicrobial Agents*, 38(1):16–26.

Specialist Advisory Committee on Antimicrobial Resistance (SACAR). (2007) Appendix 2 Specialist Advisory Committee on Antimicrobial Resistance (SACAR) Antimicrobial Framework. *Journal of Antimicrobial Chemotherapy*, 60(Suppl 1): i87–i90.

Stone, S. P., Cooper, B. S., Kibbler, C. C., et al. (2007) The ORION statement: guidelines for transparent reporting of outbreak reports and intervention studies of nosocomial infection. *Lancet Infectious Diseases*, 7(4):282–8.

## Websites

Advisory Committee on Antimicrobial Resistance and Healthcare Associated Infections (ARHAI). https://www.gov.uk/government/groups/advisory-committee-on-antimicrobial-resistance-and-healthcare-associated-infection

Centers for Disease Control and Prevention. (2014) *Get Smart for Healthcare.* <http://www.cdc.gov/getsmart/healthcare/>, accessed 29 November 2014.

Infectious Diseases Research Network. (2009) *ORION Statement.* <http://www.idrn.org/orion.php>, accessed 29 November 2014.

Scottish Medicines Consortium. (2014) *About the Scottish Antimicrobial Prescribing Group (SAPG).* <http://www.scottishmedicines.org.uk/SAPG>, accessed 29 November 2014.

World Health Organization. (2011) *The WHO Policy Package to Combat Antimicrobial Resistance.* <http://www.who.int/bulletin/volumes/89/5/11–088435/en/>, accessed 29 November 2014.

# Chapter 20

# Antimicrobial stewardship, surveillance of antimicrobial consumption, and its consequences

## Introduction to antimicrobial stewardship

Stewardship means responsible caretaking; the concept is based on the premise that we do not own the planet's resources. Rather, we are managers of resources and are responsible to future generations for their condition. Antimicrobial stewardship recognizes that there are two competing goals: first, to ensure effective treatment of patients with infection and, second, to minimize collateral damage from antimicrobial use. Both antimicrobial resistance and *Clostridium difficile* infection (CDI) are manifestations of the collateral damage to the normal flora that is an inevitable consequence of antimicrobial use. The solution to both problems lies in a combination of strategies to minimize collateral damage from use of antibiotics and promote use of infection control to minimize risk of colonization. Moreover CDI is a powerful stimulus to change because it is a very immediate threat to the patient who is receiving antibiotics, whereas selection of resistant bacteria may have no immediate impact on patients or their carers. Consequently, control of CDI is now an integral component of most national antibiotic prescribing programmes.

## Measurement of antimicrobial use

Sir William Thomson (Lord Kelvin), a nineteenth-century physicist, said 'If you cannot measure it, you cannot improve it.' Hence, surveillance of antimicrobial use is essential to improvement and to antimicrobial stewardship. Ideally, all health-care organizations should be able to measure the number of patients treated, the indication for treatment, details of therapy, including drug, dose, route, and duration, and the consequences of treatment. In reality this level of detail is only available in research databases (see e.g. Fig. 21.1). The only routine information that is available in most countries is about the total amount of antibiotic used, and most hospitals can only measure antibiotic use in terms of amount dispensed to clinical locations from the hospital pharmacy. Nonetheless, measurement of total antimicrobial consumption is a key component of clinical governance assurance on antimicrobial stewardship for all health-care organizations (Box 20.1). In order to compare between countries or organizations, a standardized method is required for estimating the number of people treated, adjusted for population size.

### Longitudinal surveillance

#### Estimating the number of people treated with antimicrobials

The origins of the World Health Organization (WHO) ATC/DDD method for surveillance of drug use can be traced to a symposium in Oslo in 1969 entitled 'The Consumption of Drugs',

## Box 20.1 Key domains for health-care organizations to assess their antibiotic stewardship

1  Antimicrobial management within the organization
  - Structures and lines of responsibility and accountability are clearly defined.
  - There is high level notification of reports on antibiotic stewardship to the board and its non-executive directors.
  - There is an antimicrobial management committee with regular, documented meetings, and action lists with clear lines of reporting to infection control, drug, and therapeutics committees and to clinical groups.

2  Operational delivery of an antimicrobial strategy
  - Antimicrobial management policies in place.
  - Restricted access to selected antimicrobials.
  - Evidence-based guidelines for treatment of common infections.
  - Frequent (at least two yearly) review of all policies and guidelines.
  - Availability of electronic versions through networked computers.
  - Availability of an easily accessible printed summary to all wards and prescribers (e.g. a pocket guide).
  - Selection for the guidelines is informed by local microbiological sensitivity patterns with selective reporting of results by a microbiology laboratory in line with formulary choices.
  - There is a policy stipulating that indication should be recorded before antimicrobials are prescribed.
  - The policy stipulates that course length or review date is recorded on the prescription chart at time of prescribing.
  - The policy stipulates that prescriptions for antimicrobials be reviewed at least every 48 hours.
  - The policy stipulates that appropriate de-escalation of therapy takes place and includes intravenous-to-oral switch guidelines.
  - The policy provides guidance on choice, dose, route, intravenous switch, and typical duration of treatment for each indication.
  - There are antimicrobial ward rounds.
  - Advice from a medical microbiologist/infectious disease physician is available by telephone.

3  Risk assessment for antimicrobial chemotherapy
  - Guidelines include advice on managing the following risks:
    - managing patients with allergies to antimicrobials;
    - safe administration of intravenous antimicrobials;
    - dosing optimization for antimicrobials with a narrow therapeutic index; and
    - therapeutic drug monitoring for high-risk antimicrobials.
  - Safety of antimicrobials is linked to incident reporting with feedback and action plans.
  - Incident reports are sent to the antimicrobial management committee.

**Box 20.1 Key domains for health-care organizations to assess their antibiotic stewardship** *(continued)*

4  Clinical governance assurance

- There is a programme for audit of the antimicrobial policy, treatment, and prophylaxis guidelines, with feedback of results to each clinical group at least once a year.
- Total antimicrobial consumption is monitored.
- Total antimicrobial consumption is reported to clinical groups.
- Attendance at audit feedback meetings is recorded.
- Action plans by clinical groups are recorded and shared with the antimicrobial management committee.

5  Education and training

- There is an antimicrobial education and training strategy.
- All antimicrobial prescribers receive printed information about antimicrobial prescribing, formulary, and guidelines at induction.
- All pharmacists receive printed information about antimicrobial prescribing, formulary, and guidelines at induction.
- An annual update on safe and effective antimicrobial prescribing is available for all prescribers, pharmacists, and staff who administer antimicrobials.
- The proportion of trainee doctors and senior doctors who attend training on safe and effective antimicrobial prescribing is recorded.
- The proportion of staff attending training on safe and effective antimicrobial prescribing is recorded.
- Competency assessment is carried out for antimicrobial prescribers.

6  Antimicrobial pharmacist

- There is a substantive antimicrobial pharmacist post in place.
- The lead antimicrobial pharmacist has a qualification higher than a first degree (e.g. Diploma/MSc).
- The lead antimicrobial pharmacist has specialist training in infection management and antimicrobial use.
- The lead antimicrobial pharmacist has written objectives with an annual appraisal.

7  Patients, carers, and the public

- There is a policy for providing information on antimicrobials to patients.
- Patients or their legal guardian are told they have been prescribed an antimicrobial, the reason why this is necessary, and the risks and side effects associated with antimicrobial treatment.
- Patients who are taking antimicrobials at home are informed about the course length, the importance of finishing the course and what to do if side effects develop at home.

where it was agreed that an internationally accepted classification system for drug consumption studies was needed. In order to measure drug use, it is important to have both a classification system and a unit of measurement. Norwegian researchers developed a system known as the anatomical therapeutic chemical (ATC) classification, and a technical unit of measurement called the defined daily dose (DDD). The Nordic Council on Medicines was established in 1975, and the Nordic Statistics on Medicines using the ATC/DDD methodology was published for the first time in 1976.

In 1981, the WHO Regional Office for Europe recommended the ATC/DDD system for international drug utilization studies, and in 1996 WHO recognized the need to develop use of the ATC/DDD system as an international standard for drug utilization studies. The aim was to support the WHO's initiatives to achieve universal access to needed drugs and rational use of drugs, particularly in developing countries. Access to standardized and validated information on drug use is essential to allow audit of patterns of drug utilization, identification of problems, educational or other interventions, and monitoring of the outcomes of the interventions.

It is important to recognize that the classification of a substance in the ATC/DDD system is not a recommendation for use, nor does it imply any judgements about efficacy or relative efficacy of drugs and groups of drugs.

The European Surveillance of Antimicrobial Consumption (ESAC) was established as a project at the University of Antwerp in 2001 and transferred to the European Centre for Disease Prevention and Control (ECDC) in 2011. ESAC-NET uses the WHO ATC/DDD system to provide publicly accessible information about antimicrobial consumption in European countries. National data come from two principal sources: wholesale supply of drugs, or national systems for the reimbursement of patients or health-care professionals for the cost of dispensing drugs from community pharmacies or doctors' offices. The 2011 report has data about the consumption of antimicrobials in ambulatory care for 29 countries, whereas hospital data were only available for 18 countries. The ESAC hospital care data come from national wholesale suppliers and only give an indication of total consumption at the national level. It is not possible to identify consumption by individual hospitals. In contrast, many countries can provide detailed regional data about consumption in ambulatory care, adjusted for regional population size. Consequently, most of the ESAC publications and reports about national consumption focus on ambulatory care.

Some countries record the number of prescriptions for antimicrobials (Fig. 20.1). For antimicrobials, this is a good indicator of the number of people treated, because most patients only receive a single prescription for each course of treatment. In the United States most hospitals have electronic records of treatment dispensed to individual patients and can provide information about actual days of treatment.

## Estimating population size

In ambulatory care, antibiotic use is usually adjusted for number of inhabitants (e.g. DDD per 1,000 inhabitants or prescriptions per 1,000 inhabitants). In hospitals, estimation of population size is more complicated. The WHO recommends that antimicrobial use is expressed per 1,000 occupied bed-days. However, the denominator (occupied bed-days) is a product of number of admissions and length of stay. In many hospitals, changes in the health-care system such as laparoscopic surgery have led to increased admissions with decreased length of stay. In these hospitals, expression of antibiotic use as DDD per 1,000 admissions would decrease over time, whereas DDD per 1,000 occupied bed-days would be stable. ESAC has established a standardized method for hospitals to compare their antibiotic use, which suggests that determination of

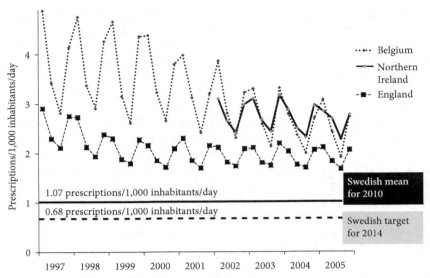

**Fig. 20.1** Use of antibiotics in ambulatory care measured in prescriptions per 1,000 inhabitants in Belgium, Northern Ireland, and England. The data show a marked downward trend in Belgium over the whole time period, with an initial downward trend in England from 1997 to 2001. Data were only available for Northern Ireland from 2002 and showed very similar levels of use to Belgium from then on. Use in England in 2005 was nearly twice as high as in Sweden in 2010. Nonetheless, the Swedish Government has set a target to reduce use to no more than 250 prescriptions per 1,000 inhabitants per year by 2014, a reduction of 36 per cent (<http://en.strama.se/dyn/84.html>).

Source: data from Davey P et al., on behalf of the ESAC Project Group, Outpatient antibiotic use in the four administrations of the UK: cross-sectional and longitudinal analysis, *Journal of Antimicrobial Chemotherapy*, Volume 62, Issue 6, pp. 1441–1447, Copyright © The Author 2008. Published by Oxford University Press on behalf of the British Society for Antimicrobial Chemotherapy.

changes in antibiotic exposure of hospital patients over a period of time is unreliable if only one clinical activity variable (such as occupied bed-days) is used as the denominator. ESAC recommends inclusion of admissions, occupied bed-days and length of stay in statistical, time-series analysis of antibiotic use in hospitals.

## Point prevalence surveys

In hospitals, point prevalence surveys have been used to estimate the prevalence of health-care associated infection and antimicrobial use. This provides additional information about indication for treatment, daily dose, and route of administration. The basic method is to collect data from every patient who is in the hospital on one day. Depending on the size of hospital and the amount of data to be collected from each patient, the survey may be completed on a single day or spread over several days. ESAC has coordinated three European point prevalence surveys, in 2006, 2008, and 2009, respectively; full reports are available on the ESAC website. The ECDC is coordinating a point prevalence survey in all European countries from 2011–2012.

The point prevalence method can be adapted for regular measurement of quality indicators in a sample of patients (see Fig. 19.5).

## Surveillance of antimicrobial prescribing in the community and hospital

The European Union, the US Food and Drug Administration, and the WHO have initiated national and regional campaigns aimed at professionals and the public to reduce the unnecessary prescribing of antibiotics. Efforts have been concentrated on prescribing in the community, not least because this accounts for 80 per cent of all human use of antimicrobial drugs. Principles such as not prescribing antibiotics for viral sore throats, or simple coughs and colds, and avoiding the unnecessary use of broad-spectrum antibacterials (e.g. quinolones and cephalosporins; see Fig. 19.6) when standard and less expensive antibiotics remain effective have been emphasized. Prescribing of antibiotics started to fall in England in 1995–1996. The decrease subsequently stabilized, with a slight rise in 2003–2004 (Fig. 20.1). However, much greater reduction in antibiotic use was achieved in Belgium (Fig. 20.1) and in France where annual, national campaigns targeted at public and professionals achieved 50 per cent reduction over 5 years. The ESAC project provides publicly accessible national comparisons of community antibiotic use in all European countries and has acted as an important stimulus to change in Belgium and France, which were among the highest users of antibiotics when ESAC began in 2001. In Sweden, use of antibiotics in 2010 was about as much as in England and Belgium in 2005 (Fig. 20.1). Nonetheless, in 2010 the Swedish Government announced a new initiative to reduce total use in the community by 36 per cent by 2014 (Fig. 20.1), In 2013 the Scottish Reduction in Antimicrobial Prescribing (ScRAP) Programme was launched, which aims to reduce total use in primary care in Scotland by 30 per cent within 2 years.

Note that measurement of antibiotic use in Fig. 20.1 is in prescriptions per 1,000 inhabitants per day. The WHO's standard measure for drug use is defined daily doses (DDD) per 1,000 inhabitants per day but this is because some national data comes from drug wholesalers, who cannot provide information about the number of prescriptions. Measurement by number of prescriptions is a better guide to the number of people treated than DDD because the WHO DDD does not always equate to the actual prescribed dose, which can vary between countries. For example, when the data used in Fig. 20.1 were expressed in DDD/1,000 inhabitants per day, use in Belgium appeared to be 66 per cent higher than in England in 2005, whereas the number of prescriptions was only 25 per cent higher (Fig 20.1). The explanation is that daily doses of penicillins in England are routinely lower than in Belgium.

It is estimated that up to 50 per cent of antibiotic usage in hospitals is inappropriate, and the problems of antimicrobial resistance and CDI are most likely to occur in hospital or in people who have recently been in hospital. Nonetheless, in comparison with the information available about community use, information about use of antibiotics in hospitals has been limited. For example, the ESAC project can obtain data about community use from 30 countries but only 19 can provide national data about hospital use. The ESAC project has therefore focused on disseminating new methods for hospitals to measure their use through point prevalence surveys of treatment of individual patients and through longitudinal analysis of data from hospital pharmacies. The ECDC coordinated the first Europe-wide point prevalence survey of antibiotic use and hospital acquired infection in 2012.

## Surveillance of antimicrobial resistance

In Europe data about resistance in invasive bacterial isolates (from blood and cerebrospinal fluid (CSF)) are made publicly available on the EARS-NET website. This is a network of national surveillance systems in the European countries. The national networks systematically collect data from clinical laboratories in their own countries. At present these include 900 public health laboratories serving over 1,400 hospitals in Europe and providing services to an estimated population of 100 million European citizens. The national networks upload the data to a central database maintained at the ECDC (The European Surveillance System (TESSy)). After the data are uploaded, each country approves its own data and the results are made available from the ECDC website. The data are externally quality assured. The data allow analysis of trends in the occurrence of antimicrobial resistance over time and between different countries (Fig. 20.2). Data are available for seven bacterial pathogens commonly causing infections in humans:

- *Streptococcus pneumoniae*;
- *Staphylococcus aureus*;
- *Enterococcus faecalis*;
- *Enterococcus faecium*;
- *Escherichia coli*;
- *Klebsiella pneumonia*; and
- *Pseudomonas aeruginosa*.

The EARS-NET data show striking differences between countries in rates and trends of resistance, which can be interpreted together with information about antibacterial use from ESAC-NET and other sources. For example, resistance to fluoroquinolones in *Escherichia coli* from blood cultures is much higher in Greece and Spain than in Sweden or the United Kingdom (Fig. 20.2), and data from ESAC-NET show that community use of fluoroquinolones is about fivefold higher in Greece and Spain than in Sweden or the United Kingdom. In the United Kingdom, resistance to fluoroquinolones was increasing until 2007 but then began to decrease at the same time as interventions in hospitals (Fig. 19.6) and the community (Fig. 19.7) targeted a reduction in use of cephalosporins

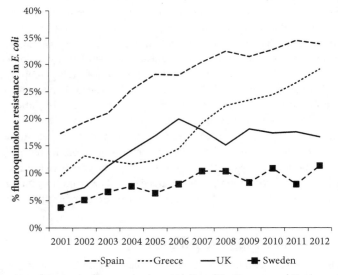

**Fig. 20.2** Increase in resistance to fluoroquinolones in *E. coli* in Greece and Spain compared with Sweden and the United Kingdom. Data are for invasive isolates (blood or CSF).

Source: data from European Centre for Disease Control, *Antimicrobial resistance interactive database (EARS-Net)*, Copyright © European Centre for Disease Prevention and Control (ECDC) 2005–2014, available from http://www.ecdc.europa.eu/en/healthtopics/antimicrobial_resistance/database/Pages/database.aspx

and fluoroquinolones to reduce risk of CDI. It is likely that reduction in use of these antibiotics was also responsible for halting the increase in fluoroquinolone resistance in *E. coli* (Fig. 20.2).

## Consequences of antimicrobial stewardship

### Control of resistance and CDI: integration of antibiotic policies with infection control

Antimicrobial stewardship is one of three pillars that support control of antimicrobial resistance (Fig. 20.3) and CDI (Chapter 25); the other two are control through prevention of transmission of infection, and environmental decontamination (Fig. 20.3). Most antimicrobials are prescribed by doctors, who have a responsibility to their patients and for public health to prescribe optimally and to minimize collateral damage (selection of drug resistant bacteria and *C. difficile*; Box 20.2, Box 20.3).

The evidence base for antibiotic stewardship and infection control interventions is steadily growing. However, this will be greatly strengthened by standardized reporting of interventions to manage

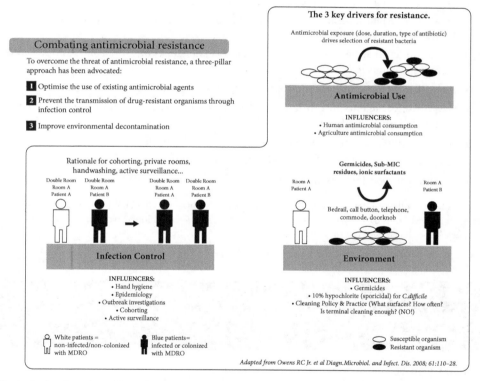

**Fig. 20.3** The three key drivers for antimicrobial resistance are, first, selection pressure from antimicrobial use; second, transmission between people in hospitals or the community; and, third, selection pressure from germicides and antimicrobial residues in the environment. It follows that these are the three targets for control of resistance; MDRO, multidrug-resistant organisms; MIC, minimum inhibitory concentration.

Reproduced with permission from Nathwani D and Sneddon J, *Practical Guide to Antimicrobial Stewardship in Hospitals*, Copyright © 2014, available from http://bsac.org.uk/wp-content/uploads/2013/07/Stewardship-Booklet-Practical-Guide-to-Antimicrobial-Stewardship-in-Hospitals.pdf

## Box 20.2 Role of the doctor in effective antibiotic prescribing as defined by the Royal College of Physicians Healthcare Associated Infections Working Group

### Effective antibiotic prescribing

Antibiotics are essential to modern medicine and may be life-saving, but their abuse leads to resistance. All physicians who prescribe antibiotics have a responsibility to their patients and for public health to prescribe optimally.

### Top 10 tips

- Institute antibiotic treatment immediately in patients with life-threatening infection
- Prescribe in accordance with local policies and guidelines avoiding broad-spectrum agents
- Document in clinical notes indication(s) for antibiotic prescription
- Send appropriate specimens to the microbiology lab, draining pus and foreign bodies if indicated
- Use antimicrobial susceptibility data to de-escalate/substitute/add agents and to switch from intravenous to oral therapy
- Prescribe the shortest antibiotic course likely to be effective
- Always select agents to minimise collateral damage (i.e. selection of multiresistant bacteria/*Clostridium difficile*)
- Monitor antibiotic drug levels when relevant (e.g. vancomycin)
- Use single-dose antibiotic prophylaxis wherever possible
- Consult your local infection experts

From Royal College of Physicians, *Effective Antibiotic Prescribing—Top Ten Tips*, London: RCP, Copyright © 2011 Royal College of Physicians, available from https://www.rcplondon.ac.uk/resources/top-ten-tips-series. Reproduced with permission.

## Box 20.3 Department of Health (England) 'Start Smart – then Focus' guidance on antimicrobial stewardship for front line clinical teams

### Start smart

- Do not start antibiotics in the absence of clinical evidence of bacterial infection.
- If there is evidence/suspicion of bacterial infection, use local guidelines to initiate prompt effective antibiotic treatment within 1 hour of diagnosis (or as soon as possible) in patients with life-threatening infections. Avoid inappropriate use of broad-spectrum antibiotics.
- Document on drug chart and in medical notes: clinical indication, duration or review date, route and dose.

**Box 20.3 Department of Health (England) 'Start Smart – then Focus' guidance on antimicrobial stewardship for front line clinical teams** *(continued)*

- Obtain cultures first.
- Prescribe single-dose antibiotics for surgical prophylaxis where antibiotics have been shown to be effective. Critical to this advice is that the single dose is administered within the 60 minutes *prior* to surgical incision or tourniquet inflation to enable peak blood levels to be present at the start of the surgical procedure.

## Then focus

- Review the clinical diagnosis and the continuing need for antibiotics by 48 hours and make a clear plan of action—the 'Antimicrobial Prescribing Decision'
  - Antibiotics are generally started before a patient's full clinical picture is known. By 48 hours, when additional information is available, including microbiology, radiographic and clinical information, it is important for clinicians to re-evaluate why the therapy was initiated in the first place and to gather evidence on whether there should be changes to the therapy.
- The five Antimicrobial Prescribing Decision options are Stop, Switch, Change, Continue and OPAT:

1 Stop antibiotics if there is no evidence of infection
2 Switch antibiotics from intravenous to oral
3 Change antibiotics—ideally to a narrower spectrum—or broader if required
4 Continue and review again at 72 hours
5 Outpatient Parenteral Antibiotic Therapy (OPAT).

It is essential that the review and subsequent decision is clearly documented in the medical notes.

Reproduced from Department of Health, *Antimicrobial Stewardship (AMS): "Start Smart - then Focus"* © Crown Copyright 2011, licensed under the Open Government Licence v.2.0, available from https://www.gov.uk/government/uploads/system/uploads/attachment_data/file/215308/dh_131181.pdf

outbreaks and to reduce endemic levels of resistance and CDI, which includes information about both infection control practices alongside changes in antimicrobial use (Figs 20.4–20.6). It is often difficult to separate the contributions of antimicrobial stewardship and infection control. The intervention to reduce fluoroquinolone use in Fig. 20.4 was accompanied by a dramatic increase in the use of alcohol-based hand rub in the post-intervention period, a factor which is likely to have contributed to the reduction in fluoroquinolone resistance in *Pseudomonas aeruginosa* as well as in methicillin-resistant *Staphylococcus aureus* (MRSA) (Fig. 20.4). Evaluation of antimicrobial stewardship and infection control is enhanced by reports that provide detail about infection control practices and patient demographics before and after the intervention, in addition to data about antimicrobial use (Figs 20.5 and 20.6).

## Clinical and cost consequences of antimicrobial stewardship

Interventions to increase the timely treatment of pneumonia are associated with a reduction in mortality (Fig. 20.7A). It is therefore important to show that interventions to reduce

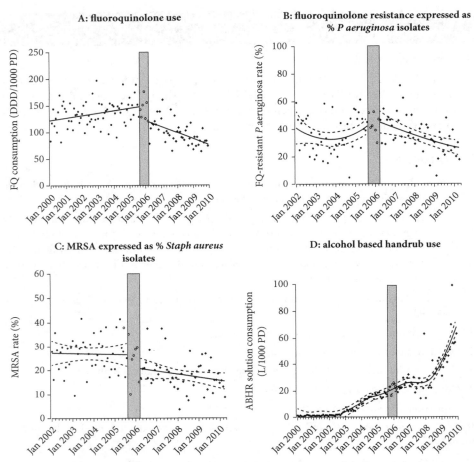

**Fig. 20.4** Impact of an intervention to reduce fluoroquinolones on use (A), fluoroquinolone resistance in *Pseudomonas aeruginosa* (B), and MRSA rates (C). Data are also provided about use of alcohol-based hand rub, because use increased sharply during the post-intervention period. In each figure, filled circles represent pre-intervention period values; open circles, intervention period values; and diamonds, post-intervention period values. The continuous line represents predictions from a model with spline smoothing, and the broken lines represent the pointwise 95 per cent confidence interval. The shaded area represents the intervention period; ABHR, alcohol-based hand rub; DDD, defined daily dose; FQ, fluoroquinolone; PD, patient-day.

Reproduced from Matthieu Lafaurie et al., Reduction of fluoroquinolone use is associated with a decrease in methicillin-resistant Staphylococcus aureus and fluoroquinolone-resistant Pseudomonas aeruginosa isolation rates: a 10 year study, *Journal of Antimicrobial Chemotherapy*, Volume 67, Issue 4, pp. 1010–1015, Copyright © 2012 British Society for Antimicrobial Chemotherapy, by permission of Oxford University Press.

excessive antibiotic use are not associated with increase in mortality (Fig. 20.7B). The 11 studies in Fig. 20.7B represent 14 per cent of 79 interventions that aimed to reduce excessive use of antibacterials from a systematic review. Nonetheless, it is reassuring that four of these studies demonstrated that it is possible to safely reduce the exposure of hospital inpatients to antibacterials by reducing the percentage treated or the total duration of treatment.

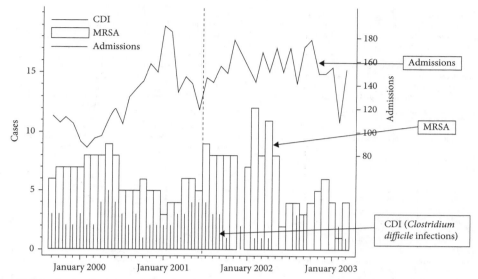

**Fig. 20.5** Reduction in CDI associated with the introduction of a conservative antibiotic policy. Infection control practices remained unchanged after the intervention (see Fig. 20.4) and there was no associated change in new cases of MRSA infection, which implies that the reduction in CDI was due to the antibiotic policy change.

Evidence about the impact of antimicrobial stewardship on mortality is important but we also need information about a wider range of potential unintended consequences of antimicrobial stewardship interventions, such as delays in treatment or increases in staff time required to implement the interventions. Very few published studies currently provide information about the cost of setting up the intervention, which can be considerable (Fig. 20.8). In addition, the estimates of savings made from the intervention often have wide confidence intervals (Fig. 20.8). Nonetheless, this analysis provides good evidence that, after the initial set-up period, savings from this intervention exceeded costs, and this was persuasive in ensuring continued support for the intervention. This intervention targeted 'alert antibacterials' (drugs that should be reserved for patients with documented or high risk of infection with resistant bacteria), which are also relatively expensive drugs. Cost savings from reducing unnecessary use of alert antibacterials and of intravenous drugs through intravenous-to-oral switch therapy (IVOST) programmes (Box 20.1) are important measures of the operational delivery of an antimicrobial strategy for ensuring the long-term sustainability of an antimicrobial management team.

Data monitoring and transparency are critical to the success of antimicrobial stewardship (Fig. 20.9). There is clear international consensus about the process and outcome measures that are required (Box 20.1, Fig. 20.9)

- ◆ Process measures of antimicrobial prescribing
  - Antimicrobial utilization and cost
  - Individual patient data about adherence to guidelines
- ◆ Outcome measures
  - Antimicrobial resistance surveillance
  - CDIs
  - Adverse drug events.

| Setting: three acute-care words for the elderly (78 beds) in 1200 bed tertiary hospital with 0.3 WTE ICD and 4.5 WTE ICNs | Dates: 1 September 1999 to 31 March 2003 | Population characteristics: 6129 unselected acute consecutive unselected elderly medical emergency admissions (80 years plus). Monthly length of stay 11.93–13.53 days. Endemic CDI and E-MRSA 15 and 16. No inter-hospital transfers. | | |
|---|---|---|---|---|
| Major infection control changes during the study: change from 'cephalosporin restrictive' antibiotic policy with audit and feedback every 2–3 months (Phase 1) to 'narrows-spectrum' antibiotic policy with audit and feedback as before and provision of laminated pocket-sized card with policy written on it (Phase 2) | | | | |
| | Antibiotic policy | Audit and feedback | Isolation policy CDI | Isolation policy MRSA |
| Phase 1: 21 months (1 September 1999 to 30 June 2001) | Cephalosporin restrictive (see below for details) | Two or three monthly feedback of antibiotic use in notional 7 day courses per 100 admissions per month and of monthly numbers of CDI and new MRSA cases | All proven cases isolated in side rooms. Aprons and gloves worn for contact | All cases of colonization or infection isolated in side rooms or four-bedded cohort in one ward. Aprons and gloves worn for contact |
| Phase 2: 21 months (1 July 2001 to 31 March 2003) | Narrow-spectrum antibiotic policy (Figure 2) Policy written on portable pocket-sized laminated card | As Phase 1 | As Phase 1 | As Phase 1 |
| Cephalosporin restrictive antibiotic policy details (phase 1): community-acquired pneumonia (CAP), amoxicillin; urinary tract infection (UTI), trimethoprim: cellulitis, flucloxacillin and benzyl penicillin; community-acquired aspiration pneumonia, benzyl penicillin and metronidazole. Ceftriaxone reserved for: (i) severe CAP; (ii) hospital-acquired aspiration pneumonia and (iii) UTI with renal failure, Gentamicin: UTI with shock, septicaemia with no apparent focus infection and intra-abdominal sepsis (with ampicillin and metronidazole); erythromycin; penicillin allergy | | | | |
| Isolation details (both phases): Ten side rooms available in the three wards. One four-bedded MRSA cohort in one ward. All other beds configured in four-bedded bays. Wall-mounted liquid soap and alcohol handrub dispenser and sink in each side room. One sink for each four-bedded bay with liquid soap and, from January 2002, one wall-mounted alcohol handrub dispenser per four-bedded bay | | | | |
| MRSA screening policy (both phases): admission screening (nose, perineum, wounds and devices) of admissions from nursing homes and of those with a past history of MRSA (both groups admitted to side room). Patients screened during admission if they had been in the same bay with a new case of MRSA | | | | |
| MRSA eradication policy (both phases): intranasal mupirocin and chlorhexidine body washes and shampoo for patient with no wounds. Clearance defined as three consecutive negative weekly swabs | | | | |
| Definition CDI (both phases): an episode of diarrhoea a sample of which was positive for toxin (I). No culture or typing performed | | | | |
| Definition of new MRSA acquisition (both phases): cases found on screening or clinical specimens taken > 48 h after admission. No routine typing performed but E-MRSA 15 and 16 endemic | | | | |

**Fig. 20.6** Description of population, clinical setting, and nature and timing of antibiotic prescribing before (Phase 1) and after (Phase 2) introduction of conservative antibiotic policy; ICD, infection control doctor; ICN, infection control nurse; WTE, whole time equivalent.

It is also important to consider balancing measures. Any improvement project, which by definition involves making changes to one or more care processes, can have unintended consequences. Balancing measures assess these potential unintended consequences and assure teams that they have indeed improved their overall system, rather than optimizing one part of the system at the expense of another. Balancing measures can also be important in helping address the concerns of those who are resistant to the proposed changes. For example, in a project to improve timely administration of treatment to patients with community-acquired pneumonia in the emergency room, a balancing measure might be the effect of intervention on misdiagnosis and unnecessary treatment of patients who do not have pneumonia. Listening to the concerns of clinicians about a stewardship intervention and including measures that address those concerns is likely to increase the success of the intervention.

A: interventions intended to increase effective treatment for pneumonia.

| Study | Intervention target | Risk ratio (95% CI) intervention *versus* standard care |
|---|---|---|
| Chu 2003 | Timely administration of antibacterials | 0.86 (0.55 -1.34) |
| Dean 2001 | Timely administration of antibacterials | 0.79 (0.63 -0.99) |
| Dean 2006 | Timely administration of antibacterials | 0.92 (0.84 -1.00) |
| Naughton 2001 | IV administration for severe infection | 0.76 (0.49 -1.19) |
| **Total** | | 0.89 (0.82 -0.97) |

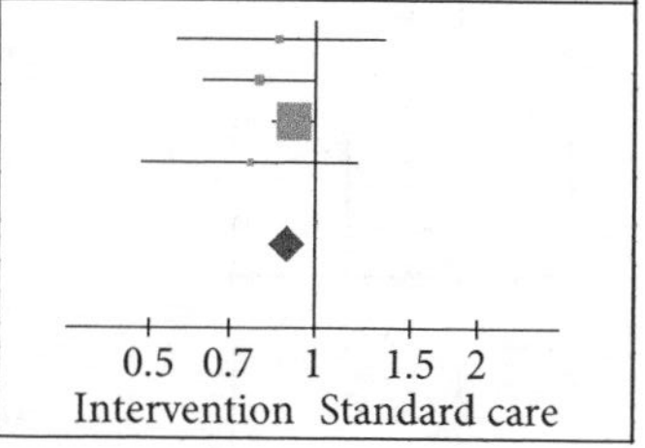

0.5 0.7 1 1.5 2
Intervention   Standard care

B: interventions intended to reduce unnecessary use of antimicrobials.

| Study | Intervention target | Risk ratio (95% CI) intervention *versus* standard care |
|---|---|---|
| Baily 1997 | Duration of IV treatment | 1.00 [0.21, 4.72] |
| Christ Crain 2004 | % patients treated | 0.96 [0.25, 3.75] |
| Christ Crain 2006 | % patients treated | 0.90 [0.50, 1.63] |
| de Man 2000 | Choice of antibacterial | 1.63 [0.90, 2.94] |
| Fine 2001 | Duration of IV administration | 0.87 [0.51, 1.48] |
| Fraser 1997 | Choice of antibacterial | 1.19 [0.59, 2.43] |
| Gums 1999 | Choice of antibacterial | 0.52 [0.23, 1.19] |
| Micek 2004 | Duration of total treatment | 0.86 [0.63, 1.18] |
| Paul 2006 | Choice of antibacterial | 0.90 [0.73, 1.12] |
| Singh 2000 | Duration of total treatment | 0.41 [0.16, 1.05] |
| Solomon 2001 | Choice of antibacterial | 1.03 [0.72, 1.49] |
| **Total** | | **0.92 [0.81, 1.06]** |

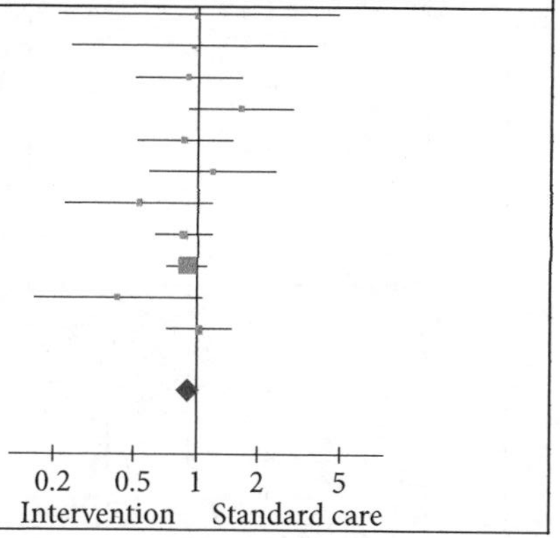

0.2 0.5 1 2 5
Intervention   Standard care

**Fig. 20.7** Forrest plots of meta-analyses of the impact on mortality of antimicrobial stewardship interventions; CI, confidence interval; IV, intravenous.

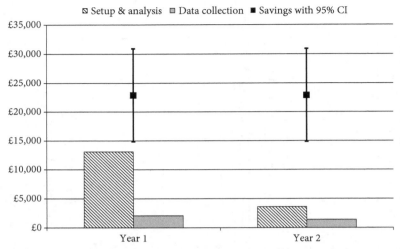

**Fig. 20.8** Cost of set-up, analysis, and data collection for an intervention to reduce unnecessary use of 'alert antibacterials' versus estimated savings with 95 per cent confidence intervals based on segmented regression analysis of monthly cost of antibacterials; CI, confidence interval.

Source: data from Ansari F et al., Outcomes of an intervention to improve hospital antibiotic prescribing: interrupted time series with segmented regression analysis, *Journal of Antimicrobial Chemotherapy*, Volume 52, Issue 5, pp. 84208, Copyright © The Author 2003. Published by Oxford University Press on behalf of the British Society for Antimicrobial Chemotherapy.

- ◆ Balancing measures of unintended consequences of interventions
  - Delay in treatment of patients with severe infection (for interventions intended to decrease excessive use of antibacterials).
  - Unnecessary treatment of patients who do not have infection (for interventions intended to increase effective antibacterial treatment).

## The antimicrobial management team

Antimicrobial management teams are multidisciplinary and acknowledge the need for a combination of expertise and roles. The role of the antimicrobial management committee is to develop and audit guidelines about antibiotic use (Box 20. 1). Doctors have a critical role in effective antimicrobial prescribing (Box 20.2) but ensuring safe and effective prescribing is also the responsibility of pharmacists and the nursing staff who dispense and administer antimicrobials (Box 20.1). There is a shortage of adequately trained specialist physicians or pharmacists, which means that their clinical role is limited to the management of complex infections or high-risk groups of patients (e.g. intensive care). Current initiatives promoting prudent antimicrobial prescribing and management have generally failed to include nurses, who potentially have key roles in starting smart and in focusing treatment through early recognition of sepsis, review of the route of administration and appropriate intravenous-to-oral switch, duration of treatment, and therapeutic drug monitoring. As nurses have the most consistent presence as patient carers, they are in an ideal

**Antibiotic Stewardship Driver Diagram**

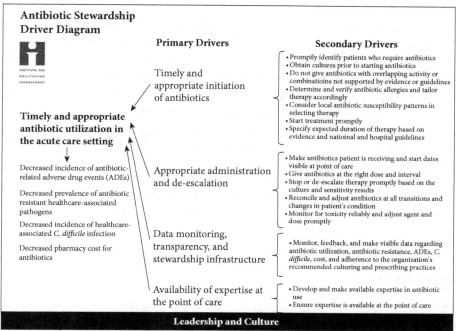

**Fig. 20.9** The Institute for Healthcare Improvement and US Centers for Disease Control and Prevention Antibiotic Stewardship Driver Diagram.

Reproduced from Centre for Disease Control and the Institute for Healthcare Improvement, *Antibiotic Steward-ship Driver Diagram*, available from http://www.cdc.gov/getsmart/healthcare/pdfs/Antibiotic_Stewardship_Driver_Diagram.pdf

position to contribute to antibiotic stewardship. Moreover, in comparison with junior doctors, nurses are more likely to remain in the same clinical team for longer, and so training of nurses in antimicrobial stewardship is a sustainable method for increasing the availability of expertise at the point of care (Fig. 20.9).

Evidence from primary care and secondary care shows that measurement and feedback of information about antibiotic prescribing does change practice (Figs. 19.6 and 19.7). Ideally, measures should be collected by clinical teams as part of their daily work, which means that they must be simple, reliable, and sustainable. Point prevalence surveys can be a sustainable method for driving change at the national level. In Scotland, progress has been achieved by clinical teams in acute admissions units with two of the key principles of effective prescribing: prescribing in accordance with local policies, and documentation in clinical notes (see Fig. 19.5). Data are collected by clinical teams on 20 patients per month. Data are shared between teams by posting on a secure website.

## Key points

◆ Surveillance of antimicrobial use and infections are critical to the control of resistance and CDI.

◆ In the last 10 years, there has been increasing evidence that both national campaigns and targeted interventions have been successful in reducing both resistance and CDI.

◆ The twin goals of antibiotic stewardship are, first, to ensure effective, timely treatment of infection and, second, to minimize collateral damage from unnecessary use.

◆ Prescribers must take responsibility for both prompt initiation of antimicrobial treatment and for review of the continuing need and outcomes of treatment.

◆ Clinical teams and health-care organizations must take responsibility for transparent data monitoring that measures antimicrobial prescribing processes and outcomes with balancing measures to address unintended consequences.

◆ There is clear international consensus about the role of doctors in antibiotic stewardship. However, sustainable increase in the availability of expertise at the point of care will require involvement and training of nurses in antimicrobial stewardship.

## Further Reading

### Surveillance

Ansari, F., Erntell, M., Goossens, H., and Davey, P. (2009) The European surveillance of antimicrobial consumption (ESAC) point-prevalence survey of antibacterial use in 20 European hospitals in 2006. *Clinical Infectious Diseases*, **49**(10): 1496–1504.

Ansari, F., Molana, H., Goossens, H., and Davey, P. (2010) Development of standardized methods for analysis of changes in antibacterial use in hospitals from 18 European countries: the European Surveillance of Antimicrobial Consumption (ESAC) longitudinal survey, 2000–2006. *Journal of Antimicrobial Chemotherapy* **65**(12): 2685–91.

European Antimicrobial Resistance Surveillance Network (EARS-Net). (2014) *European Antimicrobial Resistance Surveillance Network (EARS-Net)*. <http://www.ecdc.europa.eu/en/activities/surveillance/EARS-Net/>, accessed 30 November 2014.

European Centre for Disease Prevention and Control. (2014) *Surveillance of Antimicrobial Consumption in Europe 2011*. <http://www.ecdc.europa.eu/en/publications/Publications/antimicrobial-consumption-europe-surveillance-2011.pdf>, accessed 30 November 2014.

European Surveillance of Antimicrobial Consumption Network (ESAC-Net). (2014) *European Surveillance of Antimicrobial Consumption Network (ESAC-Net)*. <http://www.ecdc.europa.eu/en/activities/surveillance/esac-net/pages/index.aspx>, accessed 30 November 2014.

### Antimicrobial stewardship

Arnold, S. R. and Straus, S. E. (2005) Interventions to improve antibiotic prescribing practices in ambulatory care. *Cochrane Database of Systematic Reviews*, **Issue** 4: Art. No.: CD003539.pub2.

Bell, B. G., Schellevis, F., Stobberingh, E., Goossens, H., and Pringle, M. (2014) A systematic review and meta-analysis of the effects of antibiotic consumption on antibiotic resistance. *BMC Infectious Diseases*, **14**(1): 13.

Charani, E., Cooke, J., and Holmes, A. (2010) Antibiotic stewardship programmes—what's missing? *Journal of Antimicrobial Chemotherapy*, **65**(11): 2275–7.

Cooke, J., Alexander, K., Charani, E., et al. (2010) Antimicrobial stewardship: an evidence-based, antimicrobial self-assessment toolkit (ASAT) for acute hospitals. *Journal of Antimicrobial Chemotherapy*, **65**(11): 2669–73.

Davey, P., Brown, E., Charani, E., Fenelon, L., Gould, I. M., Holmes, A., Ramsay, C. R., Wiffen, P. J., and Wilcox, M. (2013) Interventions to improve antibiotic prescribing practices for hospital inpatients. *Cochrane Database of Systematic Reviews*, **Issue 4**: Art. No. CD003543.

Department of Health. Antimicrobial Stewardship (AMS). (2011) *Antimicrobial Stewardship: 'Start Smart - then Focus'*. <https://www.gov.uk/government/uploads/system/uploads/attachment_data/file/215308/dh_131181.pdf>, accessed 30 November 2014.

Duguid, M., and Cruickshank, M., eds. (2011) Antimicrobial Stewardship in Australian Hospitals. <http://www.safetyandquality.gov.au/wp-content/uploads/2011/01/Antimicrobial-stewardship-in-Australian-Hospitals-2011.pdf>, accessed 30 November 2014.

NHS Education for Scotland. (2014) *Scottish Reduction in Antimicrobial Prescribing (ScRAP) Programme*. <http://www.nes.scot.nhs.uk/education-and-training/by-discipline/pharmacy/about-nes-pharmacy/educational-resources/resources-by-topic/infectious-diseases/antibiotics/scottish-reduction-in-antimicrobial-prescribing-(scrap)-programme.aspx>, accessed 30 November 2014.

Royal College of Physicians. (2014) *Top Ten Tips Series*. <http://www.rcplondon.ac.uk/resources/top-ten-tips-series>, accessed 30 November 2014.

# 4

# Therapeutic use
# of antimicrobial agents

# Chapter 21

# Respiratory tract infections

## Introduction to respiratory tract infections

Respiratory infections are caused by viruses, or bacteria, or both. If the illness is entirely viral in origin, an antibiotic will not help. If there is a bacterial component, antibiotic treatment will sometimes help and may be vital. It is often difficult to recognize when bacteria may be involved in respiratory infection, as secondary bacterial infection may complicate viral respiratory infections. However, the key question in the decision about treatment with antimicrobials is, do the benefits to the patient outweigh the risks? It is not necessary to prescribe antimicrobials for all bacterial respiratory infections.

When considering the role of antimicrobial chemotherapy, it is important to reflect on the epidemiology of infection in the twentieth century. In the United States mortality from infection fell by 50 per cent from 1900 to 1917; then in 1918 there was a sharp spike in mortality because of the influenza pandemic. From 1919 mortality from infection declined progressively throughout the first half of the century, before the arrival of antimicrobial chemotherapy or vaccines. The introduction of antimicrobial chemotherapy did accelerate the decline in mortality from some respiratory infections (e.g. otitis media, pneumonia, and tuberculosis) but had no impact on others (e.g. bronchitis). Two conclusions can be drawn from this information. First, it is clear why there is so much concern about the possibility of an influenza pandemic, given the massive impact on mortality of the 1918 pandemic. Second, antimicrobial chemotherapy has not had the dramatic effect on mortality from infections that is popularly attributed to it. The major impact in the first half of the twentieth century came from improvements in public health, which is why death from all infections still increases with increasing socio-economic deprivation in the twenty-first century. Antimicrobial chemotherapy is just one component of an overall strategy to prevent and treat infections.

## Upper respiratory tract infection

### Antibiotic treatment of upper respiratory infection

Before discussing specific upper respiratory infections, it is important to emphasize that antibiotic treatment makes very little difference to clinical outcome. The evidence to support this statement comes from randomized controlled trials and several systematic reviews in the Cochrane Library. In the United Kingdom a large observational study of 3.36 million episodes of respiratory tract infection showed that over 2,000 people with upper respiratory tract infection would need to be treated with an antibiotic to prevent one hospitalization with complications (Fig. 21.1). In contrast, antibiotic treatment of children with respiratory tract infection in primary care significantly increases the risk of carriage of antibiotic-resistant bacteria (Fig. 21.2).

### Sore throat

This is one of the commonest acute problems seen in general medical practice, with an incidence of 100 cases per 1,000 inhabitants per year, although only a minority of these will present to a

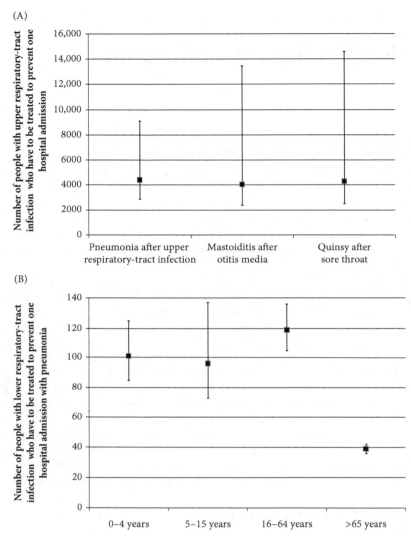

**Fig. 21.1** The number of people who need to be treated with an antibiotic to prevent one hospital admission from a complication in an observational study of 3.36 million episodes of respiratory tract infection. The risk or hospitalization was adjusted for age, sex and social deprivation. The bars are 95% confidence intervals. (a) Number of people with upper respiratory tract infection who need to be treated with an antibiotic to prevent hospitalization with specified complications. (b) Number of people with lower respiratory tract infection who need to be treated with an antibiotic to prevent hospitalization with pneumonia.

Source: data from data in Petersen I et al., Protective effect of antibiotics against serious complications of common respiratory tract infections: retrospective cohort study with the UK General Practice Research Database, *British Medical Journal*, Volume 335, Issue 7627, pp. 982–988, Copyright © 2007.

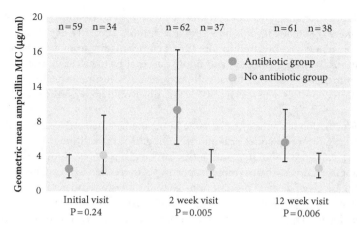

**Fig. 21.2** Geometric mean minimum inhibitory concentration for ampicillin of isolates from children according to whether or not they received antibiotics (error bars show 95% confidence intervals; *P*-values based on *t*-test); MIC, minimum inhibitory concentration.

Reproduced from *British Medical Journal*, Effect of antibiotic prescribing on antibiotic resistance in individual children in primary care: prospective cohort study, Chung A et al., Volume 355, Issue 7617, p. 429, Copyright © 2007, with permission from BMJ Publishing Group Ltd.

doctor. It is commoner in females than men. Symptoms include sore throat with anorexia, lethargy, and systemic illness. On examination, there may be inflamed tonsils or pharynx; a purulent exudate on tonsils; fever; and anterior cervical lymphadenopathy.

Sore throat may be part of the early symptom complex of many upper respiratory viral infections, in which case rhinorrhoea and/or cough are common additional features. Occasionally, it may be a presenting symptom of acute epiglottitis or other serious upper airway disease.

There is no evidence that bacterial sore throats are more severe or long-lasting than viral ones. The most commonly identified organism is *Streptococcus pyogenes*, the group A β-haemolytic streptococcus. Most other cases are caused by adenoviruses. There is no reliable way to distinguish between bacterial and viral causes based on symptoms and signs.

The gold standard for diagnosis of streptococcal infection in the throat includes a positive anti-streptolysin O (ASO) titre in addition to culture of *Str. pyogenes* from the throat. There is a high asymptomatic carrier rate for the organism (up to 40%) and it is common to culture it from sore throats when there is no serological evidence of infection. Moreover a negative culture does not rule out *Str. pyogenes* as a cause of sore throat. Neither culture of throat swabs nor rapid tests based on detection of streptococcal antigen are helpful in most cases.

Most people with sore throat manage the condition successfully without seeing a doctor. Paracetamol is an effective analgesic, with less risk of adverse effects than non-steroidal anti-inflammatory drugs. Aspirin should be avoided in children because of the risk of Reye's syndrome. The immediate benefits from antimicrobial chemotherapy are actually very meagre. Symptoms usually persist for 5–7 days with or without antibiotics, which only shorten illness by 24 hours. The same control of symptoms can probably be achieved with paracetamol.

Streptococcal sore throat is important because it may lead to serious complications, particularly rheumatic fever, which is still prevalent in many countries. Evidence about the effectiveness of antibiotics for preventing nonsuppurative and suppurative complications comes from studies on military personnel living in overcrowded barracks in the late 1940s and early 1950s. This evidence has little relevance to management of sore throat in modern communities, at least in the developed world, where rheumatic fever is now very uncommon. Similarly, experience with the use of antibiotics to prevent cross-infection in sore throat comes mainly from army barracks and other closed institutions. It is very unlikely (and unproven) that trying to eradicate *Str. pyogenes* with routine antibiotic therapy for sore throat will produce any measurable health gain in the general public in Western countries, whereas it is likely that this would increase the prevalence of antimicrobial resistance.

A patient information leaflet may be of value in the management of acute sore throat and may assist in managing future episodes at home without general practitioner involvement. Patients who are sceptical about withholding antibiotics can be given a prescription with the suggestion that they do not use it unless their symptoms persist for more than 3 days. Only about 30 per cent of patients who are given delayed prescriptions go to the pharmacy to get their antibiotics.

If antibiotics are to be prescribed, the drugs of choice are penicillin V or a macrolide, and these should be given for at least 10 days to eradicate the organism and prevent recurrence. Glandular fever commonly causes symptoms and signs that are indistinguishable from streptococcal throat infection (including a very impressive purulent exudate on the tonsils). Ampicillin, amoxicillin, and co-amoxiclav should not be used, as they will cause a rash if the sore throat is the herald of glandular fever. Tetracyclines are also inappropriate because of the high incidence of resistance among streptococci.

## Acute otitis media

Three-quarters of cases of acute otitis media occur in children; one in four children will have an episode during their first 10 years of life. Acute otitis media should be distinguished from otitis media with effusion, commonly referred to as glue ear; as many as 80 per cent of children suffer this infection at least once before the age of 4.

Acute otitis media is an inflammation of the middle ear and is of rapid onset, presenting with local symptoms (earache, rubbing or tugging of the affected ear) and systemic signs (fever, irritability, disturbed sleeping). It is often preceded by other upper respiratory symptoms such as cough or rhinorrhoea. On examination, a middle ear effusion may be present but in addition the drum looks opaque and may be bulging.

The condition is caused predominantly by *Haemophilus influenzae* and *Str. pneumoniae*. Staphylococci, *Str. pyogenes*, and α-haemolytic streptococci are less often involved. However, acute otitis media should not be treated routinely with antibiotics. As with sore throat, antibiotics only have a small impact on the duration of acute symptoms, which can be controlled equally effectively with paracetamol. If an antibiotic is to be prescribed, a 5-day course is sufficient; the antibiotic of choice is amoxicillin; erythromycin and co-amoxiclav are logical alternatives and may be necessary if β-lactamase-producing *H. influenzae* is involved. Decongestants, antihistamines, and mucolytics are not effective. As with sore throat, patient information leaflets and delayed antibiotic prescriptions are effective strategies for reducing the unnecessary use of antibiotics.

Glue ear is an inflammation of the middle ear with accumulation of fluid in the middle ear but without symptoms or signs of acute inflammation. It is often asymptomatic, and earache is uncommon. On examination, a middle ear effusion is present but with a normal looking ear drum. Antibiotics should not be given.

## Acute sinusitis

Acute sinusitis presents with pain originating in the maxillary, frontal, ethmoid, or sphenoid sinuses, with the maxillary sinus being by far the commonest. Onset of facial pain is often preceded by non-specific symptoms of upper respiratory inflammation and there may be systemic signs of inflammation. The bacterial causes of acute sinusitis are the same as acute otitis media. If X-ray or culture confirms the clinical diagnosis, then antibiotics can substantially reduce the duration of symptoms. However, neither of these investigations is routinely available in primary care. Culture of the sinuses requires percutaneous sinus puncture and aspiration, which is not a procedure that most general practitioners are trained to do (or that many patients would consent to). Unfortunately, antibiotic treatment of patients with symptoms suggestive of sinusitis but without confirmation by X-ray or culture is no more effective than symptomatic relief.

As with acute otitis media, antibiotics for acute sinusitis should be reserved for the more severe cases. Penicillin V or amoxicillin are as effective as newer antibiotics. The recommended duration of treatment is 10 days in the absence of evidence that shorter courses are as effective.

## Antibiotic treatment of lower respiratory tract infections

Acute cough is the most common symptom of lower respiratory infection, whether as a new symptom or as an exacerbation of chronic symptoms. Cough is not a universal feature: some patients with pneumonia present with pleuritic chest pain or with symptoms of systemic inflammatory response (fever, malaise, headache, or myalgia) without cough. The most important diagnosis to make is pneumonia because it can be life threatening and its outcome can be improved with antimicrobial chemotherapy. However, it is not possible to distinguish reliably between pneumonia and other causes of lower respiratory tract infection from clinical history and signs. Consequently, in primary care management must be based on an assessment of severity of illness and need for referral to hospital.

In comparison with upper respiratory tract infection, the evidence for benefits and risks of antibiotic treatment of lower respiratory tract infection is more complex. In a large observational study, the number of people who needed to be treated with antibiotics to prevent one hospitalization with pneumonia was about 100 for those aged <65, and 40 for those aged ≥65 (Fig. 21.1B). However, a cluster-randomized trial in general practice showed that two strategies (training in consultation skills or near patient testing for C-reactive protein) resulted in 50 per cent reduction in prescribing of antibiotics for lower respiratory tract infection without any measurable change in time to recovery (Fig. 21.3). This evidence shows that doctors in primary care can reliably identify patients with lower respiratory tract infection and low risk of complications. Nonetheless the risk of complications from pneumonia means that interventions to reduce prescribing need to be supported by balancing measures that will detect unintended increase in complications.

### Epidemiology

The incidence of lower respiratory tract infection in the United Kingdom is between 40 and 90 cases per 1,000 population per year, being commoner in the very young and old and in the winter months. In the United Kingdom there is about a fourfold higher incidence in the most deprived communities in comparison with the most affluent communities.

Mortality is highest in the elderly. The 30-day mortality associated with lower respiratory tract infection in people over 65 years old is 10 per cent. However, many of these elderly people die 'with' rather than 'of' the infection. Bronchopneumonia is often recorded as the immediate cause of death in people with chronic, life-threatening diseases. Mortality from 'pneumonia' has actually increased in developed countries since the introduction of antibiotics but more people are living longer and most of this mortality is from bronchopneumonia.

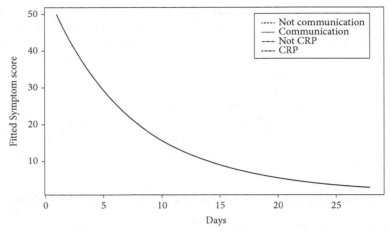

**Fig. 21.3** Corrected symptom scores for treatment groups in a cluster-randomized clinical trial of the effect of point of care testing for C-reactive protein and training in communication skills on antibiotic use in lower respiratory tract infections in general practice. The symptom scores were corrected by a four-level autoregressive-moving-averages model to account for practice, general practitioner, patient, and repeated measurements over time. The four lines in this figure are indistinguishable, meaning that treatment groups had identical clinical recovery despite fewer antibiotics prescribed in intervention groups (see Table 21.1). 'No test' and 'No training' represent usual care in the two control arms of the trial; CRP, C-reactive protein.

Most people with lower respiratory infections manage their own symptoms without seeking medical attention. Of 1 million people with lower respiratory tract infection, only 300,000 will see a primary care physician. Of these 1 in 4 (70,000) will be treated with antibiotics, although only about 1 in 10 (7,000 people) will have a diagnosis of pneumonia. From the original 300,000 people who presented to a primary care physician, only about 200 (0.7%) will be admitted to hospital with pneumonia.

## Management in primary care

The key to management of lower respiratory tract infection in primary care is to distinguish between patients who have severe infection that should be referred to hospital and the majority (99%) who can be managed safely at home. There are four questions to address:

◆ Has the patient been previously well or is there underlying chronic respiratory or other disease?

◆ Has there been the development or deterioration in either dyspnoea or sputum purulence?

◆ Are there any new localizing physical signs in the chest to suggest pneumonia?

◆ Are any features of severity present? (Box 21.1).

The answers to these questions distinguish between four broad populations of people with lower respiratory tract infection. These will be discussed starting with the most severe (but least common).

## Box 21.1 Features of severity of lower respiratory tract infection that can be easily assessed in primary care

The first three items in italics are most important, and referral to hospital should be considered for patients with any one of these three features.

- *raised respiratory rate (>30/min)*
- *low blood pressure (<90 mmHg systolic and/or <60 mmHg diastolic)*
- *confusion of recent onset*
- age >50 years
- coexisting disease present (e.g. severe chronic obstructive pulmonary disease; cardiac failure; cerebrovascular, neoplastic, renal, or liver disease)
- very high or very low temperature (<35°C or >40°C)
- tachycardia (>125/min)

## Patients with features indicating severe infection

Referral to hospital should be considered in patients who exhibit one or more of three key features of severity (Box 21.1), especially if they are over the age of 50. The three key features are

- raised respiratory rate (>30/min);
- low blood pressure (<90 mmHg systolic and or <60 mmHg diastolic); and
- confusion of recent onset.

This applies whether or not the patient has additional physical signs indicating pneumonia, because the absence of these signs is not a reliable method for excluding pneumonia. The final decision should be based on clinical judgement that includes social factors. Even a relatively well patient who lives in poor social circumstances or in an isolated rural area with no home support may require referral to hospital. Conversely, patients who are 65 years old and have signs of pneumonia can be managed safely at home if they have sufficient social support.

## Suspected community-acquired pneumonia without features of severity

These patients have new focal signs in the chest (crackles or altered breath sounds) but are not severely ill. In the absence of chest X-ray (not available in many primary care settings), pneumonia can be diagnosed from symptoms of an acute lower respiratory infection (cough, dyspnoea, or pleuritic chest pain) with at least one systemic symptom of infection (fever or tachycardia), and new focal signs on chest examination. However, only 50 per cent of those with all of these features will actually have an abnormal chest X-ray.

Below the age of 45, very few patients with pneumonia also have chronic obstructive pulmonary disease. Between the ages of 45 and 64, the proportion is up to 10 per cent and rises to 20 per cent between the ages of 75 and 84. Pneumonia in these patients is more likely to be associated with severity criteria (Box 21.1).

A wide variety of organisms can cause pneumonia, including viruses. The commonest bacterial cause is *Str. pneumoniae*, which accounts for about 70–80 per cent of cases in which a bacterial pathogen is identified. Atypical bacteria (*Mycoplasma pneumoniae, Chlamydophila (Chlamydia) pneumoniae, Chl. psittaci, Legionella pneumophila,* and *Coxiella burnetii*) collectively account for 10–20 per cent of cases, and the remainder are caused by *H. influenzae* or *Staphylococcus aureus.* The latter is particularly associated with secondary bacterial infection following influenza.

With current technology, neither sputum culture nor blood tests such as for C-reactive protein or white cell count provide sufficient added value to the diagnosis to justify routine use. Sputum culture may be recommended in areas with a high prevalence of penicillin-resistant pneumococci.

Pneumonia is a life-threatening illness. Nonetheless, patients with no features of severity (Box 21.1) can be managed safely at home with oral amoxicillin, a macrolide, or a tetracycline. There is no need to give combination therapy. A macrolide or tetracycline may be preferred if there are clinical features suggesting infection with one of the atypical bacteria (e.g. prominent upper respiratory symptoms, headache, or symptom duration for >1 week), particularly in younger patients or during an epidemic year for *Myc. pneumoniae.*

### Patients with COPD (chronic obstructive pulmonary disease) or other chronic respiratory disease

These patients often have no new signs in the chest other than dyspnoea and sputum purulence. In the absence of signs of severity (Box 21.1) or of pneumonia, the diagnosis is an acute exacerbation of the underlying condition. The likely bacterial pathogens are *H. influenzae, Str. pneumoniae,* and *Moraxella catarrhalis.* The development of green (purulent) sputum is a good indicator of a high bacterial load in the sputum. However, even in these patients antibacterial treatment has only a slight impact on the course of an acute exacerbation, shortening an illness of 5–7 days by no more than 1 day. Antibacterial treatment does not benefit patients with acute exacerbations of chronic obstructive pulmonary disease who do not have purulent sputum. The prevalence of resistance to aminopenicillins in *H. influenzae* is 10–30 per cent and is much higher in *Mor. catarrhalis.* Despite this, the clinical effectiveness of amoxicillin is just as good as co-amoxiclav or fluoroquinolones, probably because of the modest benefit from any antibacterial treatment. A macrolide or tetracycline is appropriate for patients who are allergic to penicillin or who have not responded to amoxicillin treatment. Fluoroquinolones should not be used empirically in the management of exacerbations of respiratory disease in primary care.

The duration of treatment of exacerbations of COPD should be 5 days; there is no evidence that more prolonged treatment is any more effective.

### Non-pneumonic lower respiratory infection (acute bronchitis)

Most patients with no signs in the chest, who have been previously well, and do not have other features of severity have non-pneumonic infections, most of which are caused by viruses. A few cases are caused by *Myc. pneumoniae, Bordetella pertussis, Chl. pneumoniae, Str. pneumoniae,* or *H. influenzae.* Patients will have an illness lasting several days with or without antibiotics, which should not be prescribed unless patients have signs in the chest or features of severity (Box 21.1). Sputum purulence alone is not an indication for antibiotics in a previously well patient with no chest signs. As with sore throat and acute otitis media, patient information leaflets and delayed prescriptions are effective strategies for reducing unnecessary antibiotic treatment.

### Pertussis (whooping cough)

Antibiotics are notoriously ineffective in controlling the distressing cough of pertussis; nevertheless, erythromycin has been shown to eradicate the organism from the respiratory tract and can also be used for the protection of susceptible close contacts. Vaccination is the only reliable way of preventing and controlling this early childhood infectious disease.

## Cystic fibrosis

The susceptibility of patients with cystic fibrosis to pulmonary infection is well recognized and is often the cause of early death. Most lung infections in patients with cystic fibrosis are managed in the community, usually by outreach teams from secondary care. One of the striking features of chest infections in cystic fibrosis is that relatively few pathogens are involved. Early in the disease the organisms implicated are frequently *Staph. aureus*, *H. influenzae*, or both. As patients progress through adolescence to adulthood, these pathogens are replaced by *Pseudomonas aeruginosa*. Major problems arise when *Ps. aeruginosa* is replaced by *Stenotrophomonas maltophilia* or *Burkholderia cepacia*; these organisms are often resistant to many antibiotics, and treatment should be guided by laboratory findings. The selection of antibiotics in patients with cystic fibrosis should be determined by the specialist services that manage the patient.

## Sputum samples for management of lower respiratory tract infections in primary care

Clinical guidelines do not recommend routinely sending sputum samples from children, adults, or elderly patients with suspected lower respiratory tract infections (LRTI). For patients with COPD, samples may be considered for persistently purulent sputum.

# Management in hospital

## Community-acquired pneumonia

In hospital the clinical diagnosis can be confirmed with a chest X-ray, although it should be recognized that sensitivity is not 100 per cent. The gold standard for diagnosis of bacterial pneumonia is culture of bacteria from lung tissues or a needle aspirate from the lung but these tests are too dangerous to use in routine clinical practice. The point is that some patients with pneumonia can have a normal chest X-ray at presentation; therefore, if the clinical features strongly suggest pneumonia, it is reasonable to treat and repeat the chest X-ray after 24–48 hours.

The severity criteria for community-acquired pneumonia are based on assessments of confusion, urea concentration, respiratory rate, and blood pressure for those 65 years of age and older (CURB-65 score; Table 21.1). It is similar to but importantly different from the classification of severity of sepsis (see 'Assessment of sepsis and the systemic inflammatory response' in Chapter 13). The CURB-65 score is specifically designed to be used in patients who present to hospital in order to identify low-risk patients who do not need to be admitted to hospital, whereas the classification of sepsis is intended to be used for any patient with infection (community- or hospital-acquired) to identify patients who are deteriorating and require more intensive therapy. The CURB-65 score identifies low-risk patients more accurately than the sepsis severity score. There are more complex pneumonia-specific scores (for example the pneumonia severity index used in North America) but these are no more accurate than CURB-65. In addition to considering severity of pneumonia, recent surveys about hospital antibiotic policies show increasing concern about risk of infection with *Clostridium difficile*. Pneumonia occurs commonly in older patients who are at high risk of infection with *Clo. difficile*. Consequently, some hospitals are recommending narrower spectrum therapy for high-risk and low-risk pneumonia than is recommended in national guidelines.

Between 30 and 50 per cent of patients who present to hospital with community-acquired pneumonia are found to be in the CURB-65 low-risk group. However, about half of these patients have other reasons for admission. Some will have co-morbidities that require inpatient

**Table 21.1** The CURB-65 severity score for patients presenting to hospital with community-acquired pneumonia, and the mortality range measured in two prospective cohort studies.*

| Risk | CURB-65 score | 30-day mortality(%) |
|---|---|---|
| Low risk | 0–1 | 0–1 |
| Intermediate | 2 | 8–9 |
| High risk | >2 | 22–23 |
| All patients | Not applicable | 9–10 |

* CURB-65: score one point for each of the following: confusion; urea >7 mmol/l; respiratory rate ≥30/min; low systolic (<90 mm Hg) or diastolic (≤60 mm Hg) blood pressure; age ≥65 years.

Source: data from Lim WS et al., Defining community acquired pneumonia severity on presentation to hospital: an international derivation and validation study, *Thorax*, Volume 58, Issue 5, pp. 377–382, Copyright © 2003.

management. In particular, patients with chronic obstructive pulmonary disease and pneumonia could be in respiratory failure and yet have a CURB-65 score of 0 (if they have a respiratory rate <30/min, which is likely if they have type 2 respiratory failure). In addition to medical reasons for admission, some patients will have poor social circumstances or insufficient support to be managed at home.

The management of patients admitted to hospital should be determined by their CURB-65 score. Low-risk patients who are admitted for other reasons can be managed in the same way as low-risk patients in the community, with amoxicillin, a macrolide, or a tetracycline. Some guidelines do recommend that all patients admitted to hospital with pneumonia should receive antibiotics for pneumonia caused by atypical bacteria but several clinical trials shows that treatment with an aminopenicillin alone is just as effective for patients with low- or intermediate-risk pneumonia.

At the other end of the scale, patients at high risk should be treated with intravenous antibiotics that are effective against the full range of pathogens that may cause community-acquired pneumonia. Possible regimens include benzyl penicillin or co-amoxiclav, a macrolide, or a fluoroquinolone with good activity against *Str. pneumoniae* (e.g. levofloxacin) for patients with penicillin allergy. The choice between benzylpenicillin versus co-amoxiclav for severe pneumonia is determined by hospital-specific risk of *Clo. difficile* infection; the patient must receive the antibiotic(s) immediately and certainly within 4 hours of admission, as later administration is associated with increased mortality from severe sepsis. If patients are admitted through an accident and emergency department, they must receive their first dose of antibiotics there before transfer to the ward. If they are admitted directly to a ward, the first dose must be clearly written for immediate administration, not left until the next drug round. In addition to intravenous antibiotics, patients with severe pneumonia must have their oxygen requirements assessed by pulse oximetry or blood gas measurement within 4 hours of admission and receive high-flow oxygen (5 l/minute) if they are hypoxic. Adequate fluid replacement is also essential. Patients should be referred to a high dependency or intensive care unit if their vital signs do not improve rapidly. When young patients die from community-acquired pneumonia, it is usually because of failure to recognize the need for intensive care.

The management of patients at intermediate risk falls between these two extremes and is a matter for clinical judgement. If in doubt it would be wise to treat as severe pneumonia while waiting for senior review.

## Acute exacerbations of COPD without pneumonia

The antibiotic management should be the same as in primary care. If there is no evidence of systemic inflammatory response then intravenous antibiotics are unnecessary if the patient can take oral antibiotics. Duration of treatment should be no more than 5 days.

If patients have repeated acute exacerbations requiring hospitalization, then prophylactic antibiotic treatment with a macrolide antibiotic should be considered. There is consistent evidence from randomized trials, which show that macrolides are more effective than other antibiotics. This may be due to anti-inflammatory effects of macrolides in addition to their antibacterial action. However, macrolide prophylaxis is associated with increased carriage of antibiotic-resistant bacteria, so should be used with caution.

## Hospital-acquired pneumonia

Pneumonia is the leading cause of mortality resulting from infection acquired in hospital. The incidence of hospital-acquired pneumonia in intensive care units ranges from 10 to 65 per cent, with case fatalities of 13–55 per cent. It is often associated with mechanical ventilation. The risk of hospital-acquired pneumonia can be substantially reduced by using non-invasive methods for respiratory support instead of ventilation and by having clear care protocols for protecting host defences against respiratory infection during mechanical ventilation. Chemoprophylaxis plays a role through the use of selective decontamination of the digestive tract (see Chapters 18 and 31), which reduces the numbers of Gram-negative bacilli and hence the risk of infection.

The microorganisms causing pneumonia within 5 days of admission are quite different from those seen in disease with a later onset. The bacteria responsible for early onset pneumonia are *Str. pneumoniae*, *H. influenzae*, *Staph. aureus*, and only rarely enteric Gram-negative bacilli. In contrast, late-onset infection is almost always caused by Gram-negative bacteria, mainly enterobacteria but also *Ps. aeruginosa* and *Acinetobacter* spp. Methicillin-resistant *Staph. aureus* (MRSA) is becoming increasingly common in some units. Since tracheal aspirates are poor indicators of the cause of ventilator-associated pneumonia, bronchoalveolar lavage is recommended to confirm the diagnosis.

Empirical treatment for early onset pneumonia in patients who have not received antibiotics should be with co-amoxiclav or cefuroxime. Treatment of patients who have already received antibiotics or have late-onset disease should be with a broad-spectrum cephalosporin such as cefotaxime, a fluoroquinolone, or piperacillin plus tazobactam. Combination therapy is no more effective than monotherapy. Subsequent treatment should be directed by the results of bronchoalveolar lavage.

## Other respiratory tract infections

Pneumonia developing in association with neutropenia following treatment with cytotoxic drugs, or in patients with immunosuppression, including those suffering from AIDS, may be due to *Pneumocystis carinii*, other fungi, or viruses. Appropriate treatment is discussed in Chapters 31 and 32. The treatment of tuberculosis is considered in Chapter 30; influenza and other respiratory viral infections are dealt with in Chapter 32.

# Decision making about antibacterial treatment for respiratory tract infection

Respiratory tract infection is the commonest indication for antibacterial treatment in primary and secondary care. Guidelines are required to aid decision making to initiate and discontinue antibacterials (Chapters 19 and 20). Tests of inflammatory markers have been used to guide decision making (Fig. 21.1). The strongest evidence is for procalcitonin, with a total of 14 randomized controlled trials in primary care, accident and emergency, and intensive care. Collectively these show that use of procalcitonin was associated with a mean reduction in antibiotic use by 3.5 days per patient, with no evidence of increased mortality or clinical failure.

## Key points

♦ Respiratory tract infections are the commonest indication for antibiotic treatment in primary care and in hospitals.

♦ Eighty per cent of total antimicrobial use is in primary care and 60 per cent of that is for respiratory infections that are on the whole self-limiting. Most respiratory infections in primary care are caused by viruses and will not benefit from antibiotic treatment. However, the key question in the decision about treatment with antimicrobials is, do the benefits to the patient outweigh the risks? It is not necessary to prescribe antimicrobials for all bacterial respiratory infections.

♦ Upper respiratory tract infections, sore throat, and otitis media do not benefit from antibiotic treatment, even when caused by bacteria, unless there is clinical evidence of complications.

♦ Bronchitis in adults aged <65 does not benefit from antibiotic treatment. However, in older adults it is more difficult to distinguish between bronchitis and pneumonia.

♦ Severity of suspected pneumonia should be assessed with the CRB65 score in primary care, and the CURB65 score in hospitals.

♦ Patients with severe pneumonia should be treated with intravenous antibiotics that are effective against the full range of pathogens that may cause community-acquired pneumonia. The choice of antibiotic is influenced by the risk of *Clo. difficile* infection in the hospital.

## Further reading

### All respiratory infections

**Health Protection Agency.** Management of infection guidance for primary care for consultation & local adaptation <https://www.gov.uk/government/publications/managing-common-infections-guidance-for-primary-care> (26th February 2011, date last accessed).

**Schuetz, P., Muller, B., Christ-Crain, M., et al.** (2012) Procalcitonin to initiate or discontinue antibiotics in acute respiratory tract infections. *Cochrane Database of Systematic Reviews*, Issue **9**: Art. No. CD007498.

**Scottish Antimicrobial Prescribing Group.** (2012) *Prudent Antimicrobial use in Primary Care—Respiratory.* <http://www.scottishmedicines.org.uk/files/sapg/Prudent_antimicrobial_use_respiratory.pdf>, accessed 1 December 2014.

**Scottish Intercollegiate Guidelines Network.** (2002). *SIGN 59: Community Management of Lower Respiratory Tract Infection in Adults.* <http://www.sign.ac.uk/guidelines/fulltext/59/index.html>, accessed 1 December 2014.

**Scottish Intercollegiate Guidelines Network.** (2003) *SIGN 66: Diagnosis and Management of Childhood Otitis Media in Primary Care.* <http://www.sign.ac.uk/guidelines/fulltext/66/index.html>, accessed 1 December 2014.

**Scottish Intercollegiate Guidelines Network.** (2010) *SIGN 117: Management of Sore Throat and Indications for Tonsillectomy.* <http://www.sign.ac.uk/guidelines/fulltext/117/index.html>, accessed 1 December 2014.

## Pneumonia

**Barker, B., Macfarlane, J., Lim, W. S., and Douglas, G.** (2009) Local guidelines for management of adult community acquired pneumonia: a survey of UK hospitals. *Thorax* **64**(2): 181.

**Dryden, M., Hand, K., and Davey, P.** (2009) Antibiotics for community-acquired pneumonia. *Journal of Antimicrobial Chemotherapy,* **64**(6): 1123–5.

**Harris, M., Clark, J., Coote, N., Fletcher, P., Harnden, A., McKean, M., and Thomson, A.** (2002) British Thoracic Society guidelines for the management of community acquired pneumonia in childhood. *Thorax,* **57**(Suppl 1): i1–i24.

**Lim, W. S., Baudouin, S. V., George, R. C., et al.** (2009) BTS guidelines for the management of community acquired pneumonia in adults: update 2009. *Thorax,* **64**(Suppl 3): iii1–iii55.

## Chronic obstructive pulmonary disease

**El Moussaoui, R., Roede, B. M., Speelman, P., Bresser, P., Prins, J. M., and Bossuyt, P. M.** (2008) Short-course antibiotic treatment in acute exacerbations of chronic bronchitis and COPD: a meta-analysis of double-blind studies. *Thorax,* **63**(5):415–22.

**Falagas, M. E., Avgeri, S. G., Matthaiou, D. K., Dimopoulos, G., and Siempos, I. I.** (2008) Short- versus long-duration antimicrobial treatment for exacerbations of chronic bronchitis: a meta-analysis. *Journal of Antimicrobial Chemotherapy,* **62**(3):442–50.

**Herath, S. C. and Poole, P.** (2013) Prophylactic antibiotic therapy for chronic obstructive pulmonary disease (COPD). *Cochrane Database of Systematic Reviews,* Issue **11**: Art. No. CD009764.

## Sputum samples for LRTI in primary care

**NHS Education for Scotland.** (2009) *The Knowledge Network. CLEAR: Clinical Enquiry and Response Service. Is It Appropriate To Send Sputum Samples for Microscopy, Culture and Sensitivity in Elderly Patients with a Suspected Chest Infection?* <http://www.knowledge.scot.nhs.uk/clear/answers/respiratory/is-it-appropriate-to-send-sputum-samples-for-microscopy-culture-and-sensitivity-in-elderly-patients-with-a-suspected-chest-infection.aspx>, accessed 1 December 2014.

# Chapter 22

# Topical use of antimicrobial agents

## Introduction to topical use of antimicrobial agents

The concept of applying drugs directly to clinical lesions is appealing: problems of absorption and pharmacokinetics do not apply and agents too toxic for systemic use may be safely applied to skin or mucous membranes. The major drawback is that, even in the most superficial skin lesion, there may be areas inaccessible to a topical approach. Furthermore, collections of pus may prevent the agent reaching the infecting organisms and, for this reason, the management of any abscess includes drainage of pus.

Although skin, the largest and most accessible organ of the body, is the most obvious target for topical antimicrobial agents, other sites are available for this approach to therapy: the mucous membranes of the mouth and vagina, and the external surfaces of eyes and ears. Direct application of antibiotics into normally sterile sites (e.g. joints, peritoneal cavity, spinal fluid, or the urinary bladder) or instillation into surgical wounds prior to suture may also be considered as a form of topical therapy but will not be specifically dealt with in this chapter. Application of topical agents to mucous membranes or damaged skin may lead to considerable systemic absorption, and the possibility of systemic toxicity should be borne in mind.

The chief reasons for using topical antimicrobial agents are

◆ to achieve high drug concentrations at the site of infection;

◆ to treat trivial infections where use of a systemic drug is unjustified;

◆ to prevent infection in a susceptible site (e.g. burns);

◆ to enable the use of agents that are too toxic for systemic use; and

◆ cost: topical agents are generally cheaper than systemic drugs.

## Antiseptics

Disinfectant is a general term for chemicals that can destroy vegetative (and sometimes spores of) microorganisms; those disinfectants that are sufficiently non-injurious to skin and exposed tissues to be used topically are called antiseptics. In order to achieve adequate antimicrobial activity, high concentrations of antiseptics are required and this serves to distinguish them from antibiotics in Waksman's original sense of 'substances produced by microorganisms antagonistic to the growth or life of others in high dilution'. In many cases, true antibiotics are used topically in high concentration and might thus be classed as antiseptics. In fact, antiseptics and antibiotics are often used in exactly the same situations in dermatological practice and there has been some difference of opinion as to which class of agent to use in, for example, the treatment of infected ulcers or wounds. Antiseptics are usually cheaper and have the advantage that bacterial resistance rarely develops. Preparations commonly employed include chlorhexidine, cetrimide, iodophors (non-irritant iodine complexes), triclosan, and solutions liberating hypochlorite, such as Eusol or Dakin's solution. However, recent concerns about possible toxicity, including environmental effects, associated with triclosan has led to much greater restriction of its use. Occasional reports of 'reduced susceptibility' to antiseptics (e.g. some methicillin-resistant *Staph. aureus* (MRSA) clones displaying reduced susceptibility to chlorhexidine) and cross-resistance (e.g. to benzalkonium chloride/quinolones in several bacterial species) has increased the level of debate about their widespread use.

Some concern has been expressed about the effect on tissue viability of many chemicals applied directly. There is some evidence in vitro of a direct toxic effect on epidermal cells and white blood cells of many antiseptics at concentrations well below those used topically.

## Methods of application

Drugs that are dissolved in aqueous solutions (lotions) have the disadvantage of running off the skin and cooling it by evaporation. This method of delivering antimicrobial agents to the site of infection is inefficient and not often used, except as ear or eye drops. For use in eye infections, frequent application on to the cornea and conjunctiva is necessary, because the drug is only in contact for a short time and much of the active component runs down the cheek as an expensive tear! The value of aqueous preparations resides mainly in their irrigational and cleansing action, and much of the therapeutic success may be due to these properties.

It is usual to apply drugs to the skin in a fat base, as either an oil and water cream or a largely lipid ointment. Drug solubility affects the achievable concentration in each component, and availability at the lesion depends on diffusion from the applicant and absorption from the skin. Antibiotics that are lipid soluble and freely diffusible, for example, fusidic acid, are at an advantage in this respect.

Sticky ointments may remain in contact with the infected site for a considerable time, and application may be needed only once daily but this obviously depends on the frequency of washing or removal of dressings.

Some of the commonly used topical preparations are listed in Tables 22.1 and 22.2. Many of the formulations designed for topical use contain combinations of antimicrobial agents. Mixtures are intended to cover a wide antibacterial spectrum and to be compatible.

## Choice

The results of laboratory tests may be helpful if adequate specimens are sent to the laboratory but swabbing chronic ulcers or other skin wounds is not helpful (Chapter 29). Frequently, colonizing microbes are isolated from the surface of deep lesions, leaving the true underlying pathogen undetected. The clinician must be careful not to use a battery of antimicrobials to treat harmless commensals colonizing an unoccupied niche. The golden rule is 'treat the patient, not the wound'.

Conventional antimicrobial sensitivity testing is often irrelevant, because susceptibility of organisms to antiseptics can usually be assumed. Moreover, laboratory criteria of susceptibility to antibiotics usually apply to systemic use, not the high concentrations achievable by topical application. Nevertheless, complete resistance in laboratory tests is a contraindication to use of a particular agent. Regular monitoring of hospital patients with large skin lesions such as ulcers and burns may sometimes be used to determine the nature and prevalence of resistant organisms, as well as the extent of cross-infection.

Choice, if not based on microbiological evidence, must include agents active against all likely pathogens. Topical antiseptics and hydroxyquinolines are to be preferred to antibiotics on microbiological grounds of avoidance of resistance but many users prefer antibiotics because it is claimed that a quicker response is generally obtained. Tetracyclines are not a good choice given

**Table 22.1** Commonly used topical antimicrobial agents for skin infections (the numerous topical antiseptics available are omitted).

| Infection | Agent | Application | Comments |
|---|---|---|---|
| Bacterial | Chloramphenicol[a] | Ointment | Very broad spectrum |
| | Clindamycin[a] | Ointment | Used for acne |
| | Erythromycin[a] | Ointment | Used for acne |
| | Fusidic acid[a] | Ointment | Only active against *Staphylococcus aureus* and *Streptococcus pyogenes* |
| | Gentamicin[a] | Cream/ointment | Ototoxic and nephrotoxic if used over large areas of broken skin |
| | Metronidazole[a] | Gel | Used in rosacea and acne |
| | Mupirocin | Ointment | Macrogol-based ointment or nasal cream; only active against Gram-positive cocci and mainly used for eradication of methicillin-resistant *Staph. aureus* (MRSA) carriage |
| | Neomycin | Cream/ointment/powder | Often combined with gramicidin or bacitracin and/or polymyxin B; ototoxic and nephrotoxic if used over large areas of broken skin |
| | Polymyxins[a] | Ointment/powder | Nephrotoxic and neurotoxic if used over large areas of broken skin |
| | Silver sulfadiazine (sulphonamide) | Cream | May cause sensitization |
| | Tetracycline[a] | Ointment/cream/drops | Broad spectrum; resistance common |
| Fungal | Imidazoles (clotrimazole, etc.) | Cream/powder | For dermatophyte or yeast skin infections but ineffective against nail infections |
| | Nystatin (and other polyenes) | Cream | For dermatophyte or yeast skin infections but ineffective against nail infections |
| | Tioconazole and amorolfine | Nail lacquer/cream | For limited dermatophyte nail infections |
| Viral | Aciclovir[a] and penciclovir[a] | Ointment/cream | Antiviral agents; for use on herpes lesions |
| | Idoxuridine | Ointment/drops | |

[a] Compounds that are also used systemically.

the prevalence of tetracycline resistance and the readiness with which this increases under selective pressure. Combinations of antibiotics, such as bacitracin and neomycin, or bacitracin, neomycin, and polymyxin, are often used and a corticosteroid is sometimes added for good measure. These antibiotics are not usually used for systemic therapy, so possible problems of compromising the activity of systemically useful agents by encouraging the emergence of resistance are minimized (see below). Nevertheless, it should be remembered that the topical use of neomycin might generate strains of bacteria cross-resistant to other aminoglycosides such as gentamicin.

**Table 22.2** Commonly used topical antimicrobial agents for other sites (the numerous topical antiseptics available are omitted).

| Site | Agent | Application | Comments |
|------|-------|-------------|----------|
| Ear, bacterial | Chloramphenicol[a] | Ear drops | For otitis externa |
| | Aminoglycosides (framycetin, gentamicin[a] and neomycin) | Ear drops | For otitis externa; should not be used in otitis media because of risk of ototoxicity with a perforated ear drum |
| | Polymyxins[a] | Ear drops | For otitis externa; should not be used in otitis media because of risk of ototoxicity with a perforated ear drum |
| | Fluoroquinolones (ciprofloxacin and ofloxacin)[a] | Ear drops | For otitis externa and otitis media; not licensed in the United Kingdom |
| Ear, fungal | Clotrimazole | Ear drops | For fungal otitis externa |
| Eye, bacterial | Aminoglycosides (framycetin, gentamicin[a], and neomycin) | Eye and ear drops | |
| | Chloramphenicol[a] | Eye drops or ointment | Drug of choice for superficial eye infections |
| | Fusidic acid[a] | Eye drops | For staphylococcal infections only |
| | Polymyxins[a] | Eye drops or ointment | |
| | Fluoroquinolones (ciprofloxacin and ofloxacin)[a] | Eye drops | |
| Eye, viral | Aciclovir[a] | Eye ointment | For local treatment of superficial herpes simplex (dendritic ulcer) |
| | Ganciclovir[a] | Eye drops | For treatment of herpes keratitis |
| Mouth, fungal | Amphotericin[a] | Lozenges or suspension | For mild oral candida (thrush); not absorbed |
| | Miconazole | Oral gel | For mild oral candida (thrush); enough oral absorption to cause drug interactions; check before use |
| | Nystatin | Pastilles or suspension | For mild oral candida (thrush); not absorbed |
| Vaginal, fungal | Imidazoles (e.g. clotrimazole, econazole) | Creams, ointments and pessaries | Vaginal candidiasis (thrush) |
| | Nystatin | | |

[a] Compounds that are also used systemically.

One antibiotic, mupirocin (pseudomonic acid), has been marketed solely for topical use. The spectrum of activity of this agent is virtually restricted to Gram-positive cocci. Mupirocin is unsuitable for systemic use since it is quickly metabolized in the body. It has a unique mode of action (on protein synthesis) and cross-resistance is not a problem. However, prolonged and/or repeated administration of mupirocin, most often to suppress/eradicate MRSA in the nose, is associated with the emergence of resistant strains.

In practice, one of the most important limitations to choice is the availability of a particular drug as a topical product. Manufacturers are well aware that it makes little commercial sense to market a relatively cheap topical formulation if it is going to encourage resistance that diminishes the usefulness of more expensive parenteral forms of the drug. Here, at least, the interests of industry and the consumer coincide.

## Bacterial skin infections

Trivial skin sepsis, often due to staphylococci, is common but usually self-limiting in healthy individuals. In general, mild infections of the skin respond to local measures involving cleansing of the crusted areas and application of topical agents, such as fusidic acid or mupirocin, to the raw surfaces. More severe staphylococcal and streptococcal skin lesions may require systemic therapy (Chapter 29).

### Nasal carriage

In recurrent sepsis with *Staph. aureus*, it may be necessary to attempt to eradicate the organism from the body. This is also desirable in patients and staff colonized with antibiotic-resistant strains, particularly MRSA, which can cause serious cross-infection problems. The external surface of the skin can be washed in antiseptics but nasal carriage of staphylococci is often resistant to this treatment. For this purpose, nasal creams should be applied at least twice a day for 5 days. Chlorhexidine/neomycin cream (Naseptin) has been widely used but does not appear to be as effective as mupirocin in the eradication of nasal carriage of MRSA. The normal dermatological preparation of mupirocin, which is in a macrogol (polyethylene glycol) excipient, is unsuitable for nasal application, and a paraffin-based ointment should be used for this purpose. Antibiotic application to the nares is usually carried out in combination with use of topical skin/hair washing, typically with chlorhexidine preparations. Without the latter, recurrence of MRSA colonization is more common.

### Acne

The role of bacteria in the pathogenesis of acne vulgaris is still under debate, although commensal diphtheroids, such as *Propionibacterium acnes*, are thought to play some part. Systemic antibiotics, including tetracycline and erythromycin, do improve severe intractable cases, and success has also been claimed for topical antimicrobial agents, in particular, for clindamycin. Treatment with any of these agents needs to be prolonged and is an adjunct to other measures aimed at improving the condition.

### Burns

The treatment of burns is a very specialized topic that cannot be covered adequately in this chapter. However, topical agents do have definite value in the prevention of infection in patients with burns, so it is appropriate that their use should be mentioned.

Initially, a thermal burn renders the skin sterile but bacterial colonization is inevitable, even with scrupulous aseptic technique. Indeed, infection, usually with *Streptococcus pyogenes*, *Staph. aureus*, or *Pseudomonas aeruginosa*, is an important determinant in the outcome of extensive burns, since it is a major cause of delay in skin healing and of death.

Prophylaxis with topical antibiotics and antiseptics has been shown significantly to reduce colonization and sepsis. Mafenide, a sulphonamide derivative, was widely used but has been largely replaced in the United Kingdom by silver sulphadiazine or chlorhexidine. None of these agents will reliably prevent infection by multiresistant Gram-negative rods, especially *Ps. aeruginosa* (an organism that has replaced *Str. pyogenes* as the major scourge of burns units), or fungi. Aggressive surgical approaches, including early wound closure by skin grafting after debridement, have reduced the requirement for topical applications to burned tissues.

In cases in which infection becomes established, systemic drugs will often have to be employed, the choice being dictated by laboratory tests. However, since the penetration of antibiotics to surface lesions with a poor blood supply may be inadequate, topical dressings are additionally required. Urinary and respiratory infections are commonly encountered in the burned patient and may result in bacteraemia with sepsis, which has a poor prognosis. These infections require, of course, systemic therapy but choice may be limited by bacterial resistance, since many burns units are notorious for the prevalence of highly resistant strains, especially of *Ps. aeruginosa*.

## Skin ulcers

Ulceration of the skin of the leg or the area overlying the sacrum may arise from a variety of pathological states, and colonization is usually a sequela, not an initiating event. Disorders of the circulation, including obliterative arterial disease, small-vessel damage consequent on diabetes mellitus, and varicose veins, are the most common underlying conditions; correction of the underlying cause is essential to the healing of any ulcer. Continuous pressure is another common factor in the formation of a break in the skin, particularly in the bed ridden. Such pressure sores (bed sores) are difficult to prevent without scrupulous nursing care. This problem has led to the development of special air beds and cushions to minimize local vascular occlusion to the skin overlying bony areas such as the sacrum.

The presence of colonization in a skin ulcer may be detected by odour and appearance of pus, which in the case of pseudomonas infection may be characteristically green. However, colonization is not an indication for antibacterial treatment, which should be reserved for patients with spreading cellulitis or systemic inflammatory response (Chapter 29). Swab reports showing the presence of potential pathogens do not prove infection since colonization of a large raw skin area is inevitable. *Staph. aureus*, environmental bacteria, and gut bacteria are the organisms most commonly found in these sites. *Ps. aeruginosa* is frequently found in long-standing ulcers because of its intrinsic resistance to many antibiotics and chemical agents used as antiseptics. There is some evidence that deep swabs (after debridement) or tissue samples (e.g. punch biopsies) may yield more useful microbiological information but it is impractical to obtain these frequently from a patient.

Some chemical antiseptics are cytotoxic and impair wound healing; consequently, older remedies such as honey, sugar, and vinegar may be as effective as modern antiseptics. Topical antibiotics should be avoided. Many weeks of regular dressing combined with bed rest may be required to heal large ulcers; admission to hospital often speeds up the process. Skin grafting or vascular surgery (to improve the blood supply) can be considered for the most recalcitrant cases.

## Superficial fungal infections

Confirmation of the diagnosis of superficial fungal infections such as ringworm and tinea pedis of the skin, or thrush of the mouth or vagina, depends on laboratory investigation of appropriate specimens from the affected area (nail, hair, skin scrapings, swabs of lesions of mucous membranes). Microscopy alone will be sufficient to establish a fungal cause in most cases but culture is necessary to identify the aetiological agent. Susceptibility testing presents technical difficulties but dermatophytes may usually be assumed to be susceptible to appropriate agents (see Table 4.1).

*Candida albicans* may acquire resistance to some drugs but this is of great importance only in invasive candidiasis.

The limiting factor in treating dermatophyte infections is penetration of the agent. For superficial skin infections, old-fashioned remedies, such as benzoic acid-containing ointments (e.g. Whitfield's ointment) are perfectly effective but for hair and nail infections, agents that penetrate into keratinized tissue are needed. Oral griseofulvin and terbinafine are suited to this purpose, since they are absorbed from the gastrointestinal tract and are preferentially concentrated in keratin. Because of the slow turnover of nail and hair, treatment for several months may be required; indeed, fungal infections of toenails may not completely clear even after a year's treatment with griseofulvin, despite susceptibility of the infecting fungus. In such cases terbinafine (see Chapter 8) may be successful. Topical treatment with amorolfine or tioconazole, which are formulated to penetrate nails, are less effective than terbinafine.

Thrush responds in most cases to an appropriate antifungal agent, applied topically (e.g. nystatin or an imidazole), but precipitating factors such as diabetes or antibiotic therapy must also be corrected if they are present. If there is clinical evidence for invasive infection as, for example, *Candida* oesophagitis, appropriate systemic drugs, such as amphotericin, 5-fluorocytosine, fluconazole, ketoconazole, or itraconazole must be added.

## Disadvantages of topical therapy

Topical therapy is not without its hazards. Although the direct toxic effects of drugs given systemically are reduced, exposed tissues and mucous membranes offer a fairly efficient site for drug absorption. For example, aminoglycoside ototoxicity has been reported following local application of neomycin, especially in the newborn. A more frequently observed effect is sensitization to the agent so that subsequent use of the drug, either topically or parenterally, produces a hypersensitivity reaction. Penicillin, in particular, is prone to sensitize the host and, because of possible anaphylactic reactions, it is not advisable to use any β-lactam antibiotic on the skin. A further hazard of topical therapy is that local irritation may lead to a delay in wound healing, even though the actual infection is controlled.

Superinfection with resistant bacteria or with fungi is a common consequence of using any topical antibiotic for a prolonged period. Widespread use of one particular agent will lead to a larger reservoir of resistant organisms and the possibility of cross-infection. This is particularly likely to occur in burns units and dermatology wards, where there are many patients with large open skin lesions. Prevention of infection and cross-infection by aseptic methods is desirable, but often difficult in practice.

Of equal concern is the development of bacterial resistance during therapy. It has been shown that topical neomycin can select resistant *Staph. epidermidis* strains, which can transfer resistance to *Staph. aureus* on the skin. The emergence of gentamicin-resistant *Ps. aeruginosa* and coliforms has been associated with topical use of that aminoglycoside, particularly on leg ulcers. In some instances, the resistance is plasmid mediated. In this manner, topical agents select multiresistant organisms, which may subsequently cause systemic infection in the patient or, by cross-infection, others.

Tetracycline eye drops select for tetracycline-resistant bacteria in the mouth flora when used for mass population treatment of trachoma. The explanation is likely to be that medications administered to the eye can readily reach the nasopharynx via the naso-lachrymal duct. Selection of resistant bacteria is the most powerful argument against the indiscriminate use of topical antibiotics and, since antiseptics lack this disadvantage, they are to be preferred wherever possible.

## Key points

♦ Although skin, the largest and most accessible organ of the body, is the most obvious target for topical antimicrobial agents, other sites are available for this approach to therapy: the mucous membranes of the mouth and vagina, and the external surfaces of eyes and ears.

♦ The major drawback to topical treatment of skin infections is that, even in the most superficial skin lesion, there may be areas inaccessible to a topical approach. Furthermore, collections of pus may prevent the agent reaching the infecting organisms and, for this reason, the management of any abscess includes drainage of pus.

♦ Application of topical agents to mucous membranes or damaged skin may lead to considerable systemic absorption, and the possibility of systemic toxicity should be borne in mind.

♦ Superinfection with fungi/resistant bacteria and selection of resistant strains during treatment are both common consequences of using any topical antibiotic for a prolonged period.

♦ Widespread use of one particular agent will lead to a larger reservoir of resistant organisms and the possibility of cross-infection. This is particularly likely to occur in burns units and dermatology wards, where there are many patients with large open skin lesions.

## Further reading

Harbarth S, Tuan Soh S, Horner C, Wilcox MH. Is reduced susceptibility to disinfectants and antiseptics a risk in healthcare settings? A point/counterpoint review. J Hosp Infect. 2014;87:194–202.

O'Meara S[1], Al-Kurdi D, Ologun Y, Ovington LG, Martyn-St James M, Richardson R. Antibiotics and antiseptics for venous leg ulcers. Cochrane Database Syst Rev. 2014;1:CD003557.

# Chapter 23

# Urinary tract infections

## Introduction to urinary tract infections

Urinary tract infection is the second most common clinical indication for empirical antimicrobial treatment in primary and secondary care; respiratory tract infections are the commonest clinical indication in both settings. Urine samples constitute the largest single category of specimens examined in most medical microbiology laboratories. Health-care practitioners regularly have to make decisions about prescription of antibiotics for urinary tract infection. Criteria for the diagnosis of urinary tract infection vary depending on the patient and the context.

## Diagnostic methods

### Culture of bacteria from urine

The laboratory confirmation of bacteriuria is made by quantitative culture of an uncontaminated urine specimen. The most reliable methods for obtaining a urine sample without contamination by skin or perineal flora are by suprapubic aspiration of the bladder with a syringe and needle or by urethral catheterization. Neither of these is practical or acceptable in clinical practice, so urine samples are collected during micturition. The practice of cleansing the perineum and taking the specimen in the middle of micturition minimizes the risk of contamination by the perineal flora. However, it is critical that cultures of urine are done as quickly as possible; otherwise, a few contaminating bacteria from skin and perineal flora will multiply in a few hours at room temperature and give false positive results. Refrigeration and rapid processing in the laboratory can reduce this problem. Alternatively, culture of urine as soon as it is passed can circumvent the possibility of contaminants growing in the urine during transit. This is achieved by using dip-inoculum methods, which consist of agar attached to slides or spoons that are dipped in the urine, drained, and transported in a stoppered bottle to the laboratory, where any bacterial colonies are counted after overnight incubation at 37°C.

When more than $10^5$ organisms/ml ($10^8$/l) of a single bacterial species are cultured from a freshly voided midstream specimen of urine, the term 'significant' bacteriuria is used, because it is highly unlikely that such a large number of bacteria could be the result of contamination of the sample. In other words, the laboratory finding of 'significant' bacteriuria means that it is very likely that the bacteria were present in the urine in the body before micturition. The symptoms of urinary tract infection can be associated with lower counts of bacteria: $10^3$ organisms/ml in men and $10^2$ organisms/ml in women. However, most clinical laboratories cannot detect such low levels of bacteria with routine methods, so in practice the threshold for significant bacteriuria remains at $10^5$ organisms/ml.

### Urine dipstick testing

Urine dipsticks use reagents to detect the presence of chemicals in the urine. The presence of nitrites in urine is associated with bacteriuria as they are products of bacterial metabolism;

however, nitrites can be found in sterile urine as well. The presence of leucocyte esterase is associated with the presence of white blood cells in the urine, which may in turn be associated with urinary tract infection. However, any cause of inflammation of the urinary tract will result in white cells in the urine. Other substances (blood or protein) can be present in the urine of patients with symptomatic urinary tract infection but they are even less specific to the diagnosis than nitrites or leucocyte esterase.

## Management of common clinical problems

### Asymptomatic bacteriuria

Although normal urine is sterile some healthy people have bacteriuria without any symptoms. Most information comes from women, in whom the prevalence of bacteriuria increases with age (Fig. 23.1). The prevalence at any given age is related to sexual activity: 5 per cent of married women aged 24–44 are likely to have asymptomatic bacteriuria, compared with <1 per cent of nuns of the same age. There is less information about men. As with women, the prevalence of bacteriuria in men increases with age but it is always lower than in women of the same age. In the elderly the prevalence in men and women increases with deterioration of health and reaches 100 per cent in anybody who has an indwelling urinary catheter present for >4 weeks (Table 23.1).

There are only two groups of patients in whom asymptomatic bacteriuria should be treated with antibiotics:

1 In very young children whose kidneys are still growing, there is evidence that asymptomatic bacteriuria is associated with scarring of the kidney and predisposes to hypertension or chronic

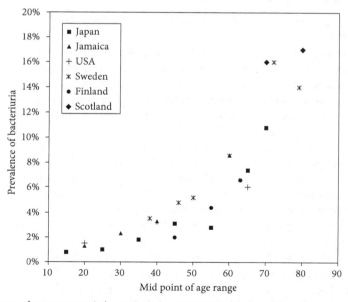

**Fig. 23.1** Presence of asymptomatic bacteriuria in non-pregnant women by age in six countries.
Source: data from Scottish Intercollegiate Guidelines Network, *Management of suspected bacterial urinary tract infection in adults*, Sign Guidelines 88, Copyright © 2006, available from http://www.sign.ac.uk/pdf/sign88.pdf

**Table 23.1** Prevalence of bacteriuria in men and women aged 70 years or greater.

| Category | Men (%) | Women (%) |
| --- | --- | --- |
| Healthy, ambulatory | 7 | 17 |
| Institutionalized | 37 | 57 |
| Indwelling urinary catheter for >4 weeks | 100 | 100 |

renal impairment. Young children who have had symptomatic urinary tract infection are therefore followed up after treatment to ensure that they do not have continuing bacteriuria.

2 In pregnancy, asymptomatic bacteriuria is associated with increased risk of pyelonephritis later in pregnancy and with preterm delivery. Moreover, there is good evidence that antibiotic treatment of asymptomatic bacteriuria reduces the risk of both these outcomes. Consequently, all pregnant women should be screened in the first trimester of pregnancy, and women with bacteriuria should be treated.

Asymptomatic bacteriuria should not be treated with antibiotics in any other people. Placebo-controlled trials have failed to show convincing benefit in patients with diabetes, in institutionalized elderly men or women, or in those with long-term indwelling catheters, whereas the same trials did show increased risk of adverse events in the treated patients, including colonization with antibiotic-resistant bacteria.

The important point to remember is that bacteriuria is not diagnostic of urinary tract infection, which only occurs once bacteria invade the tissues of the urinary tract. Bacteriuria is a laboratory finding, not a disease.

## Symptomatic urinary tract infection

### Lower urinary tract infection in non-pregnant women (uncomplicated urinary tract infection)

Infection of the tissues of the bladder or urethra causes increased frequency of micturition with severe burning pain on passing urine (dysuria). The walls of the bladder and urethra have a relatively poor blood supply and so bacteria are not able to penetrate into the blood; people with lower urinary tract infection do not have a systemic inflammatory response. In fact, if a patient presents with dysuria, frequency, and symptoms of systemic inflammatory response, it should be assumed that they have upper urinary tract infection.

The symptoms of lower urinary tract infection can be very severe and make it impossible for patients to continue their normal lives without effective treatment.

Cystitis means inflammation of the bladder and is sometimes used as a pseudonym for lower urinary tract infection, although strictly the term should be bacterial cystitis to distinguish from other causes of cystitis (e.g. chemical cystitis or interstitial cystitis).

Uncomplicated urinary tract infection is defined as lower urinary tract infection in non-pregnant women with no underlying anatomical abnormalities that predispose to recurrent urinary tract infection. The adjective 'uncomplicated' is being used in two different ways:

1 The likelihood that the infection can be resolved successfully with a short (3-day) course of antibiotics. This is why lower urinary tract infection in men is classified as complicated, because it is likely to be associated with prostatitis, in which case it is likely to relapse unless antibiotics are continued for 2 weeks.

2   The likelihood that there will be no clinical complications from the infection. This is why all upper urinary tract infections and also symptoms of lower urinary tract infections in pregnant women are classed as complicated, because both problems are associated with immediate risk to the patient from sepsis or severe sepsis.

Clinical diagnosis of lower urinary tract infection is reliable in young adult women who have dysuria and frequency but no history of vaginal discharge. Neither dipstick tests nor urine culture are necessary to confirm the diagnosis, and empiric antibiotic treatment (3 days of trimethoprim or nitrofurantoin) should be given on the basis of these symptoms alone (Fig. 23.2). If the symptoms are less clear-cut, then urine dipstick testing should be done. If this is positive then 3 days of trimethoprim or nitrofurantoin should be given; but, if it is negative, bacteriuria should be confirmed with culture before treatment is given (Fig. 23.2).

Urinary tract infection is difficult to diagnose in older women because it is more likely to present with vague, generalized symptoms. Moreover the prevalence of asymptomatic bacteriuria increases steadily with age and with increasing co-morbidity. Over 50 per cent of institutionalized elderly women have asymptomatic bacteriuria all of the time. The decision to give antibiotic treatment should be based on clinical diagnosis of infection, supported by acute local or systemic symptoms of inflammation. Smelly urine just means that the patient has bacteriuria, which is not unusual and does not require antibiotic treatment.

In domiciliary practice, *Escherichia coli* predominates, accounting for at least 80 per cent of isolates. Resistance to trimethoprim and co-trimoxazole is increasingly common and is

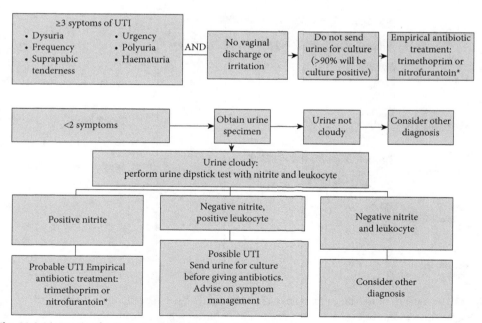

**Fig. 23.2** Diagnosis of urinary tract infection in adult women.

Adapted from Health Protection Agency, Diagnosis of UTI, *Quick Reference Guide for Primary Care 2011*, © Crown Copyright, licence under the Open Government Licence v2.0, available from http://www.hpa.org.uk/webc/HPAwebFile/HPAweb_C/1194947404720

>30 per cent in some countries (Fig. 23.3). However, in countries with lower antibiotic use, such as the Netherlands and the United Kingdom, resistance to trimethoprim remains at about 20 per cent; guidelines recommend empirical treatment without urine culture for women with obvious symptoms because trimethoprim is extremely well tolerated (Table 23.2). However, the risk of infection with trimethoprim-resistant bacteria is increased in women who have been exposed to co-trimoxazole or trimethoprim in the past three months, and these women should be treated with nitrofurantoin. Most *E. coli* remain sensitive to nitrofurantoin (Fig. 23.3) but the drug is not as well tolerated as trimethoprim and is also ineffective if the patient has upper urinary tract infection. The use of co-trimoxazole is not recommended in the treatment of urinary infection in the United Kingdom, since the sulphonamide component plays an insignificant role and trimethoprim alone is less toxic.

For bacteria that are resistant to nitrofurantoin and trimethoprim, or for patients who cannot tolerate these drugs, there is a range of alternative oral agents, including co-amoxiclav, ciprofloxacin, and pivmecillinam. The reason that these drugs are not used first line is that they are no more effective than nitrofurantoin or trimethoprim and have more adverse effects (Table 23.2). They should be reserved for patients in whom these first line agents are ineffective or contraindicated.

The prevalence of resistance in *E. coli* is variable between countries (Fig. 23.3). The prevalence of multiresistant *E. coli* with extended spectrum β-lactamases (also known as ESBLs) has been increasing in all European countries over the past 10 years, and even in primary care patients

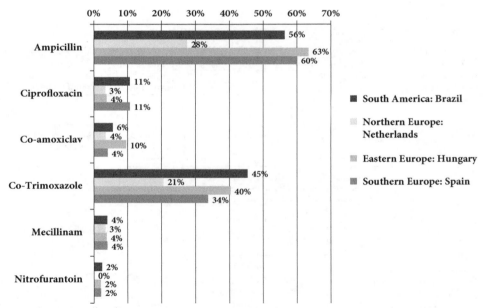

**Fig. 23.3** Prevalence of resistance to antibiotics in urinary isolates of *E. coli* from women aged 18–65 with symptoms of uncomplicated cystitis and consecutively enrolled in four countries.

Source: data from *European Urology*, Volume 54, Issue 5, Naber KG, et al., 'Surveillance study in Europe and Brazil on clinical aspects and Antimicrobial Resistance Epidemiology in Females with Cystitis (ARESC): implications for empiric therapy', pp. 1164–75, Copyright © 2008 European Association of Urology. Published by Elsevier B.V. All rights reserved.

**Table 23.2** Treatment regimens and expected early efficacy rates for acute uncomplicated cystitis.*

| Drug | Mean clinical efficacy (%) | Mean microbiological efficacy (%) | Common side effects |
|---|---|---|---|
| Nitrofurantoin for 3 days | 93 | 88 | Nausea, headache |
| Trimethoprim for 3 days | 93 | 94 | Nausea |
| Fosfomycin, single dose | 91 | 80 | Nausea, diarrhoea, headache |
| Pivmecillinam for 3 days | 73 | 79 | Nausea, vomiting, diarrhoea |
| Ciprofloxacin for 3 days | 90 | 91 | Nausea, vomiting, diarrhoea, headache, insomnia |
| Co-amoxiclav for 3 days | 89 | 82 | Nausea, vomiting, diarrhoea, rash |

* Efficacy rates refer to cure rates on the visit closest to a 5- to 9-day period following treatment and are averages from clinical trials published since 1999 so as to represent efficacy rates that account for contemporary prevalence of antibiotic-resistant uropathogens. Note that efficacy rates may vary geographically depending on local patterns of antimicrobial resistance among uropathogens.

Source: data from Gupta K et al., International clinical practice guidelines for the treatment of acute uncomplicated cystitis and pyelonephritis in women: A 2010 update by the Infectious Diseases Society of America and the European Society for Microbiology and Infectious Diseases, *Clinical Infectious Diseases*, Volume 52, Issue 5, e-103–120m Copyright © The Authors 2011. Published by Oxford University Press on behalf of the Infectious Diseases Society of America; and Health Protection Agency, *Management of infection guidance for primary care for consultation and local adaptation*, Copyright © 2012 available from http://www.hpa.org.uk/webc/HPAwebFile/HPAweb_C/1279888711402

may present with infections caused by bacteria that are resistant to all available oral antibiotics. Fosfomycin is an antibiotic that was discovered over 35 years ago but until recently was only used in a few European countries. An oral formulation is available, and fosfomycin may provide the only option for oral treatment of some urinary tract infections in primary care. Fosfomycin can be obtained on a named patient basis in countries such as the United Kingdom; however, while it has a UK marketing authorization for treating acute lower uncomplicated urinary tract infections, it is currently not distributed here by the manufacturer.

## Recurrent symptomatic infections in women

Recurrent urinary tract infection in healthy non-pregnant women is defined as three or more episodes during a 12-month period. Antibiotics can be used to reduce the frequency of recurrent infection in two ways. A single dose of either trimethoprim or nitrofurantoin taken at night reduces the risk of symptomatic infection to about one-fifth of the risk with no treatment. However, the risk of recurrent urinary infection may return to pretreatment levels as soon as treatment is stopped. An alternative, equally effective strategy for women with infection associated with sexual intercourse is to take a single post-coital dose of antibiotic. Prophylactic antibiotics for recurrent infection have side effects (oral or vaginal candidiasis and gastrointestinal symptoms) but infection by bacteria resistant to the prophylactic antibiotic does not appear to be a significant risk.

In postmenopausal women, oestrogen replacement is not consistently effective in preventing recurrent urinary tract infection and is less effective than antibiotic prophylaxis.

Cranberry products (juice and capsules or tablets containing concentrated extracts) are effective for preventing recurrent infection in women after antibiotic treatment of an acute attack. The effectiveness of prophylaxis with antibiotics or cranberry products against recurrent urinary tract infections decreases with age. Cranberry products are nearly as effective as trimethoprim in preventing urinary tract infection and have significantly fewer adverse effects.

## Upper urinary tract infection (pyelonephritis)

Infection of the kidney causes loin pain and flank tenderness but these are likely to be accompanied by symptoms of lower urinary tract infection as well. The kidney has an excellent blood supply so, in contrast to lower urinary tract infection, patients with upper urinary tract infection commonly have a systemic inflammatory response and may develop bacteraemia with severe sepsis or even septic shock.

Nitrofurantoin is not an effective treatment for upper urinary tract infection because it does not achieve effective concentrations in the blood. Resistance to trimethoprim is too common to recommend this drug for empirical treatment of a life-threatening infection. Consequently, empirical treatment should be with a broad-spectrum antibiotic such as co-amoxiclav or ciprofloxacin.

Because of the potentially serious consequences of upper urinary tract infections, it is recommended that urine cultures should be obtained before starting antibiotic treatment in all patients. This is because community-acquired infection can be caused by pathogens that are resistant to co-amoxiclav, ciprofloxacin, or any of the other oral antibiotics used in general practice and this is not an acceptable risk with a serious infection.

## Acute symptomatic infections in children

Diagnosis of symptomatic urinary tract infection is rarely straightforward, especially in younger children. They may present with generalized symptoms (fever, vomiting, general malaise) rather than with symptoms in the urinary tract. Consequently, clinically, suspicion should be confirmed by urine culture. If it is difficult to obtain a high-quality clean-catch midstream specimen of urine, then diagnosis may have to rely on obtaining urine by catheterization or suprapubic needle aspirate. In a child with a low clinical suspicion of urinary tract infection in whom these tests are considered unnecessarily invasive, urine dipstick testing can be used, followed by culture of urine only if the dipstick results suggest bacteriuria. However, false negative dipstick tests do occur.

## Acute symptomatic infections in men

Uncomplicated lower urinary tract infection does not occur in men. Urinary tract infections in men are generally viewed as complicated because they result from an anatomic or functional anomaly or instrumentation of the genito-urinary tract. Consequently, urine cultures should be obtained before antibiotic treatment is started. It is impossible to distinguish reliably between urinary tract infection and prostatitis; consequently, 2 weeks' empirical treatment with a fluoro-quinolone is recommended.

## Catheterized patients

Between 2 per cent and 7 per cent of patients with indwelling urethral catheters acquire bacteriuria each day, even with the application of best practice for insertion and care of the catheter. All patients with a long-term indwelling catheter are bacteriuric, often with two or more organisms. The presence of a short- or long-term indwelling catheter is associated with a greater incidence of fever of urinary tract origin. Fever without any localizing signs is a common occurrence in catheterized patients, and urinary tract infection accounts for about a third of these episodes.

In catheterized patients the common occurrence of fever, the consistent presence of bacteriuria, and the variable presence of a broad range of other associated clinical manifestations (new onset confusion, renal angle tenderness or suprapubic pain, chills, rigours, etc.) makes the diagnosis of symptomatic urinary tract infection difficult.

The presence of one of the following symptoms is an indication for empiric antibiotic treatment:

- new costovertebral tenderness;
- rigours;
- new onset confusion; or
- fever greater than 37.8°C or 1.5°C above baseline on two occasions during a 12-hour period.

Urine culture should be used to test the susceptibility of the bacteria that are inevitably present in the urine. Antibiotic treatment should never be given simply because of change in the smell or appearance of the urine in patients with indwelling urinary catheters.

## Key points

- Bacteriuria is not a disease; it is a laboratory finding.
- Tests for bacteriuria do not establish the diagnosis of urinary tract infections, as diagnosis should be based on symptoms and signs.
- Treatment of asymptomatic bacteriuria is indicated only in children and pregnant women.
- The main value of urine culture is to identify the bacteria responsible for an infection and their sensitivity to antibiotics.
- Urine dipstick tests have a very limited role in the diagnosis of urinary tract infection. They are not sufficiently accurate to be used for screening of asymptomatic bacteriuria in pregnancy and are only helpful in the management of patients who do not have clear symptoms of lower urinary tract infection.
- Trimethoprim for 3 days is the treatment of choice for uncomplicated urinary tract infections, with nitrofurantoin as second choice in women who have received trimethoprim or co-trimoxazole in the previous three months.

## Further reading

Gupta, K., Hooton, T. M., Naber, K. G., et al. (2011) International clinical practice guidelines for the treatment of acute uncomplicated cystitis and pyelonephritis in women: a 2010 update by the Infectious Diseases Society of America and the European Society for Microbiology and Infectious Diseases. *Clinical Infectious Diseases*, **52**(5): e103–e20.

Public Health England. (2014) *Urinary Tract Infection: Diagnosis Guide for Primary Care.* <http://www.hpa.org.uk/webc/HPAwebFile/HPAweb_C/1194947404720>, accessed 1 December 2014.

Public Health England. (2014) *Managing Common Infections: Guidance for Primary Care.* <http://www.hpa.org.uk/webc/HPAwebFile/HPAweb_C/1279888711402>, accessed 1 December 2014.

McMurdo, M. E. T., Argo, I., Phillips, G., Daly, F., and Davey, P. (2009) Cranberry or trimethoprim for the prevention of recurrent urinary tract infections? A randomized controlled trial in older women. *Journal of Antimicrobial Chemotherapy*, **63**(2):389–95.

Naber, K. G., Schito, G., Botto, H., Palou, J., and Mazzei, T. (2008) Surveillance study in Europe and Brazil on clinical aspects and Antimicrobial Resistance Epidemiology in Females with Cystitis (ARESC): implications for empiric therapy. *European Urology*, **54**(5): 1164–75.

Scottish Intercollegiate Guidelines Network. (2012) *SIGN 88: Management of Suspected Bacterial Urinary Tract Infection in Adults.* <http://www.sign.ac.uk/pdf/sign88.pdf>, accessed 1 December 2014.

Turner, D., Little, P., Raftery, J., Turner, S., Smith, H., Rumsby, K., and Mullee, M. (2010) Cost effectiveness of management strategies for urinary tract infections: results from randomised controlled trial. *BMJ*, **340**: c346.

Wang, C.-H., Fang, C.-C., Chen, N.-C., Liu, S. S., Yu, P.-H ., Wu, T.-Y., Chen, W.-T., Lee, C.-C., and Chen, S.-C. (2012) Cranberry-containing products for prevention of urinary tract infections in susceptible populations: a systematic review and meta-analysis of randomized controlled trials. *Archives of Internal Medicine*, **172**(13): 988–96.

# Chapter 24

# Sexually transmitted infections

## Introduction to sexually transmitted infections

Sexually transmitted infections (Table 24.1), formerly referred to as venereal diseases, are common (Fig. 24.1) but remain underdiagnosed because of the reluctance of some to seek medical help when genital symptoms develop. Some, such as syphilis and human immunodeficiency virus (HIV) infection (see Chapter 33), are potentially serious and have life-threatening complications; others, such as trichomonal vaginal discharge, are merely a nuisance. The stigmatization of sexually transmitted infections has been reduced in many societies, particularly following the rapid emergence of HIV infection in the last two decades of the twentieth century. Realization that prevention of transmission of pathogens, notably by practising safe sex, is of paramount importance has eroded taboos that have existed for centuries. The explosive increase in sexually transmitted diseases worldwide makes it important for all doctors to have knowledge of their treatment. While genito-urinary medicine clinics specialize in their diagnosis, management, and follow-up, community-based doctors deal with an increasingly large proportion of cases.

## Laboratory diagnosis

Direct microscopic examination is of utmost importance in genito-urinary medicine, as it confirms many clinical diagnoses and, for this reason, many clinics have some laboratory function on site. In most cases, a sufficiently accurate microbiological diagnosis can be made to enable specific chemotherapy to be given. Microscopy of a genital discharge can give accurate, rapid confirmation of a clinical diagnosis in many cases. Typical Gram-negative intracellular diplococci in a Gram-stained film of a urethral discharge are strongly supportive of the diagnosis of acute gonorrhoea in a man. Conversely, in a patient with dysuria and discharge, large numbers of neutrophils (pus cells), but no diplococci, in 'threads' of urethral discharge that are present in an early stream urine sample suggest chlamydial (formerly referred to as 'non-specific') urethritis. The examination of exudate from a syphilitic chancre must be done by dark-ground microscopy within a few minutes of collecting the specimen; the presence of motile spirochaetes confirms the diagnosis; it is not possible to cultivate these organisms in artificial media. The unstained 'wet' film of vaginal secretions can be used to diagnose trichomoniasis, by virtue of seeing the motile *Trichomonas vaginalis* protozoa, and may also reveal *Candida* or bacteria-studded epithelial cells ('clue' cells) suggestive of bacterial vaginosis.

For several reasons, culture and other methods of detection of the presence of sexually transmitted pathogens should also be attempted. Multiple infections may be present simultaneously and it is routine practice therefore to screen patients with symptoms or signs of genital infection for the common causes. The antimicrobial susceptibility of pathogens can give important case-specific and epidemiological information (see 'Gonorrhoea'). Culture of cervical swabs and from extragenital sites in both sexes is necessary because examination of Gram-stained smears is unreliable. Few genital pathogens can be cultivated easily. The most commonly sought, *Neisseria*

**Table 24.1** Common genital tract infections and their treatment.*

| Condition | Pathogen | Antimicrobial agent (second-line agent) |
|---|---|---|
| **Urethral discharges** | | |
| Gonorrhoea | *Neisseria gonorrhoeae* | Ceftriaxone |
| Non-specific urethritis | *Chlamydia, Ureaplasma*, or *Mycoplasma* spp. | Azithromycin (tetracyclines) |
| **Vaginal discharges** | | |
| Thrush | *Candida albicans* | Nystatin (clotrimazole) |
| Trichomoniasis | *Trichomonas vaginalis* | Metronidazole |
| Non-specific vaginosis | *Gardnerella vaginalis* and *Mobiluncus* spp. | Metronidazole |
| **Genital sores** | | |
| Syphilis | *Treponema pallidum* | Penicillin (doxycycline) |
| Chancroid | *Haemophilus ducreyi* | Erythromycin (tetracyclines) |
| Lymphogranuloma venereum | LGV (chlamydia) | Tetracyclines (erythromycin) |
| Herpes | Herpes simplex virus | Aciclovir |
| **Warts** | Human papillomaviruses | Local podophyllin (cryotherapy) |

* Compounds in brackets are examples of alternative drugs.

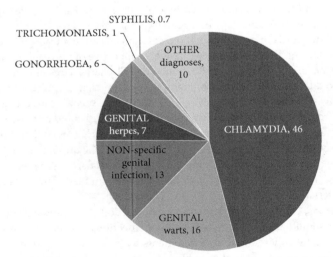

**Fig. 24.1** Relative proportions (%) of new diagnoses of sexually transmitted infection made in genito-urinary medicine clinics and community settings in England in 2012

Source: data from Public Health England, *Sexually transmitted infections (STIs): Annual data tables*, © Crown Copyright 2015, available from https://www.gov.uk/government/statistics/sexually-transmitted-infections-stis-annual-data-tables. Reproduced under the Open Government Licence v3.0.

*gonorrhoeae*, is a fastidious organism requiring special media and growth conditions. Selective media containing antibiotics to inhibit commensal bacteria are used. Isolation of *Chlamydia trachomatis* requires cell culture, as this is an obligate intracellular pathogen. The laborious steps required to culture and then visualize *Chl. trachomatis* led to the development of enzyme immunoassays to detect antigenic chlamydial particles. Both of these detection methods have been displaced in favour of more rapid and sensitive DNA amplification methods. The latter methods can be applied to urine samples and/or (self-taken) vulvo-vaginal swabs, and so diagnosis is not reliant on invasive sampling, such as inserting a swab into the urethra; such approaches make it more likely that a patient will (re)seek medical help.

# Genital tract infections and their treatment

Some patients with sexually transmitted infections either default treatment or do not remain abstinent until the antimicrobial treatment course has been completed, risking disease transmission and/or re-infection. It is therefore important to render as many patients as possible non-infectious after a single visit to the clinic. Short-course or ideally single-dose treatment, where therapy compliance is directly observed, is therefore increasingly preferred. Concomitant treatment of the sexual partner(s) is essential to prevent re-infection, and the value of contact tracing has been shown, particularly in the control of spread of antibiotic-resistant strains of *N. gonorrhoeae*.

## Gonorrhoea

Acute gonococcal urethritis occurs 2–10 days after contact and in men is nearly always obvious, presenting as a visible thick yellow discharge accompanied by dysuria. Asymptomatic cases represent less than 5 per cent of male infections but about 50 per cent of female infections. Prompt treatment with appropriate antibiotics will cure patients with no residual effects: it is hard to imagine that gonorrhoea was once treated by weeks of local irrigation and that many sufferers were left with urethral strictures. Nowadays, the major problems of the disease are seen in women, especially with disseminated gonococcaemia. It is one of the main causes of infertility in the world.

*N. gonorrhoeae* was originally sensitive to many antimicrobial agents. However, the emergence of resistance has led to changes in the recommended treatment options. Penicillin replaced sulphonamides as the drug of choice once it became available in the later stages of the Second World War. In the late 1950s, in vitro testing showed that some strains of *N. gonorrhoeae* were becoming less sensitive to penicillin. Increasing the dose of penicillin to keep ahead of bacterial resistance worked successfully until the emergence of high-level, plasmid-mediated resistance in the 1970s.

In acute disease, in areas in which resistance is uncommon or when susceptibility is already known, a single dose of a penicillin giving high tissue concentrations for 12 hours is sufficient. Intramuscular injections of procaine penicillin were often used for this purpose but these have been largely replaced by single oral doses of amoxicillin together with probenecid to delay renal excretion. In the 1980s and 1990s, widespread penicillin resistance led to a switch in empirical therapy to a fluoroquinolone, such as a single dose (250–500 mg) of ciprofloxacin. As happened with penicillin, disseminated resistance to fluoroquinolones occurred, leading to many clinics having again to alter empirical therapy for gonorrhoea in the late 1990s and early part of this century (Fig. 24.2). β-Lactamase-producing strains of *N. gonorrhoeae* still respond to intramuscular treatment with cephalosporins such as ceftriaxone or to oral therapy with cefixime. If there is known hypersensitivity to penicillin, cephalosporins may be used but, if the reaction was

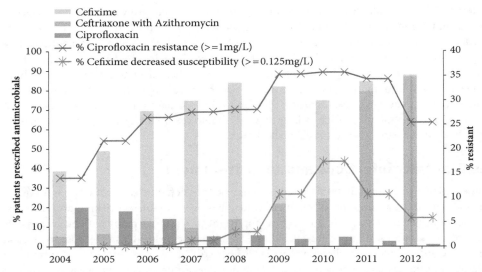

**Fig. 24.2** Prescribing for the treatment of gonorrhoea in genito-urinary medicine clinics in England and Wales and resistance trends. Gonococcal Resistance to Antimicrobial Surveillance Programme (Public Health England), 2004–2012.

Reproduced from Public Health England, *Trends in Antimicrobial Resistant Gonorrhoea Data from 2012 Report*, © Crown Copyright, licence under the Open Government Licence v2.0, available from http://www.hpa.org.uk/webc/HPAwebFile/HPAweb_C/1317140533438. Source: data from: Gonococcal Resistance to Antimicrobial Surveillance Programme (GRASP).

previously severe, the danger of cross-allergy is too great and a non-β-lactam alternative (e.g. ciprofloxacin, azithromycin, or spectinomycin) can be employed.

Data on the prevalence of antibiotic resistance in *N. gonorrhoeae* (Table 24.2) show that the great majority of isolates remain susceptible to ceftriaxone and cefixime but occasional strains are now being seen with increased minimum inhibitory concentrations (MICs) to these agents and, more worryingly, treatment failures have been reported. UK data for 2009 show that 1.2 per cent of gonococcal isolates demonstrated decreased susceptibility to cefixime (MIC ≥ 0.25 mg/l), and 0.3 per cent to ceftriaxone (MIC ≥ 0.125 mg/l). Using a slightly lower cut off of MIC ≥ 0.125 mg/l, 10.6 per cent of isolates showed decreased susceptibility to cefixime. Isolates with decreased susceptibility to cefixime and ceftriaxone were predominantly found among men who have sex with men of white ethnicity, who reported having frequent new partners. Notably, all isolates with decreased susceptibility to cefixime and ceftriaxone were also found to be ciprofloxacin (MIC ≥ 1 mg/l) and tetracycline (MIC ≥ 2 mg/l) resistant. The lower susceptibility of *N. gonorrhoeae* to cefixime (and reduced activity of ceftriaxone) led to a recommended switch to use of ceftriaxone plus azithromycin (Figure 24.2).

Azithromycin-resistant strains remain uncommon but reduced susceptibility has been documented and there is increasing use of this antibiotic for the treatment of chlamydial infection detected via screening programmes. Unfortunately, such intensive antibiotic prescribing may well compromise the utility of azithromycin in the future.

Antibiotic treatment usually results in a rapid and complete cure in acute gonorrhoea. Occasional complications such as epididymitis, arthritis, and pelvic infection in women require

**Table 24.2** Prevalence of resistance in *Neisseria gonorrhoeae* isolates from laboratories in England and Wales, 2003 and 2009.

| Antimicrobial agent (breakpoint concentration) | Prevalence of resistance (%) | |
|---|---|---|
| | 2003 | 2009 |
| Penicillin (≥1 mg/l or β-lactamase positive) | 10.0 | 22.0 |
| Tetracycline (≥2 mg/l) | 38.0 | 53.0 |
| Ciprofloxacin (≥1 mg/l) | 9.0 | 35.0 |
| Azithromycin (≥1 mg/l) | 0.9 | 1.3 |
| Spectinomycin (≥128 mg/l) | 0.0 | 0.0 |
| Ceftriaxone (≥0.125 mg/l) | 0.0 | 0.3 |
| Cefixime (≥0.25 mg/l) | 0.0 | 1.2 |

Source: data from Health Protection Agency, *Gonococcal Antimicrobial Resistance Surveillance Programme (GRASP)*, © Crown Copyright, licensed under the Open Government Licence v2.0, available from http://webarchive. nationalarchives.gov.uk/20140714084352/http://www.hpa.org.uk/Topics/InfectiousDiseases/InfectionsAZ/Gonorrhoea/ AntimicrobialResistance/

admission to hospital and prolonged antibiotics. Non-genital gonococcal infection also requires more than a single dose of penicillin to achieve cure (see 'Pelvic inflammatory disease').

## Non-gonococcal urethritis or cervicitis

After penicillin became available for the treatment of gonorrhoea, it was evident that some treated individuals still had symptoms of urethritis, cervicitis, or both. The terms 'non-specific' or 'non-gonococcal urethritis' were used to refer to such cases or when gonococci could not be demonstrated despite symptoms. It is now clear that most of these infections are caused by *Chl. trachomatis*. Indeed, numbers of *Chl. trachomatis* sexually transmitted infections now far exceed cases of gonorrhoea in most developed countries. Of great concern, *Chl. trachomatis* is a major cause of pelvic inflammatory disease in women (see below), which can lead to infertility. Some cases of non-gonococcal urethritis are probably due to ureaplasmas or mycoplasmas but, as these cell-wall deficient bacteria may be found in some healthy individuals, diagnosis of infection is difficult and not routinely practised. *Tri. vaginalis*, herpes simplex virus, urinary tract infection, and local causes such as trauma also account for some cases of urethritis/cervicitis.

The now widespread availability of nucleic acid tests for *Chl. trachomatis* infection means that cumbersome invasive sampling, and internal examination in females, is no longer mandatory. Furthermore, screening of urine samples from young sexually active people, particularly those frequently changing sexual partners, is increasingly used to detect subclinical chlamydia infection.

Tetracyclines, especially doxycycline, given for at least 7 days are effective. Failure of therapy occurs and may reflect poor compliance or re-infection. A single dose of azithromycin is as effective as one to two weeks of tetracycline therapy and clearly overcomes compliance problems. It is considerably more expensive than tetracyclines but improved overall compliance and efficacy has led to increasing preference for this treatment option. Erythromycin can also be used for one to two weeks but the relatively poor gastrointestinal side-effect profile does not encourage compliance. Genuine relapses of infection are possibly due to latent phase chlamydial infection. Antimicrobial resistance is thought to be rare but, as routine culture and susceptibility testing of *Chl. trachomatis* is not practised, limited data are available. Chlamydiae are eukaryotic cells and, although these bacteria lack a peptidoglycan cell wall, ampicillin and penicillin still achieve some cellular penetration. In pregnancy, erythromycin is the preferred treatment option for *Chl. trachomatis* infection but amoxicillin or clindamycin can be used if it is not tolerated. Azithromycin has not been approved for use in pregnancy.

## Pelvic inflammatory disease

In women, upper genital tract infection with sexually transmitted pathogens, anaerobes, streptococci, or Gram-negative bacilli commonly results in pelvic inflammatory disease, which gives rise to serious complications of tubal blockage or dysfunction. The condition is difficult to diagnose because of the variety of symptoms, its often chronic nature, and difficulty in obtaining microbiological confirmation of the presence of pathogens in the peritoneal cavity. The disease is becoming more common, primarily because of the increases in sexually transmitted infections: it develops in 10–40 per cent of women with inadequately treated chlamydial or gonococcal cervicitis. Pelvic inflammatory disease increases the chance of ectopic pregnancy sevenfold, as a result of tubal damage. Also, the risk of subsequent infertility increases with each episode. Chronic disease, a condition with considerable morbidity, commonly occurs, typified by chronic lower abdominal or pelvic pain.

Unless there is a known cause, combination antimicrobial therapy is usually prescribed to cover the many different pathogens. In severe cases intravenous therapy with a cephalosporin such as cefotaxime or ceftriaxone, combined with a tetracycline with or without metronidazole is used. Oral therapy can comprise a fluoroquinolone, such as levofloxacin, moxifloxacin, or gatifloxacin with or without metronidazole. Therapy duration is usually two weeks.

Throughout the world, chlamydiae cause substantial morbidity in terms of pelvic infection and infertility as well as the blinding eye disease, trachoma. Trachoma is treated using 1 per cent tetracycline eye ointment (applied twice daily for six weeks), oral erythromycin, or, if affordable, with single-dose azithromycin.

## Neonatal gonococcal or chlamydial infection

Ophthalmia neonatorum occurs within the first month, and usually a few days after birth, in babies born to infected mothers. Gonococci in the female genital tract are implanted in the conjunctivae during delivery and the neonate develops a purulent discharge from one or both eyes. There may be considerable cellulitis and, if untreated, the infection may lead to destruction of the cornea. Treatment should be prompt, with parenteral penicillin if the strain is sensitive and frequent local instillations of saline. Silver nitrate drops placed in the eyes immediately after birth may prevent the condition but this has no activity against chlamydiae (see below). This therapy (Credé's method) is still used in areas where the danger of infection is high, but carries a risk of inducing a chemical conjunctivitis, especially if the concentration of silver nitrate is too high. Topical povidone iodine (Betadine) is an inexpensive alternative used to prevent eye infection in developing countries and has the advantage of broader antimicrobial activity than silver nitrate.

Neonatal conjunctivitis due to chlamydiae is a less severe form of ophthalmia neonatorum than gonococcal infection. It may be so mild as to be unsuspected clinically and, like all the conditions due to chlamydiae, it is underdiagnosed. In spite of its mild, self-limiting course, it can cause permanent eye damage and, whenever suspected, chlamydial conjunctivitis should be treated. Erythromycin or tetracycline eye ointment can be used but, as local treatment can be difficult to apply adequately, many clinicians also advise giving erythromycin orally to prevent the development of chlamydial pneumonia. Erythromycin is used to treat infants because systemic tetracycline stains teeth and bones. Therapy needs to be for at least two weeks, as with all complicated chlamydial infections. It is self-evident that the parents should be examined and treated as for non-specific urethritis (see above).

## Syphilis

Syphilis may manifest as a primary illness, typified by the painless ulcer (chancre), or in more chronic forms (secondary or tertiary syphilis) that can affect nearly every organ. The old student adage 'know syphilis and you will know medicine' reflects the many ways in which syphilis can present and how it can mimic many other conditions. The progression of the infection varies greatly; even in untreated cases, latent periods of many years frequently occur. A diagnosis of syphilis used to be viewed with dread, in a similar way to identifying HIV infection, at least prior to the discovery of effective and non-toxic antimicrobial options. The incidence of syphilis is now increasing again, primarily in men who have sex with men (MSM).

Heavy metals, in particular mercury, were used for many centuries to treat syphilis. The development early in the twentieth century of arsenicals such as Salvarsan heralded the start of modern chemotherapy. Penicillin has been the mainstay of therapy since 1943, when the drug was first used to treat the disease. *Treponema pallidum* is exquisitely sensitive to penicillin: as little as 0.002 mg/l is bactericidal. There is no evidence of resistance to penicillin but occasional treatment failures do occur. The aim of treatment is to maintain tissue levels of penicillin above 0.03 mg/l to ensure treponemal killing. Early syphilis is treated with intramuscular procaine penicillin, usually given with probenecid for 2 weeks. In countries where it is still available, benzathine penicillin is used. Doxycycline, azithromycin, or ceftriaxone are alternatives in patients hypersensitive to penicillin. Erythromycin is associated with treatment failure and should not be used. Many antimicrobial agents may only suppress the disease, which can reappear in its later manifestations. This danger exists in treating a patient with non-syphilitic sexually transmitted infections who may also be incubating syphilis. For this reason, serological tests for syphilis should be done on all high-risk patients.

In tertiary syphilis, treatment for several weeks is necessary. Slow-release penicillins do not achieve adequate cerebrospinal fluid concentrations, and frequent high doses of benzylpenicillin are recommended in the treatment of neurosyphilis. Similarly, high doses and longer duration of penicillin administration are recommended in patients co-infected with HIV, as a higher incidence of treatment failure has been noted in these patients. This presumably reflects the importance of the natural T-cell response in combating syphilis infection.

A common hazard of syphilis therapy is the Jarisch–Herxheimer reaction observed within a few hours of treatment with penicillin (or arsenicals). This is a hypersensitivity reaction due to spirochaetal endotoxin and is not related to penicillin allergy. The Herxheimer response is of little significance in primary cases but may occasionally be fatal in some tertiary or late cases.

## Genital herpes simplex virus

Herpes simplex virus types 1 and 2 generally cause infection 'above and below the belt' respectively, although sexual practices obscure this association. Genital infection is characterized by vesicles, usually on the penis or labia, similar to 'cold sores' found around the mouth. Proctitis is common in MSM. The painful vesicles burst to form superficial erosions, which can be secondarily infected. Virus goes latent in the dorsal root ganglia of the lumbo-sacral spinal cord and may reactivate, causing recurrent disease. The presence of virus in the genital tract of a pregnant woman at the time of delivery may lead to infection of the neonate, which is potentially catastrophic. Treatment of genital herpes is with oral aciclovir (or derivatives) for severe attacks or to reduce the frequency of recurrence. Topical aciclovir is available over-the-counter for treatment of mild recurrent disease.

## Vaginal discharge

The normal bacteria flora of the adult vagina before the menopause consists of numerous lactobacilli, diphtheroids, and anaerobes. These maintain a local pH of 4–5, which is inhibitory to coliforms. However, yeasts can flourish in such relatively acidic conditions.

## Candidiasis

*Can. albicans*, the commonest pathogenic yeast, may be found in up to a quarter of healthy women of child-bearing age and frequently the delicate balance between the resident flora and intruding *Candida* is disturbed to produce clinical 'thrush'. Oral antibiotics, in particular tetracyclines, are prone to produce this side effect, which is also more common in pregnancy. Men, especially if uncircumcised, may occasionally have clinical balanitis caused by *Candida*, and healthy individuals frequently carry the organism. Sexual transmission is probable in these circumstances but thrush can occur without intimate contact. Local applications of nystatin or one of the imidazoles such as clotrimazole are sufficient but prolonged and repeated courses are required. Persistent infections are sometimes treated with oral fluconazole, along with therapy for the partner.

## Trichomonal infection

*Tri. vaginalis* is a flagellate protozoon commonly found throughout the world. It favours a more alkaline pH than *Candida* and causes a foul-smelling yellow vaginal discharge often noticed because of staining of clothes and itching. It has been found in a high proportion of asymptomatic women in antenatal clinics but may cause symptoms subsequently, especially after menstruation. In some patients the organism invades the anterior urethra, and symptoms of dysuria and frequency may lead the clinician to make a tentative diagnosis of urinary tract infection. Some patients labelled as having 'urethral syndrome' may be suffering from trichomoniasis. The organism is sometimes carried transiently and asymptomatically by men but a low-grade non-specific urethritis may occur.

Trichomonal infection is treated with a single oral high dose (2 g) of metronidazole or tinidazole. Longer courses of therapy are not more effective. Treatment of partners is required to reduce the risk of recurrence. Metronidazole used to be avoided during pregnancy because of a possible, albeit unproven, teratogenic effect. However, a possible association between trichomoniasis and premature rupture of membranes means that its use can be justified in this setting.

## Bacterial vaginosis

This is a term employed for a symptomatic discharge for which no obvious cause can be found. As with non-specific urethritis, there are likely to be many possible aetiological agents, not all microbial. Bacterial vaginosis is now known to be associated with an increased risk of premature delivery and with pelvic inflammatory disease in women undergoing termination of pregnancy. There is evidence that a proportion of these cases are associated with a pleomorphic, Gram-variable rod, *Gardnerella* (formerly *Haemophilus*) *vaginalis*, although the bacterium can be found in normal healthy individuals. Oral metronidazole given for 7 days is the treatment of choice for bacterial vaginosis, even though *G. vaginalis* is relatively resistant to this agent; its role may be to inhibit associated anaerobic, curved bacteria called *Mobiluncus*. Topical metronidazole or clindamycin can also be used. In treatment-resistant cases, intravaginal boric acid has been successful. In recurrent infection of women, male partners are sometimes treated.

## Warts

Genital (condylomata acuminata) and common skin warts are caused by human papillomavirus (HPV). Importantly, certain types of virus (e.g. types 16 and 18) are carcinogenic and can cause cervical, vulval, penile, or anal cancer in some infected individuals. The treatment of genital warts occupies a good part of the work of genito-urinary medicine clinics and is often unrewarding. A long course of chemical applications such as podophyllin, trichloroacetic acid, or salicylic acid, or burning the lesions with diathermy or liquid nitrogen, is often required; in some patients the warts disappear spontaneously. Imiquimod cream may be helpful by inducing the production of interferon-α and other cytokines. Genital warts in immunocompromised patients, including HIV-infected individuals, are relatively refractory to treatment; combinations of the above options are often required.

Two vaccines are now available: one covering HPV types 16 and 18, and the other additionally confers protection against types 6 and 11, which cause 90 per cent of genital warts. Mass population HPV vaccination campaigns in most countries currently target prepubertal girls and there is already evidence that a reduction in the incidence of associated cancers is occurring. Public health decisions about which vaccine to use and whether only to vaccinate girls will continue to be scrutinized to determine the most efficacious approach.

## Chancroid (soft sore)

Chancroid is caused by *Haemophilus ducreyi* but is rarely seen in the United Kingdom. In tropical and subtropical countries, epidemics occur and the infection enhances the spread of HIV. The genital lesions are painful and often multiple with large associated inguinal glands, which may suppurate to form a 'bubo'. Erythromycin, for 7 days, or single-dose azithromycin is usually effective. Ceftriaxone can also be used but may be less efficacious in HIV-infected individuals. Tetracyclines and co-trimoxazole work in most cases unless bacterial resistance is common. Short courses (3 days) of co-amoxiclav or fluoroquinolones have also been used successfully.

## Lymphogranuloma venereum

This is also a predominantly tropical condition, caused by specific serovars of *Chl. trachomatis*. It starts as a small ulcer, which may be unnoticed until inguinal glands enlarge and become matted together. Associated inflammation may give the appearance of elephantiasis as a late complication and breakdown of abscesses may give rectovaginal fistulae. Tetracyclines, sulphonamides, or erythromycin may be used but, as with other chlamydial infection, two to three weeks of therapy is required.

## Key points

- Directly observed, stat, oral treatment is preferable for sexually transmitted infections.
- The recommended treatment of gonorrhoea has changed from penicillin to ciprofloxacin, then to cefixime or ceftriaxone, and now to ceftriaxone plus azithromycin because of resistance emergence.
- Azithromycin is increasingly used to treat *Chl. trachomatis* infection but occasional reports of resistance are starting to appear.
- Two HPV vaccines are available: one covers the oncogenic types (16 and 18), and the other additionally confers protection against types 6 and 11, which cause 90 per cent of genital warts.

## Further reading

**Centers for Disease Control and Prevention.** (2014) *Sexually Transmitted Diseases (STDs).* <http://www.cdc.gov/STD/>, accessed 1 December 2014.

**Public Health England.** (2014) *Sexually transmitted infections (STIs): Surveillance, Data, Screening and Management.* <http://www.hpa.org.uk/Topics/InfectiousDiseases/InfectionsAZ/STIs/>, accessed 1 December 2014.

**World Health Organization.** (2014) *Health topics: Sexually Transmitted Infections.* <http://www.who.int/topics/sexually_transmitted_infections/en/>, accessed 1 December 2014.

# Chapter 25

# Gastrointestinal infections

## Introduction to gastrointestinal infections

Gastrointestinal disease caused by bacteria, viruses, protozoa, and helminths are among the commonest infections suffered by mankind. Worldwide it has been estimated that on any one day 200 million people are suffering from acute infective gastroenteritis. Over two million children in Asia, Africa, and Latin America die each year of gastrointestinal infection. The very young, elderly, and malnourished are particularly at risk from the electrolyte and fluid losses that complicate severe diarrhoea or vomiting. Restoration of fluids and electrolytes is the mainstay of treatment; oral rehydration therapy has had a significant impact in reducing mortality in developing countries. For every one case of intestinal infection identified by laboratory testing, many more people have symptoms of this infection (Fig. 25.1).

## Transmission and acquisition

Gastrointestinal pathogens are transmitted directly from person to person or indirectly through faecal contamination of the environment, food, or water supply. Viral gastroenteritis, which is highly infectious and affects all ages, is often transmitted by aerosols from vomit or possibly from explosive diarrhoea. Some pathogens, most notably salmonellae, are common to human beings and animals. The high frequency of gastroenteritis in developing countries reflects the scarcity of clean water supplies or safe sewage disposal, the close proximity of human beings living with animals, and the extent of poverty and malnutrition.

Travel-associated diarrhoea often affects residents of industrial countries travelling to developing countries. The onset is usually within 5–15 days of arrival and generally follows ingestion of salads, raw vegetables, and/or untreated water (or ice). Enterotoxigenic *Escherichia coli* is the most common cause.

Viral gastroenteritis has become much more common in recent years in the United Kingdom and Europe, typically among people in close contact, such as children in nurseries, patients and health-care workers in hospitals, and holidaymakers on cruise ships. Hospital outbreaks can force wards closures and cancellations of operations.

Food may be contaminated by various gut pathogens or their toxins at source, in the abattoir, subsequent to marketing, or during preparation. When illness occurs as a sudden outbreak that can be traced to a common foodstuff, the term 'food poisoning' is used. Non-microbial food poisoning occasionally results from the ingestion of chemicals, fungi, and other toxins such as scombrotoxin and ciguatoxin.

## Clinical manifestations

The incubation period of gastrointestinal infections varies according to the ingested dose, the site of infection in the gut, and the pathogenic mechanism of diarrhoea. The shortest incubation

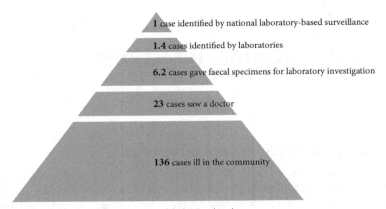

**1** case identified by national laboratory-based surveillance

**1.4** cases identified by laboratories

**6.2** cases gave faecal specimens for laboratory investigation

**23** cases saw a doctor

**136** cases ill in the community

**Fig. 25.1** Underascertainment of gastroenteritis in England.
Reproduced with permission from Handysides S., Underascertainment of infectious intestinal disease, Communicable Disease and Public Health Volume 2, Issue 2, pp. 78–79, Copyright © 1999, available from http://webarchive.nationalarchives.gov.uk/20140714084352/http://www.hpa.org.uk/Publications/HealthProtection/HealthProtectionReport/CommunicableDiseaseandPublicHealthCDPH/

periods are seen with *Staphylococcus aureus* food poisoning, where a preformed toxin produces symptoms within 0.5–8 hours of ingestion. Longer incubation periods are associated with salmonellosis and shigellosis, in which microbial replication within the bowel may take a day or so before symptoms occur. The severity of illness is essentially dictated by the degree of fluid loss and the capacity of some pathogens to cause invasive infection. Once fluid loss exceeds 10 per cent body weight, oliguria and cardiovascular collapse develop and may be fatal unless rapidly corrected. Bacteraemia may complicate salmonellosis and *E. coli* infection.

## General management

### Fluid replacement

The management of acute gastroenteritis is largely dictated by the severity of the illness. Most attacks are self-limiting, and adequate oral fluid replacement is usually possible. Admission to hospital may be required if vomiting persists or clinical dehydration develops from severe or protracted diarrhoea. Other indications include extremes of age, fever, abdominal pain, and other significant pre-existing disease. In most instances, oral fluid replacement is successful. In infants oral treatment with a glucose–electrolyte solution is usually given; milk feeding is temporarily stopped as lactose deficiency frequently complicates gastroenteritis in early childhood. Gut bacteria break down unhydrolysed lactose remaining in the bowel to lactic and acetic acid, which produce diarrhoea through the effects of an osmotic load. Older children and adults can usually replace fluid losses by drinking water, fruit juices, or soft drinks. Few patients require intravenous fluid and electrolyte replacement. However, under such circumstances normal saline and bicarbonate are usually rapidly effective in the severely dehydrated.

The glucose-salts solution recommended for oral rehydration by the World Health Organization and the United Nations Children's Fund (UNICEF) is shown in Table 25.1. Over-the-counter preparations available in the United Kingdom generally contain less sodium chloride and more glucose. They may be useful in moderate attacks of diarrhoea, but are not as effective as the World Health Organization formulation in severe dehydration. Glucose facilitates the absorption of

**Table 25.1** Formula for oral rehydration glucose–salts solution recommended by the World Health Organization (updated 2003).*

| Substance | Weight (g) |
|---|---|
| Sodium chloride | 2.6 |
| Potassium chloride | 1.5 |
| Sodium citrate | 2.9 |
| Glucose (anhydrous) | 13.5 |

* To be dissolved in 1 litre of clean drinking water.

Source: data from World Health Organization, Essential Medicines and Health Products Information Portal, *WHO Drug Information*, Volume 16, Number 2, Copyright © 2002, available from http://apps.who.int/medicinedocs/en/d/Js4950e/2.4.html#Js4950e.2.4

sodium (and hence water) on a 1:1 molar basis in the small intestine; sodium and potassium are needed to replace the body losses of these essential ions during diarrhoea (and vomiting); and citrate corrects the acidosis that occurs as a result of diarrhoea and dehydration.

## Use of antibiotics in gastrointestinal infections

Since most episodes of acute gastroenteritis are self-limiting, antibiotics are not generally indicated. Furthermore, the use of antibiotics carries the risk of directly irritating an inflamed bowel mucosa or of inducing diarrhoea due to *Clostridium difficile* infection (CDI; see 'Antibiotic-associated diarrhoea and CDI). In addition, their use may encourage transferable drug resistance (see Chapter 10).

There are some specific circumstances where antibiotics are appropriate for gastrointestinal infections and associated with clear benefits. Table 25.2 summarizes the chief indications for antimicrobial therapy.

## Gut sedatives and adsorbents

These agents act by slowing gastrointestinal motility or fluid adsorption. Diphenoxylate with atropine, loperamide, and codeine slow gastrointestinal motility and may have an additional mild analgesic effect. Adsorbants include kaolin, chalk, aluminium hydroxide, and cellulose, which tend to increase the stool bulk. Their use should not minimize the importance of adequate fluid and electrolyte replacement. This is especially important in infancy and early childhood, where bowel sedatives may induce an ileus and mask fluid loss. Moreover, excessive dosing with diphenoxylate may induce respiratory depression in the young child. Bowel sedatives should also be used cautiously in those with fever or bloody diarrhoea, since it is possible to potentiate toxin-mediated or invasive bacterial disease.

# Specific infections

## Virus infections

Viral infections of the bowel commonly cause sporadic and epidemic disease in the community and in health-care institutions. Numerically, the most important are infections with norovirus (including 'Norwalk' virus) and rotavirus, which often causes diarrhoea in infants and young children. Several other viruses, including enteric adenoviruses, caliciviruses, and astroviruses may

**Table 25.2** Major gastrointestinal infections and appropriate antimicrobial therapy.

| Organism | Site of infection | Disease produced | Antimicrobial therapy | Comments |
|---|---|---|---|---|
| *Bacillus cereus* | Small bowel | Food poisoning | None | Reheated rice often incriminated |
| *Campylobacter jejuni (coli)* | Small bowel | Enteritis | Erythromycin,[c] ciprofloxacin[c] | Antibiotics in severe cases only |
| *Clostridium botulinum* | Central nervous system | Botulism (neural paralysis) | Penicillin | Antitoxin more important than antibiotics |
| *Clo. difficile* | Large bowel | Antibiotic-associated diarrhoea; pseudomembranous colitis | Metronidazole; vancomycin | Antibiotic associated; stop offending antibiotic(s) if possible |
| *Clo. perfringens* | Small bowel | Food poisoning | None | Due to toxin production |
| *Entamoeba histolytica* | Large bowel[b] | Amoebic dysentery | Metronidazole | See Chapter 35 |
| *Escherichia coli* | Small/large bowel | Traveller's diarrhoea | (Ciprofloxacin)[c] | Mostly self-limiting |
| *Escherichia coli* serotype O157[a] | Small/large bowel; kidneys | Haemolytic uraemic syndrome | None | Antibiotics contraindicated |
| *Giardia lamblia* | Small bowel | Giardiasis | Metronidazole | See Chapter 35 |
| Norovirus | Small bowel[b] | 'Winter vomiting disease' | None | Outbreaks occur |
| Rotavirus | Small bowel[b] | Diarrhoea | None | Outbreaks occur |
| *Salmonella enterica* serotypes Typhi and Paratyphi | Extra-intestinal | Enteric fever | Ciprofloxacin, chloramphenicol, or co-trimoxazole | Antibiotic treatment mandatory; resistance occurs |
| Other salmonellae | Small bowel[b] | Diarrhoea | None | Ciprofloxacin in systemic infection |
| *Shigella sonnei* | Large bowel[b] | Sonnei dysentery | None | Usually self-limiting |
| Other shigellae | Large bowel[b] | Bacillary dysentery | Ciprofloxacin, co-trimoxazole | Antibiotics in severe cases only |
| *Staphylococcus aureus* | Small bowel | Food poisoning (vomiting) | None | Due to enterotoxin |
| *Vibrio cholerae* | Small bowel | Cholera | Doxycycline, ciprofloxacin | Fluid replacement essential |
| *Yersinia enterocolitica* | Small bowel | Mesenteric adenitis/ileitis | Ciprofloxacin, co-trimoxazole | Antibiotics in severe cases only |

[a] Other serotypes are sometimes involved.

[b] Mucosal invasion.

[c] Routine use not recommended.

also be involved. The infections are usually self-limiting and there is currently no effective anti-viral therapy. Rotavirus vaccines are becoming available and should prove especially beneficial in reducing mortality in children in developing countries.

## Cholera

Cholera is prevalent throughout the Indian subcontinent and South-East Asia, from where it has spread to many parts of Africa and central and South America. *Vibrio cholerae* multiplies and survives, possibly for years, in the environment, and as such does not require a human host to maintain its life cycle. *V. cholerae* is present in large numbers in the stools of infected patients and is spread primarily by faecal contamination of water supplies.

The onset of cholera is sudden with the development of profuse, pale, watery diarrhoea, which may reach several litres a day; the classical rice-water stools that are isotonic with plasma. The patient rapidly becomes dehydrated and, unless fluid and electrolytes are replaced, becomes apathetic and confused with subsequent hypotension and death. Mortality is highest in old, very young, or malnourished people.

Cholera is one of the few gastrointestinal infections for which there is little argument concerning the merits of antibiotic treatment as an adjunct to fluid and electrolyte replacement therapy. The duration of diarrhoea is decreased and the volume of stool is reduced by almost half by the use of an oral tetracycline such as doxycycline, prescribed as a single dose of 300 mg in adults. Resistance to tetracyclines is, unfortunately, increasing. Alternatives include co-trimoxazole, azithromycin, or ciprofloxacin (although fluoroquinolone resistant strains have emerged in India).

## Campylobacter infection

*Campylobacter jejuni* (or occasionally *Campylobacter coli*) is among the commonest causes of sporadic acute gastrointestinal infection throughout the world. The organism produces infection in all age groups, but most frequently in young adults and preschool children. Epidemics have occurred involving several thousand people following the ingestion of contaminated milk or water supplies. Campylobacters cause infection in domestic and farm animals, poultry, and wild birds, and hence there are many opportunities for spread to humans. Campylobacter gastroenteritis generally lasts for a few days but may occasionally be more protracted, with marked abdominal symptoms of colicky pain and tenderness as well as profuse diarrhoea. Acute appendicitis may be mimicked. Attacks are self-limiting and managed mainly by increasing the oral fluid intake. Although campylobacter infection is common, fatalities are rare. Excretion ceases soon after clinical recovery. Antibiotic therapy is not beneficial in most cases. Cases with severe or prolonged symptoms may benefit from oral therapy with erythromycin or a fluoroquinolone such as ciprofloxacin. Importantly, campylobacter infection is occasionally complicated by the development of Guillain–Barré syndrome or reactive arthritis.

## Helicobacter infection

*Helicobacter pylori* is an important cause of chronic gastritis and gastroduodenal ulceration. It is also likely to be responsible for some cases of gastric carcinoma. Treatment of *H. pylori* infection usually involves 7 days' therapy with two antibiotics (various combinations of clarithromycin, metronidazole, and amoxicillin are often used) together with a proton pump inhibitor such as omeprazole. Treatment fails in approximately 10 per cent of patients. Resistance to metronidazole occurs in approximately 50 per cent of infected individuals in many European countries, with levels of up to 90 per cent in developing countries. Resistance to clarithromycin is currently below 10 per cent in many European countries but rates may be increasing. Pretreatment resistance to clarithromycin can reduce the effectiveness of therapy by about 50 per cent. Resistance to amoxicillin or tetracycline is presently uncommon.

## Salmonellosis

### Intestinal salmonellosis

Gastrointestinal salmonellosis is second only to campylobacter as a bacterial cause of community-acquired gastrointestinal infection; several thousand cases are reported annually in the United Kingdom. There are more than 2,400 different serotypes of *Salmonella enterica*, although relatively few regularly cause human disease. Frozen poultry and eggs are a common source of infection, which is easily transmitted among battery hens and during the evisceration of carcasses. Measures to control infection in chickens have markedly reduced the incidence of salmonella infection in the United Kingdom.

Illness is commonly associated with systemic features of fever and malaise, in addition to the gastrointestinal symptoms. Bloodstream invasion may occur following mucosal penetration. Bloodstream infection complicating salmonella gastroenteritis is more likely in the very young and the elderly, and in those with underlying diseases such as alcoholism, cirrhosis, and AIDS. Achlorhydria from pernicious anaemia, atrophic gastritis, gastrectomy, or therapy with $H_2$-receptor antagonists or proton pump inhibitors enhances the risk of salmonellosis by eliminating the protection afforded by the normal gastric acid so that the number of bacteria needed to be ingested to cause infection is reduced.

Treatment of acute gastrointestinal salmonellosis is essentially directed at the replacement of any lost fluid or electrolytes, either by mouth or intravenously. Antibiotics are usually unnecessary unless there is secondary bloodstream invasion, since they do not reduce the duration of illness. Antibiotic treatment may also be associated with increased incidence of carriage of salmonellae. For severe or invasive infections, fluoroquinolones are useful, although resistance is becoming more common. Co-trimoxazole or a cephalosporin such as ceftriaxone provides an alternative choice. The emergence of multiresistant strains, some with transferable genes, compromises treatment choices in some parts of the world. Local epidemiological surveillance data can help guide empirical therapy.

### Enteric (typhoid and paratyphoid) fever

Enteric fever is caused by *Sal. enterica* serotypes Typhi or Paratyphi A, B, or C. This is primarily a bacteraemic illness but the bowel is also involved since the lymphoid tissue in Peyer's patches is inflamed and often ulcerates. Notably, constipation is more common than diarrhoea. Perforation and peritonitis are not uncommon in untreated cases. Enteric fever is potentially fatal and, unlike gastrointestinal salmonellosis, should always be treated with antibiotics. The bacteria are often located intracellularly and drugs active in vitro may not evoke a satisfactory clinical response.

The antibiotic of choice for enteric fever is ciprofloxacin, which produces the most rapid resolution of fever and best cure rates. Treatment must be continued for 2 weeks and, even so, relapse may occur. Relapses should be treated for a further 2 weeks. Resistance to fluoroquinolones has emerged. Alternative agents with variable activity include chloramphenicol, co-trimoxazole, and high-dose amoxicillin. For multiresistant strains, cephalosporins such as ceftriaxone or cefixime (which can be given orally) have proved useful. Because of the threat of multiresistant strains, the susceptibility of clinical isolates should be tested in the laboratory whenever possible. In severe infection, steroids given in the first 48 hours may be beneficial.

### Salmonella carriage

Salmonellae may be excreted in faeces for several weeks after clinical recovery. If this continues for more than 3 months, it is likely that the patient will become a persistent carrier. Chronic carriage is uncommon (< 5%) but more frequent in infants and in people with biliary disease (including bile stones) or schistosomal bladder infection. The chronic carrier is normally harmless to the individual but may be a threat to the household and the community if lapses in personal hygiene cause contamination of food or water supplies. Importantly, humans are the only natural host for *Salmonella* Typhi and so it is important to identify and treat carriers as a public health control measure. Chronic excretion precludes employment as a food handler. Ciprofloxacin is the preferred treatment for carriers; alternatively, prolonged high-dosage ampicillin may be curative.

## Shigellosis

Shigellosis in its most severe form is characterized by profuse diarrhoea with blood and pus; that is, classic bacillary dysentery. Infection is more common in underdeveloped countries, where sanitation and levels of hygiene are low. In developed countries shigellosis occurs particularly among young children in nurseries and schools and also in long-stay institutions. The spectrum of illness ranges from mild diarrhoea to a fulminating attack of dysentery. The more severe forms of disease are associated with *Shigella dysenteriae*, whereas milder symptoms are caused by *Shigella sonnei*. *Shigella* spp. are among the most virulent gastrointestinal pathogens, requiring only few bacteria to produce disease. The bacteria multiply in the small bowel, with subsequent invasion of the mucosa of the terminal ileum and colon. The intense inflammatory response produces a hyperaemic bowel which readily bleeds, although bloodstream invasion is uncommon. Occasionally, haemolytic uraemic syndrome (see below) occurs.

Treatment of shigellosis is dependent on the severity of the diarrhoea and blood loss. Mild attacks, including most *Sh. sonnei* cases, may be managed by oral rehydration. More severe cases may require admission to hospital and intravenous fluids. Antibiotic treatment is used in severe shigellosis and to shorten symptoms and bacterial excretion, particularly in outbreaks. Three days of treatment with oral ciprofloxacin, co-trimoxazole, ampicillin, or tetracycline have been widely used. However, resistance to each of these agents occurs, and laboratory testing of susceptibility is important.

## *E. coli*

Distinct types of *E. coli* cause a wide spectrum of gastrointestinal infection.

- *Enterotoxigenic E. coli* cause most cases of traveller's diarrhoea. The toxins have many similarities to cholera toxin, and the pathophysiology of the illness is similar, although fatalities are uncommon.

- *Entero-invasive E. coli* can produce severe invasive (dysentery-like) infection of the bowel but are fortunately uncommon.

- *Enterohaemorrhagic E. coli* (principally *E. coli* O157) produce a shiga-like toxin. In addition to haemorrhagic colitis, these strains can cause renal impairment and haemolysis (haemolytic uraemic syndrome); this develops in approximately 5% of affected children during outbreaks.

Antimicrobial therapy is usually unnecessary in the treatment of gastrointestinal infections with *E. coli*. Indeed, in haemolytic uraemic syndrome, antibiotic administration is usually contraindicated because of the chance of exacerbating symptoms, presumably because of antibiotic-mediated bacterial cell lysis and toxin release.

The use of antibiotics to prevent traveller's diarrhoea is not recommended because of the possibility of encouraging the emergence of multiresistant strains, the risk of side effects, and the generally mild nature of the infection. If diarrhoea develops, fluoroquinolones can alleviate symptoms within 24 hours.

## Intestinal parasites

Some protozoa and helminths may cause symptoms ranging from mild diarrhoea to severe dysentery. These are considered in Chapters 9 and 35.

## Antibiotic-associated diarrhoea and CDI

The use of antimicrobial agents is sometimes complicated by diarrhoea. This is most often due to a direct effect on gut motility or the bowel mucosa. However, about 20 per cent of cases are caused by toxin-producing strains of *Clo. difficile*. Less commonly, *Clo. perfringens*, *Staph. aureus*, and *Klebsiella oxytoca* may also cause antibiotic-associated diarrhoea/colitis. Colitis and occasionally pseudomembranous colitis can complicate CDI. Colonic perforation is the major cause of death and severe cases may require surgical intervention (colectomy). Some *Clo. difficile* strains are associated with epidemic infection, especially in hospitals, and strains with increased virulence have spread rapidly in North America and Europe. Such strains cause more severe disease and decrease the chances of survival, especially in the elderly.

All antibiotics may induce CDI and toxin production, but clindamycin, broad-spectrum β-lactam antibiotics, and fluoroquinolones are most commonly incriminated. CDI should be suspected in any patient with diarrhoea in hospital (Fig. 25.2). However, CDI is increasingly being seen in the community and should be suspected in any patient who has recently been in hospital or received antibiotics (Fig. 25.2). When CDI is community acquired, only 30–50 per cent of cases have received antibiotics within the previous 3 months. This condition is, ironically, treated with antibiotics after stopping the causative agent. Oral metronidazole, vancomycin, or fidaxomicin are usually effective; recurrence occurs less often following fidaxomicin treatment. Metronidazole is recommended for non-severe cases, and vancomycin or fidaxomicin are reserved for severe cases (Fig. 25.3). The risk of recurrent infection is increased if other antibiotics are continued.

Between 15–30 per cent of patients may have recurrent symptoms. Metronidazole should not be used for the management of a recurrent episode; instead, either vancomycin or fidaxomicin is used. Sometimes a tapering/pulsed dose regimen of vancomycin is used (Fig. 25.4). The rationale for this is that *Clo. difficile* forms spores that are resistant to treatment, and interruption of therapy allows the spores to become (antibiotic-susceptible) mature bacteria. Thereafter, there are several options that have been tested in case series but not in randomized controlled trials (Fig. 25.4). For extreme cases with multiple recurrences of CDI, faecal microbiota transplant therapy has been used with success, although there are considerable logistical and possible ethical issues here.

Oral metronidazole, vancomycin, or fidaxomicin are usually effective but recurrence is common (less so with the latter option).

If a patient has diarrhoea (Bristol Stool Chart types 5–7) that is not clearly attributable to an underlying condition (e.g. inflammatory colitis, overflow) or therapy (e.g. laxatives, enteral feeding) then it is necessary to determine if this is due to CDI. If in doubt please seek advice.

This pathway relates to the diagnosis of CDI. Patients should be considered for treatment of CDI *before* test results are available, particularly if symptoms / signs indicate severe infection. Patients with suspected infectious diarrhoea should be isolated to prevent the transmission of *C. difficile*, norovirus or other transmissible pathogens.

**Ideally isolate patient in a single room** - if unable to do this within 2 hours escalate the problem.

**Collect stool specimen & send to Microbiology**
In order for the specimen to be processed for *C. difficile* the sample must take on the shape of the container and ideally be at least 1/4 filled (to indicate the patient has diarrhoea).

Diarrhoeal samples should be tested for *C. difficile* from:
* hospital patients aged ≥2 years, and,
* community patients, aged ≥65 years, and
* community patients aged <65 years wherever clinically indicated.

**GDH EIA (or NAAT) positive, toxin EIA or cytotoxin positive:**
CDI is likely to be present,
- *for mandatory reporting to HPA;*
OR
**GDH EIA (or NAAT) positive, toxin EIA negative:**
*C. difficile* could be present i.e. potential *C. difficile* excretor,
- *not for mandatory reporting (but may have transmission potential and be suitable for local reporting);*
OR
**GDH EIA (or NAAT) negative, toxin EIA negative: C.** difficile or CDI is very unlikely to be present,
- *not for mandatory reporting but may have transmission potential (other pathogens)*

* Please note other Indications for mandatory reporting of CDI at;
http://www.hpa.org.uk/web/HPAweb&HPAweb Standard/HPAweb_C/117 9746015058
NB: A cytotoxin assay may be considered as an alternative to a sensitive toxin EIA, but it yields slower results and this will need to be taken into account when making management decisions on infection control.

**Refer to the following local policies:**
• Remember the **SIGHT** list (see bottom of page)
• *Clostridium difficile* Infection Policy
• *Clostridium difficile* Treatment Guideline
• Source Isolation Policy
• Source Isolation Cleaning Policy
• Inform patient, relative/carer of test result

Consider other causes of diarrhoea.
Consider continuation of single room isolation and other measures to reduce risk of CDI.

Consider other causes of diarrhoea; if not infective may consider ending single room isolation.

| S | Suspect that a case may be infective when there is no clear alternative cause for diarrhoea |
|---|---|
| I | Isolate the patient within 2 hours |
| G | Gloves and aprons must be used for all contacts with the patient and their environment |
| H | Hand washing with soap and water should be carried out before and after each contact with the patient and the patient's environment |
| T | Test the stool for *C. difficile* by sending a specimen immediately |

**Fig. 25.2** Algorithm for a patient with unexplained diarrhoea; EAI, enzyme immunoassay; GDH, glutamate dehydrogenase assay; HPA, Health Protection Agency; NAAT, *Clo. difficile* nucleic acid amplified test.

Reproduced from Department of Health, *Updated guidance on the diagnosis and reporting of Clostridium difficile 2012*, © Crown Copyright 2012, licensed under the Open Government Licence v2.0, available from https://www.gov.uk/government/uploads/system/uploads/attachment_data/file/215135/dh_133016.pdf

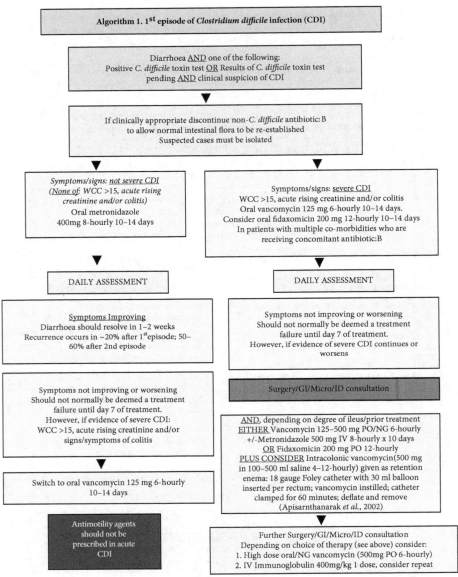

**Fig. 25.3** Treatment algorithm for initial episode of CDI; ID, infectious diseases; GI, gastrointestinal; IV, intravenous; Micro, microbiology; NG, nasogastric; PO, per orem; WCC, white cell count.

Reproduced from Public Health England, *Updated guidance on the management and treatment of* Clostridium difficile *infection guidance*, © Crown Copyright 2013, licensed under the Open Government License v2.0, available from https://www.gov.uk/government/uploads/system/uploads/attachment_data/file/321891/Clostridium_difficile_management_and_treatment.pdf

**Algorithm 2 Recurrent *Clostridium difficile* infection (CDI)**
Recurrent CDI occurs in ~15–30% of patients treated with metronidazole or vancomycin

Recurrence of diarrhoea (at leaset 3 consecutive type 5–7 stools) within ~30 days of a previous CDI episode <u>AND</u> positive *C. difficile* toxin test

Must discontinue non- *C. difficile* antibiotics if at all possible to allow normal intestinal flora to be re-established
Review all drugs with gastrointeatinal activity or side effects
(stop PPIs unless required acutely)
Suspected cases must be isolated

Symptoms/signs: <u>not life-threatening CDI</u>
Oral fidaxomicin 200 mg 12-hourly for 10–14 days
(efficacy of fidaxomicin in patients with multiple recurrences is unclear)
Depending on local cost-effectiveness decision making.
Oral vancomycin 125 mg 6-hourly 10–14 days is an atternative

Daily Assessment
(Include review of severity markers, fluid/electrolytes)

<u>Symptoms improving</u>

Diarrhoea should resolve in 1–2 weeks

IF MULTIPLE RECURRENCES ESPECIALLY IF EVIDENCE OF MALNUTRITION, WASTING, etc.

1. Review ALL antibiotic and other drug therapy (consider stopping PPIs and/or other GI active drugs)
2. Consider supervised trial of anti-motility agents alone (<u>no</u> abdominal symptoms or signs of severe CDI)

*Also consider on discussion with microbiology:*
3. Fidaxomicin (if not received previously) 200 mg 12-hourly for 10–14 days
4. Vancomycin tapering/pulse therapy (4–6 week regimen)
   (*Am J Gastroenterol* 2002; 07:1709-75)
5. IV Immunoglobulin, especially if worsening albumin status (*J Antimicrob Chemother* 2004:53:852-4)
6. Donor stool transpiant (*Clin infect Dis* 2011;53:994-1002. *Van Nood et al., NEJM* 2013)

**Fig. 25.4** Treatment algorithm for recurrent CDI; GI, gastrointestinal; IV, intravenous; PPIs, proton pump inhibitors.

## Key points

- On any one day 200 million people are suffering from acute infective gastroenteritis.
- The very young, elderly, and malnourished are particularly at risk from the electrolyte and fluid losses that complicate severe diarrhoea or vomiting.
- Restoration of fluids and electrolytes is the mainstay of treatment; oral rehydration therapy has had a significant impact in reducing mortality in developing countries.
- Gastrointestinal pathogens are transmitted directly from person to person or indirectly through faecal contamination of the environment, food, or water supply.
- Since most episodes of acute gastroenteritis are self-limiting, antibiotics are not generally indicated. Furthermore, the use of antibiotics carries the risk of directly irritating an inflamed bowel mucosa, or of inducing diarrhoea due to CDI.
- About 20 per cent of cases of antibiotic-associated diarrhoea are caused by toxin-producing strains of *Clo. difficile*.
- All antibiotics may induce CDI and toxin production but clindamycin,and broad-spectrum β-lactam antibiotics (especially amoxicillin, ampicillin, cephalosporins, and fluoroquinolones) are most commonly incriminated.
- CDI should be suspected in any patient with diarrhoea in hospital, in any patient who has recently been in hospital, or any patient who has recently received antibiotics in the community.

## Further reading

A wide variety of information about specific gastrointestinal pathogens is available from the UK Government at: https://www.gov.uk/government/collections/gastrointestinal-infections-guidance-data-and-analysis

**Department of Health.** (2012) *Updated Guidance on the Diagnosis and Reporting of* Clostridium difficile. <https://www.gov.uk/government/uploads/system/uploads/attachment_data/file/215135/dh_133016.pdf>, accessed 2 December 2014.

**Kelly, C. P. and LaMont, J. T.** (2014) Clostridium difficile *in Adults: Treatment*. <http://www.uptodate.com/contents/topic.do?topicKey=ID/2698>, accessed 2 December 2014.

**Public Health England.** (2013) Clostridium difficile *Infection: Guidance on Management and Treatment*. <http://www.hpa.org.uk/webc/HPAwebFile/HPAweb_C/1317138914904>, accessed 2 December 2014.

World Health Organization information about their recommended new formulation for oral rehydration with glucose-salts solution is available at: <http://apps.who.int/medicinedocs/en/d/Js4950e/2.4.html#Js4950e.2.4>

# Chapter 26

# Serious bacterial bloodstream infections

## Introduction to serious bacterial bloodstream infections

The blood is normally sterile in health. Bacteria can invade the blood stream, however, either by infecting tissue with secondary spread into the bloodstream (e.g. cellulitis, dental abscess, gastroenteritis); or by direct inoculation into the bloodstream by a medical device (e.g. infected intravenous catheter). The consequences of bloodstream infections are dependent upon the virulence of the bacterial species and the susceptibility of the host and can range from a mild systemic inflammatory response to severe sepsis and dissemination of the bacteria to infect other organs and tissues, including heart valves.

## Bacteraemia

Bacteraemia simply refers to the presence of viable bacteria in the blood. The patient may be completely asymptomatic or present with fever, rigours, tachycardia, shock, and multi-organ failure, sometimes leading to death. When bacteraemia is associated with clinical signs and symptoms, it was often referred to as 'septicaemia'; however, this term is imprecise and should no longer be used. Bacteraemia is a laboratory finding. The clinical features of systemic response to infection should be described using objectively defined criteria to distinguish between systemic inflammatory response syndrome (SIRS), sepsis, severe sepsis, and septic shock (Fig. 26.1). SIRS is a consequence of the release of cytokines (inflammatory mediators such as tumour necrosis factor, interleukin-1, and interleukin-6) stimulated by microbial products (structural component of organisms, such as lipopolysaccharide, teichoic acid, or exotoxins). SIRS may also be triggered by non-infective causes.

## Assessment of sepsis and the systemic inflammatory response

Sepsis is defined as the combination of symptoms or signs of a localized primary site of infection plus SIRS (Fig. 26.1). The presence of systemic inflammatory response is often the first sign that infection is spreading from the primary site and that the patient may be bacteraemic.

Severe sepsis is defined as sepsis plus evidence of organ dysfunction (Fig. 26.1). Evidence of perfusion abnormalities affecting the vital organs (brain, heart, kidneys, and lungs) includes acute confusion, hypotension, oliguria, and hypoxia or lactic acidosis. The CURB criteria provide relatively simple thresholds for definition of dysfunction of the brain, kidneys, lungs, and heart (Box 26.1). The CURB criteria were originally designed and tested as a prognostic marker for community-acquired pneumonia but have subsequently been shown to predict mortality in patients with sepsis from any source (Fig. 26.2). In this study the presence of any one of the four CURB criteria was associated with a similar risk of 30-day mortality as severe sepsis defined by

### 1. SIRS*

*American College of Chest Physicians and the Society of Critical Care Medicine (ACCP/SCCM) 1990 Consensus Conference

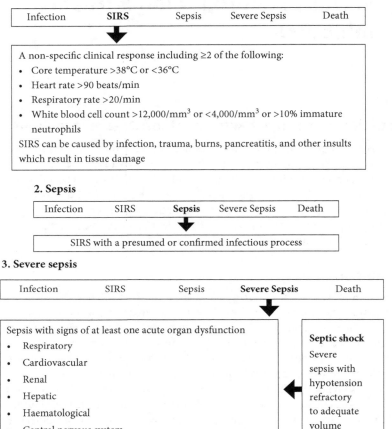

| Infection | **SIRS** | Sepsis | Severe Sepsis | Death |

A non-specific clinical response including ≥2 of the following:
- Core temperature >38°C or <36°C
- Heart rate >90 beats/min
- Respiratory rate >20/min
- White blood cell count >12,000/mm$^3$ or <4,000/mm$^3$ or >10% immature neutrophils

SIRS can be caused by infection, trauma, burns, pancreatitis, and other insults which result in tissue damage

### 2. Sepsis

| Infection | SIRS | **Sepsis** | Severe Sepsis | Death |

SIRS with a presumed or confirmed infectious process

### 3. Severe sepsis

| Infection | SIRS | Sepsis | **Severe Sepsis** | Death |

Sepsis with signs of at least one acute organ dysfunction
- Respiratory
- Cardiovascular
- Renal
- Hepatic
- Haematological
- Central nervous system
- Unexplained metabolic acidosis

**Septic shock**
Severe sepsis with hypotension refractory to adequate volume resuscitation

**Fig. 26.1** Progression of clinical features in the diagnosis and severity assessment of sepsis. Reproduced with permission from Scottish Intensive Care Society, *Identifying Sepsis Early Course*, Copyright © 2006 Identifying Sepsis Early Group, available from: http://www.knowledge.scot.nhs.uk/media/CLT/Resource Uploads/4029646/IdentifyingSepsisEarlySICS.pdf

the more complex 'Surviving Sepsis' criteria (Fig. 26.2) or the Institute for Healthcare Improvement's severe sepsis criteria. Serum lactate is increasingly used as an objective measure of vital organ function; however, in most hospitals this test is reserved for patients with sepsis, so clinical criteria are vital for the initial assessment of sepsis severity. The presence of organ dysfunction doubles the risk of mortality, from 15 per cent for sepsis to 30 per cent with severe sepsis.

Septic shock is defined as sepsis with hypotension that persists despite adequate fluid resuscitation, along with the presence of perfusion abnormalities. The more severe is the host response to the trigger of sepsis, the higher is the mortality (see Chapter 13).

## Box 26.1 CURB score for severity assessment

CURB was developed as a clinical score to predict mortality in patients with community-acquired pneumonia. However, it is also a good predictor of mortality in patients with sepsis arising from any site of infection (see Fig. 26.2).

Score 1 for any of these variables:

**C**onfusion: MSQ (Mental State Questionnaire) $\leq 8/10$

**U**rea >7 mmol/l

**R**espiratory rate $\geq 30$ breaths per minute

**B**lood pressure <90 systolic or $\leq 60$ diastolic

Reproduced with permission from *Thorax*, BTS Guidelines for the Management of Community Acquired Pneumonia in Adults, WS Lim, Volume 56, Supplement 4, pp. 1–64, Copyright © 2001, with permission from BMJ Publishing Group Ltd.

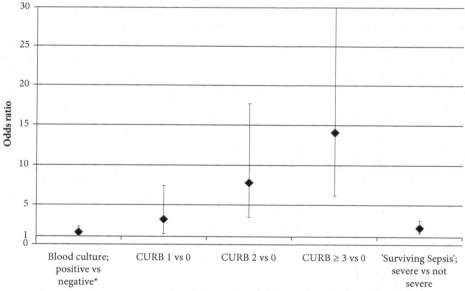

*Blood cultures were taken from 633 patients and grew bacteria that were considered clinically significant in 150 (24%). "Blood culture positive" refers to these 150 patients. Blood cultures from an additional 65 patients grew bacteria that were considered to be contaminants.

**Fig. 26.2** Association of positive blood cultures and clinical risk scores with 30-day mortality (odds ratio with 95% confidence interval) in a multivariate analysis of data from 640 patients with sepsis recruited from general wards in 1 hospital (excluding high dependency units, intensive care units and haematology/oncology). Other independent risk factors for mortality were age, co-morbidity, admission type (emergency higher than elective), ward type (medical higher than other wards) and length of stay prior to sepsis onset. The y-axis has been truncated at an odds ratio of 30.

Source: data from Marwick CA et al, Identifying which septic patients have increased mortality risk using severity scores: a cohort study, *BMC Anaesthesiology*, Volume 14, Issue 1, Copyright © 2014 Marwick et al.; licensee BioMed Central Ltd.

## Epidemiology of bacteraemia and sepsis

Any traumatic procedure that facilitates entry of organisms from healthy skin, an infected cutaneous lesion, or bacteria-laden mucosal surface in the gastrointestinal or gynaecological systems may cause bacteraemia. In addition, invasive infections such as pneumococcal pneumonia, meningitis, or osteomyelitis may be associated with bacteraemia.

In the last 50 years, changes have taken place in the type of organism most frequently encountered. In the pre-antibiotic era *Streptococcus pyogenes* and *Str. pneumoniae* accounted for most positive blood cultures and fatalities but by 1960 *Staphylococcus aureus* had become dominant. Today, staphylococci and pneumococci are still important but are outnumbered by Gram-negative bacilli as causes of sepsis and death. Anaerobes such as *Bacteroides fragilis* are also encountered more frequently, perhaps because of improved anaerobic techniques. The commonest causes of community-acquired bacteraemia are *Escherichia coli* and *Staph aureus*.

The increase in bacteraemic infections due to Gram-negative bacilli follows the success of antibiotics in controlling many Gram-positive infections but advances in medical and surgical expertise have also played an important part: Gram-negative sepsis is a complication of severe urinary tract infections. It is also common in patients undergoing intra-abdominal surgery or aggressive immunosuppressive therapy and invasive procedures and in those whose normal defences are already compromised by underlying disease. These infections are mostly hospital acquired and, because of the widespread use of antibiotics, the infecting organisms are often multiresistant.

Vascular catheters are widely used in medical management and have resulted in an increase in bacteraemia caused by Gram-positive cocci, notably *Staph. aureus* and *Staph. epidermidis*. Polymicrobial bacteraemia and recurrent bacteraemia have also become more common in recent years.

Bacteraemia may be transient (lasting for several minutes), intermittent, or continuous (lasting for several hours to days). The danger of transient bacteraemia depends on the host and the organism. Thus, transient bacteraemia due to viridans streptococci after dental extraction is of no consequence in an otherwise healthy individual but, in those patients with abnormal heart valves, it may produce endocarditis (see 'Infective endocarditis'). *Staph. aureus* may localize in the metaphyses of long bones in children or the vertebrae in adults and lead to osteomyelitis. Transient bacteraemia with Gram-negative bacilli following instrumentation of an infected urinary tract may produce rigour and fever.

Continuous bacteraemia is the hallmark of intravascular infection and also occurs in infections in patients with neutropenia, overwhelming sepsis, acute haematogenous osteomyelitis, and infections with intracellular organisms such as *Salmonella enterica* serotype Typhi.

Most other bacteraemias are intermittent and are characteristic of abscesses and certain types of chronic infection such as meningococcal or gonococcal sepsis.

Sepsis is common in acute hospitals. In a large (>500 bed) secondary care hospital, there will be at least 50 cases of sepsis per month, of which half present from the community and half arise in patients who are already in the hospital. Hospital-onset sepsis is more challenging because the cases are diffused across several continuing care wards, whereas sepsis on arrival at hospital is channelled through emergency medicine and acute admissions units. It is important to recognize that about 25 per cent of patients who have SIRS in the first 24 hours of hospital admission do not have SIRS on arrival at the hospital.

## Blood cultures

There are no specific clinical findings that are diagnostic of bacteraemia or fungaemia, or, for that matter, that differentiate between Gram-negative and Gram-positive sepsis. Hence, blood cultures are important, so that the pathogen is identified and specific therapy instituted as soon as possible.

**Table 26.1** Criteria influencing the likelihood of blood cultures being positive; data about management of patients with cellulitis are from a prospective study of patients with community-acquired skin and soft-tissue infections.

| Pretest probability of positive blood culture | 2% with cellulitis69% with septic shock |
|---|---|
| Influence of clinical variables | Likelihood ratio (95% confidence interval) |
| Temperature ≥38°C | 1.90 (1.40–2.40) |
| Leukocytosis | <1.70 |
| Shaking chills | 4.70 (3.00–7.20) |
| SIRS* <2 | 0.09 (0.03–0.26) |
| Management of patients with cellulitis | |
| SIRS ≥2 on admission | 38/79 (48%) |
| Blood cultures on admission if SIRS <2 | 23/41 (56%) |
| Blood cultures on admission if SIRS ≥ 2 | 29/38 (76%) |

* SIRS, systemic inflammatory response score.

Source: data from Coburn B et al., Does this adult patient with suspected bacteremia require blood cultures?, *Journal of American Medical Association*, Volume 308, Number 5, pp. 502–511, Copyright © 2012 American Medical Association; and Marwick C et al., Prospective study of severity assessment and management of acute medical admissions with skin and soft tissue infection, *Journal of Antimicrobial Chemotherapy*, Volume 76, Issue 4, pp. 1016–9, Copyright © The Author 2012. Published by Oxford University Press on behalf of the British Society for Antimicrobial Chemotherapy.

Most episodes of bacteraemia are intermittent; hence it is important to perform more than one set of blood cultures before starting antibiotics. In addition, the presence of bacteria from the normal flora of the skin (e.g. *Staph. epidermidis)* in a single blood culture always raises the possibility of contamination of the blood sample from bacteria on the skin, whereas growth from two or more cultures is strong evidence of bacteraemia. Ideally, at least two sets should be taken from separate venepunctures. Since bacteraemias are usually low-grade, the volume of blood drawn at each venepuncture is important: in adults at least 10 ml should be taken; in infants and young children, 1–3 ml.

Blood cultures should be taken from all patients with sepsis. However, blood cultures should not be taken from patients with either fever or leukocytosis alone. For example, the pretest probability that a patient with cellulitis has bacteraemia is 2 per cent. This is not greatly increased by the presence of fever alone and not at all by the presence of leukocytosis alone (Table 26.1). In fact, if a patient with cellulitis does not have SIRS, then the probability that they have bacteraemia is only about 0.5 per cent at most (Table 26.1). Taking blood cultures from patients at such low risk of bacteraemia means that most positive cultures are false positives caused by contamination from bacteria on the skin and thus lead to the unnecessary investigation and treatment of patients who do not have bacteraemia. In practice, far too many blood cultures are done on patients without SIRS, whereas not all patients with sepsis have blood cultures (Table 26.1).

## The neonate

The newborn baby is more susceptible to bacterial invasion of the bloodstream. However, the recognition and localization of infection may be difficult because the manifestations are frequently non-specific. However, it is imperative that the diagnosis is made early, specimens collected, and antibiotic treatment started at once.

**Table 26.2** Clinical management quality indicators for *Staphylococcus aureus* bacteraemia.*

| | Indicator | Documented evidence in patient record | Rationale/evidence for Indicator |
|---|---|---|---|
| 1 | **Source of SAB** Is the confirmed or likely source documented or Is there a clearly documented plan of investigation? | Source of infection documented: skin, wound infection, IV line, endocarditis, spinal infection, deep abscess, respiratory tract, septic arthritis, other<br><br>**OR** Unknown source and plan of investigation clearly recorded; includes clinical examination of skin, heart sounds, respiratory system, abdomen and musculoskeletal system (joints and spine)<br><br>**AND** Documentation of further planned investigations including imaging (e.g. MRI, CT, USS, ECHO) or specialist (surgical) review | Site of infection determines duration of therapy, need for surgical intervention and prognosis.<br><br>Relapse in SAB is predicted by an unidentified or inadequately managed deep source [1–6] |
| 2 | **Antibiotic therapy** Is the patient receiving appropriate IV antibiotic therapy (based on the organism sensitivities and likely source of infection) at time of SAB review? | If MSSA and no penicillin allergy: IV Flucloxacillin 2g 4–6 hourly (reduced to 1g 6 hourly if documented evidence of renal Impairment).<br><br>If MRSA or MSSA and penicillin allergy: Vancomycin as per local guidelines | IV therapy Is standard of care for SAB for at least the first 10–14 days of therapy. Site/source or infection determines duration of therapy and potential for IV to oral switch. IV therapy should therefore continue until the source and severity of the infection is determined and for at least for 10–14 days.<br><br>Flucloxacillin is more effective than glycopeptides in sensitive organisms and therefore is the preferred antibiotic [1, 2, 7 ,8] |
| 3 | **Vascular device** If vascular line-related SAB has the IV catheter(s) been removed? | Documentation of line removal in medical record **OR** documentation of reason for line retention | Not removing an infected IV device is a strong predictor of SAB relapse [6, 9, 10] |
| 4 | **Infection specialist** Has an infection specialist reviewed the patient? | Case record documentation of review by or telephone advice from a microbiologist or infectious diseases physician | Review by an infection specialist has been associated with more appropriate investigation, treatment and improved outcome in patients with SAB [6] |

References

1. Thwaites GE,Edgeworth JD,Gkrani klostas E et al. Clinical management of SAB.Lancet Inf Dis 2011; 11: 208–222.

2. Gould FK, Brindle R,Chadwick PR etal. Guidelines(2008) for the prophylaxis and treatment of methicillin-resistant Staphylococcus aureus(MRSA) infections in the United Kingdom,. Journal of Antimicrobial Chemotherapy (2009) 63, 849–861.

3. Fernandez Guerrero ML, Gonzalez Lopez JJ, Goyenechea A. et al. Endocanditis caused byStaphylococcus aureus: a reappraisal of the epidemiologic, clinical pathologic manifestations with analysis of factors determining outcome. Medicine(Baltimore) 2009; 88: 1–22.

4. Bradbury T, Fehring TK, Taunton M et al. The fate of acute MRSA periprosthetic knee infections treated by open debridement and retention of components. J Arthroplasty 2009; 24(6 suppl) 101–104.

5. Davis JS. Management of bone and joint infections due to Staphylococcus aureus. Int Med J 2005; 35 (supply 2): 579–96.

6. Fowler VG Jr, Sanders LL., Sexton DJ. et al. Outcome of SAB accoring to compliance with recommendations of infectious diseases specialists: experience with 244 patients. Clin Infect Dis 1998; 27: 478–86.

7. Fortun J, Navas E, Martinez Beltran J et al. Short course therapy for right sided endocarditis caused by Staphylococcus aureus in drug abusers: cloxacillin versus glycopeptides in combination with gentamicin. Clin Infect Dis 2001; 33: 10–125.

8. Fortun J, Penez Mollina JA, Anon MT et al. Right sided endocarditis caused by Staphylococcus aureus in drug abusers. Antimicrob Ag Chemather 1995; 163: 2006–72.

9. Jenson AG, Wachmann CH., Esperson F. et al. Treatment and outcome of SAB: a prospective study of 278 cases. Arch Interm Med 2003; 30: 525 28.

10. Johnson LB, Almoujahed MO., Ilg K. et al. SAB: compliance with standard treatment, long term outcome and predictors of relapse. Scan J Infect Dis 2003; 35: 782–89.

* CT, computed tomography; ECHO, echocardiogram; IV, intravenous; MRI, magnetic resonance imaging; MSSA, methicillin-sensitive Staphylococcus aureus; SAB, Staphylococcus aureus bacteraemia; USS, ultrasound scan.

Reproduced with permission from Scottish Antimicrobial Prescribing Group (SAPG), Staphylococcus aureus bacteraemia (SAB) clinical management quality indicators, Copyright © SAPG 2012, available from http://www.scottishmedicines.org.uk/files/sapg/SAB_Quality_Indicators_December_2012.pdf

## Management of sepsis

Sepsis is a medical emergency. Early recognition and severity assessment reduce mortality by preventing progression (Fig. 26.3). Unstable patients with evidence of organ dysfunction must be identified with consideration of referral for advice from microbiology, the need for surgical control of the source of infection, and for supportive care (Fig. 26.3). The 'Sepsis Six' is a set of interventions that can be delivered by any health-care professional at the point of care (Box 26.2). Responsibility for recognition of severe sepsis and escalation of care often falls on relatively junior members of the clinical team, so the development of communication skills related to calling for help early is as important as skills related to identification and management of sepsis.

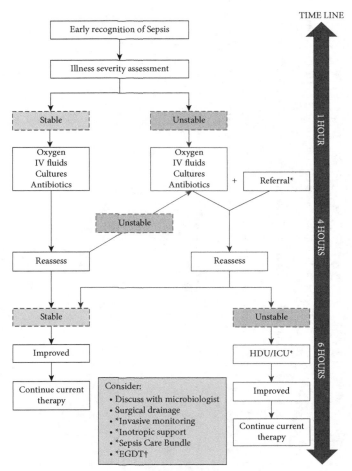

**Fig. 26.3** Fundamental sepsis management; HDU/ICU, high dependency unit/intensive care unit; IV, intravenous.

Reproduced with permission from Scottish Intensive Care Society, *Identifying Sepsis Early Course*, Copyright © 2006 Identifying Sepsis Early Group, available from: http://www.knowledge.scot.nhs.uk/media/CLT/ResourceUploads/4029646/IdentifyingSepsisEarlySICS.pdf

## Box 26.2 The Sepsis Six: a set of interventions that can be delivered by any junior health-care professional working as part of a team

1 Administer high flow oxygen.

2 Take blood cultures.

3 Give broad-spectrum antibiotics.

4 Give intravenous fluid challenges.

5 Measure serum lactate and haemoglobin.

6 Measure accurate hourly urine output.

Reproduced with permission from The UK Sepsis Trust, *The Sepsis Six*, Copyright © 2012 Survive Sepsis, available from http://survivesepsis.org/the-sepsis-six/

The outcome of severe sepsis has been greatly improved by early goal-directed therapy that defines specific targets for fluid replacement based on measurement of central venous pressure, with criteria for escalation of care to include mechanical ventilation and invasive cardiovascular support. Hence the need for early recognition of sepsis on continuing care wards and discussion with high dependency or intensive care units.

Antimicrobial treatment of sepsis depends on the identification of a likely source but guidelines recommend initial broad-spectrum regimens with review and de-escalation of treatment after 48 hours. Identification of a source of infection is particularly important for *Staph. aureus* bacteraemia (SAB; Fig. 26.4). In comparison with patients with identifiable sources of infection, mortality is substantially greater in patients with no established source, because many of these patients have endocarditis. Guidelines recommend at two weeks of intravenous treatment for all patients with SAB, with consideration of echocardiography for patients with no identified source (Fig. 26.5). Four key quality criteria for the management of SAB are source identification,

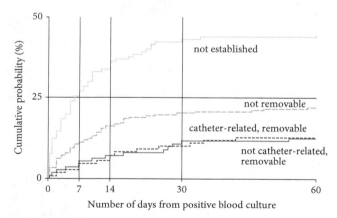

**Fig. 26.4** Cumulative incidence of inpatient mortality for patients with *Staph. aureus* bacteraemia from date of positive blood culture, by focus of infection.

Reproduced from Thwaites GE, The management of Staphylococcus aureus bacteremia in the United Kingdom and Vietnam: a multi-centre evaluation, *PLoS One*, Volume 5, Issue 12, e14170, Copyright © 2010 Thwaites, under Creative Commons Attribution 2.5 Generic (CC BY 2.5).

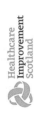
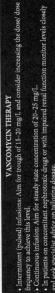

**Fig. 26.5** Algorithm for management of proven or suspected *Staph. aureus* bacteraemia in adults; CT, computed tomography; DVT, deep venous thrombosis; IV, intravenous; MIC, minimum inhibitory concentration; MRI, magnetic resonance imaging; MSSA, methicillin-sensitive *Staph. aureus*; MSSU/CSU, midstream specimen of urine/catheter specimens of urine; MRSA, methicillin-resistant *Staph. aureus* SAB, *Staph. aureus* bacteraemia; SSI, surgical site infection; SSTI, skin and soft-tissue infections.

Reproduced with permission from Scottish Antimicrobial Prescribing Group (SAPG), *Guidance on management of proven or suspected Staphylococcus aureus bacteraemia in adults 2013, Copyright © SAPG 2013*, available from http://www.scottishmedicines.org.uk/files/sapg/StaphAureusBacteraemia_algorithm_January_2013.pdf

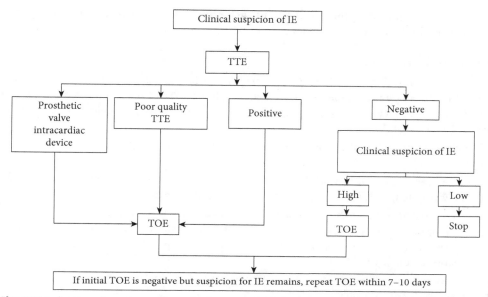

**Fig. 26.6** Indications for echocardiography in suspected infective endocarditis; IE, infective endo-carditis; TTE, transthoracic echocardiography; TOE, transoesophageal echocardiography. TOE is not mandatory in isolated right-sided native valve IE with good quality TTE examination and unequivocal echocardiographic findings.

Reproduced from Gould FK et al., Guidelines for the diagnosis and antibiotic treatment of endocarditis in adults: a report of the Working Party of the British Society for Antimicrobial Chemotherapy, *The Journal of Antimicrobial Chemotherapy*, Volume 62, Issue 2, pp. 269–89, Copyright © 2012 British Society for Antimicrobial Chemotherapy, by permission of Oxford University Press.

intravenous antibiotic therapy, removal of vascular devices, and referral of the patient to an infection specialist (Table 26.2). The criteria for use of transthoracic and transoesophageal endocarditis in the diagnosis of endocarditis (Fig. 26.6) also apply to the investigation of patients with SAB of unknown source, particularly if the SAB is persistent (Fig. 26.5).

# Infective endocarditis

Endocarditis is inflammation of the endocardial surface of the heart and usually involves the heart valves. When caused by microorganisms it is known as 'infective' endocarditis and may be caused by bacteria, including rickettsiae and chlamydiae, and also fungi. The terms acute and subacute endocarditis originated in the pre-antibiotic era, when nearly all patients with endocarditis died. Those who died in less than six weeks due to infection of normal valves by virulent organisms such as *Staph. aureus*, *Str. pneumoniae*, or *Neisseria gonorrhoeae* were said to have acute bacterial endocarditis. In contrast, those who suffered a more indolent course due to infection of abnormal valves by organisms of relatively low virulence (e.g. viridans streptococci), died much later and were said to have subacute bacterial endocarditis.

Nowadays, the majority of patients with infective endocarditis are cured, provided they are diagnosed and treated early. It is also more useful to classify endocarditis according to the infecting organism and the underlying site of infection (e.g. *Staph. aureus* tricuspid endocarditis). In addition, distinguishing native from prosthetic valve infection is also important. These definitions are of relevance in predicting the probable course of the disease and also have therapeutic implications with regard to the optimal antibiotic regimen.

## Epidemiology

Infective endocarditis affects about 2,000 people per year in England and Wales and has a mortality of 15–30 per cent. With the decline in rheumatic heart disease (in the developed world) and the increase of endocarditis complicating degenerative heart disease, the epidemiology of this disease has changed.

- ◆ The mean age of the patient has increased; it is now over 50 years of age for the following reasons.
  - People with congenital heart disease or rheumatic heart disease survive longer because of advances in medical and surgical expertise to correct valve dysfunction.
  - Increased life expectancy is associated with a raised incidence of degenerative valve disease. Minor degenerative changes produce valvular lesions that serve as a nidus for infection; even so, almost 30 per cent of elderly patients who develop endocarditis do not have a pre-existing cardiac condition.
  - Infectious complications of genito-urinary and gastrointestinal disease predispose to bacteraemia in elderly people.
- ◆ Acute *Staph. aureus* endocarditis is an important complication of intravenous drug use.
- ◆ Mitral valve prolapse with regurgitation predisposes to endocarditis and is now recognized more frequently.
- ◆ Prosthetic valve endocarditis has increased in proportion to cardiac valve surgery.
- ◆ The 'classic' physical signs of subacute bacterial endocarditis are seen in fewer patients as a result of earlier diagnosis.

## Pathogenesis

Infective endocarditis is the consequence of several events (Fig. 26.7):

- ◆ haemodynamic or disease-associated damage to the endothelial surface of the valve;
- ◆ deposition of platelets and fibrin on the edges of the valve or other damaged endothelial surfaces, initially resulting in the formation of sterile or non-bacterial thrombotic vegetation; and
- ◆ colonization by microorganisms transiently circulating in the blood to produce an infected vegetation.

Transient bacteraemia is common. A wide variety of trivial events (e.g. chewing and toothbrushing) can induce bacteraemia with oral streptococci. Some 85 per cent of cases of streptococcal endocarditis cannot be related to any medical or dental procedure. To cause endocarditis, organisms must also be able to survive natural complement-mediated serum bactericidal activity and adhere to thrombotic vegetations. Certain streptococci produce extracellular dextran, which promotes adherence to fibrin–platelet vegetations. These strains cause endocarditis more frequently than non-dextran-producing streptococci. However, organisms such as enterococci and *Staph. aureus* that do not produce dextran are also important causes of endocarditis. In these cases, host proteins such as fibronectin and fibrinogen may mediate adherence.

Once valve colonization occurs, there is rapid deposition of additional layers of platelets and fibrin over and around the growing colonies, causing the vegetation to enlarge. Within 24–48 hours, marked proliferation of bacteria occurs, leading to dense populations of organisms

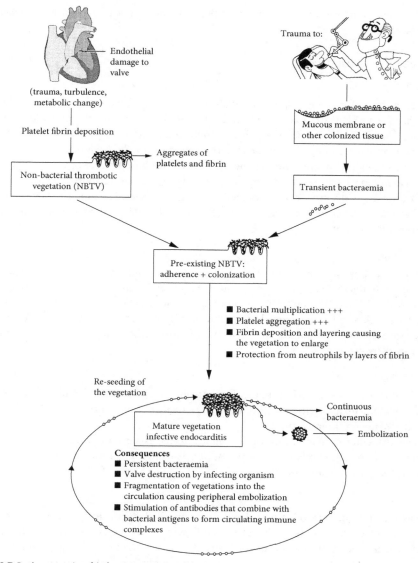

**Fig. 26.7** Pathogenesis of infective endocarditis.

($10^9$–$10^{10}$ bacteria/g tissue). Microorganisms deep within the vegetations are often metabolically inactive, whereas the more superficial ones proliferate and are shed continuously into the bloodstream. Fresh vegetations are composed of colonies of microorganisms in a fibrin–platelet matrix with very few leucocytes.

## Aetiological agents

Any organism can cause infective endocarditis but streptococci and staphylococci account for more than 90 per cent of culture-positive cases. However, the frequency with which various organisms are involved differs not only for the type of valve that is infected (native or prosthetic) but also with the causative event (e.g. dental manipulation, intravenous drug abuse, or a hospital-acquired infection).

## Native valve endocarditis

### Streptococci

Streptococci account for about 65 per cent of all cases of native valve endocarditis. Most common of all are the 'viridans streptococci', which include *Str. mitis*, *Str. sanguis*, *Str. mutans*, the *Str. milleri* group, and *Str. salivarius*, all of which are mouth commensals; most are highly sensitive to penicillin and cause infections primarily on abnormal heart valves. *Str. bovis* is an important cause of endocarditis in elderly people and may be associated with bowel pathology, notably colonic polyps and carcinoma. Recovery of this organism should prompt investigation for colonic disease.

Enterococci are gut streptococci and cause 10 per cent of cases. Haemolytic streptococci of Lancefield groups B and G are occasional causes of endocarditis. Diabetic patients are particularly at risk of group B infections.

### Staphylococci

Staphylococci account for 25 per cent of cases of native valve endocarditis but over 90 per cent are due to *Staph. aureus*, which is the leading cause of acute endocarditis. The course is frequently fulminant, with widespread metastatic abscesses and death in about 40 per cent of cases. The organism can attack normal or damaged valves and cause rapid destruction of the affected valves. Emergency surgery is often required. *Staph. epidermidis*, in contrast, causes an indolent infection on previously damaged valves.

### Other bacteria

Other occasional causes are the fastidious, slow-growing Gram-negative bacilli of the HACEK group (*Haemophilus* spp., *Actinobacillus actinomycetemcomitans*, *Cardiobacterium hominis*, *Eikenella corrodens*, and *Kingella* spp.).

Gram-negative enteric bacteria rarely cause endocarditis, except in intravenous drug abusers and patients with prosthetic valves. However, salmonellae have an affinity for abnormal cardiac valves and aneurysms of major vessels.

### Fungi

Fungi are an uncommon cause of native valve endocarditis. Risk factors include major underlying illnesses, prolonged courses of broad-spectrum antibiotics, corticosteroids, or cytotoxic agents, and an infected central venous line in situ for a considerable length of time. Fungal endocarditis is more often seen in intravenous drug abusers or after reconstructive cardiovascular surgery. *Candida* and *Aspergillus* species are usually implicated. The course is indolent but grave. Large vegetations frequently embolize, occluding major vessels in the lower extremities. Culture of material obtained at embolectomy may yield the offending organism when blood cultures are negative.

## Prosthetic valve endocarditis

Endocarditis complicating prosthetic valve or other devices is divided into 'early' and 'late' onset disease. Early-onset disease usually reflects contamination during the peri-operative period. Despite prophylactic antibiotics, staphylococci account for 50 per cent of all cases; *Staph. epidermidis* is more common than *Staph. aureus*. Early-onset infection is a serious complication and is often associated with valve dehiscence, a fulminant course, and a high mortality. Late-onset prosthetic valve endocarditis occurs after the valve has become endothelialized. The source of infection, as in native valve endocarditis, is seeding of the valves following transient bacteraemia so that viridans streptococci again become the commonest organism. Late-onset disease caused by *Staph. epidermidis*, diphtheroids, or other organisms of the early-onset type may just reflect a delayed manifestation of infection acquired in the peri-operative period.

## Infective endocarditis and intravenous drug use

The skin is the commonest source of microorganisms responsible for infective endocarditis in intravenous drug users, although contaminated drug and syringes are other possibilities. *Staph. aureus* is the predominant cause but other organisms, including *Pseudomonas* spp., group A haemolytic streptococci, other streptococci, and fungi, are also important. Endocarditis often involves the tricuspid valve, especially when *Staph. aureus* is the causative agent.

## Culture-negative endocarditis

Blood culture may be persistently negative in some patients with suspected endocarditis. Likely explanations are

- prior administration of antibiotics (the most common cause);
- infection with fastidious organisms, including those of the HACEK group, *Coxiella burnetii*, *Chlamydia psittaci*, or *Brucella* spp.;
- infection with *Candida* spp., as only 50 per cent of blood cultures may be positive;
- infection of the right side of the heart, which is occasionally accompanied by negative blood cultures; or
- cardiac disease other than infective endocarditis (e.g. left atrial myxoma).

When blood cultures are negative, paired samples of sera (one taken on admission and another 10–14 days later) should be examined for antibodies against other infective causes of endocarditis.

Echocardiography (transthoracic and transoesophageal) is key to the diagnosis, assessment, and management of patients with suspected infective endocarditis but negative results do not exclude the diagnosis, especially in those with prosthetic valves.

## General principles of therapy

The chief aims of management are to sterilize the vegetation and to ensure that relapse will not occur.

## Bactericidal antibiotics

In endocarditis, organisms reach extremely high densities within the vegetation and are encased in layers of fibrin, where they are free to divide without interference from phagocytic cells or humoral defences. Hence, bactericidal antibiotics are considered essential to sterilize the vegetation. The most commonly used bactericidal agents are the penicillins, in particular, benzylpenicillin. In penicillin-hypersensitive patients, vancomycin or a cephalosporin is a suitable alternative.

In nearly all cases, treatment duration is a minimum of four to six weeks of parenteral antibiotics; the treatment of fungal and coxiella endocarditis may need to be much longer. In all cases, expert help should be sought and current national treatment guidelines consulted.

**Table 26.3** Antibiotic regimens for empirical treatment of patients with suspected endocarditis.

| Antimicrobial | Dose/route | Comment |
|---|---|---|
| **1. NVE—Indolent presentation** | | |
| Amoxicillin° AND (optional) | 2 g q4h iv | If patient is stable, ideally await blood cultures. |
| | | Better activity against enterococci and many HACEK microorganisms compared with benzylpenicillin. |
| gentamicin° | 1mglkg ABW | The role of gentamicin is controversial before culture results are available. |
| **2. NVE, severe sepsis (no risk factors for Enterobacteriaceae, *Pseudomonas*)** | | |
| Vancomycin° AND | dosed according to local guidelines | In severe sepsis, staphylococci (including methicillin-resistant staphylococci) need to be covered. |
| | | If allergic to vancomycin, replace with doptomycin 6 mg/kg q24h iv. |
| gentamicin° | 1 mg/kg IBW q12h iv | If there are concerns about nephrotoxicity/acute kidney injury use ciprofloxacin place of gentamicin° |
| **3. NVE, severe sepsis AND risk factors for multiresistant Enterobacteriaceae, *Pseudomonas*** | | |
| Vancomycin° AND | dosed according to local guidelines, iv | Will provide cover against staphylococci (including methicillin-resistant staphylococci), streptococci, enterococci, HACEK, Enterobacteriaceae and *P. oeruginoso.* |
| Meropenem° | 2 g q8h iv | |
| **4. PVE pending blood cultures or with negative blood cultures** | | |
| Vancomycin° AND | 1g q12h iv | |
| gentamicin° AND | 1mg/kg q12h iv | Use lower dose of rifampicin in severe renal impairment. |
| rifampicin° | 300--600 mg q12h po/iv | |

NVE, native valve endocarditis; PVE, prosthetic valve endocarditis; ABW, actual body weight: IBW, ideal body weight; iv, intravenous; pa, orally; q4h, every 4 h;q8h, every 8 h; q12h, every 12 h.

°Doses require adjustment according to renal function.

## Empirical therapy

Empirical antimicrobial therapy should be guided by the distinction between native versus prosthetic valve endocarditis, by sepsis severity, and by risk factors for infection with multiresistant bacteria (Table 26.3). The management of patients with established endocarditis requires multidisciplinary specialist input and is beyond the scope of this book. The reader is referred to the most recent national treatment guidelines, which provide detailed recommendations for the most effective antibiotic treatment of all the commonly implicated organisms.

## Key points

- Bloodstream infections are usually secondary to infection at another body site.
- The pathogens vary by age, underlying disease, and risk factors such as recent surgery, intravascular lines, or bladder catheterization.
- Early recognition and assessment of severity of sepsis are vital to reducing mortality. Responsibility often falls on junior members of clinical teams. Key skills are
  1 differentiating between the different forms of sepsis syndromes (simple, severe, and septic shock);
  2 applying the fundamentals of sepsis management using the 'Sepsis Six';
  3 describing priority actions for establishing and implementing early goal-directed therapies for septic patients along the continuum of care; and
  4 developing and applying communication skills related to calling for help early.
- Blood cultures should be taken from all patients with sepsis but should be used selectively in patients who do not have SIRS.
- In patients with *Staph. aureus* bacteraemia, identification of a source is associated with reduced mortality. All patients should receive at least two weeks of intravenous antibacterial therapy.
- Infective endocarditis is a serious life-threatening infection of the heart valves (native or prosthetic) and adjacent endocardium. All prescribers should be aware of criteria for appropriate empirical antibacterial treatment but management of patients requires multiprofessional specialist input.

## Further reading

### Sepsis

Department of Health Advisory Committee on Antimicrobial Resistance and Healthcare Associated Infection (ARHAI). (2011) *Antimicrobial Stewardship: 'Start Smart—Then Focus'*. <https://www.gov.uk/government/uploads/system/uploads/attachment_data/file/215308/dh_131181.pdf>, accessed 2 December 2014.

Identifying Sepsis Early Group. (2006) *Identifying Sepsis Early*. <http://www.knowledge.scot.nhs.uk/media/CLT/ResourceUploads/4029646/IdentifyingSepsisEarlySICS.pdf>, accessed 2 December 2014.

NHS Education for Scotland. (2014) *Introducing the NHSScotland NEWS and Sepsis Screening Tool App.* <http://www.nes.scot.nhs.uk/about-us/whats-new/introducing-the-nhsscotland-news-and-sepsis-screening-tool-app.aspx>, accessed 2 December 2014.

Stanford School of Medicine. (2014) *Septris.* <http://med.stanford.edu/septris/>, accessed 2 December 2014.

Survive Sepsis. (2012) *The Sepsis Six.* <http://survivesepsis.org/the-sepsis-six/>, accessed 2 December 2014.

## Blood cultures

Coburn, B., Morris, A. M., Tomlinson, G., and Detsky, A. S. (2012) Does this adult patient with suspected bacteremia require blood cultures? *JAMA*, **308**(5): 502–11.

## Bacteraemia

Scottish Antimicrobial Prescribing Group. (2012) Staphylococcus aureus *Bacteraemia (SAB) Clinical Management Quality Indicators.* <http://www.scottishmedicines.org.uk/files/sapg/SAB_Quality_Indicators_December_2012.pdf>, accessed 2 December 2014.

Scottish Antimicrobial Prescribing Group. (2013) *Guidance on Management of Proven or Suspected* Staphylococcus aureus *Bacteraemia in Adults.* <http://www.scottishmedicines.org.uk/files/sapg/Staph AureusBacteraemia_algorithm_January_2013.pdf>, accessed 2 December 2014.

Thwaites, G. E., Edgeworth, J. D., Gkrania-Klotsas, E., et al. (2011) Clinical management of *Staphylococcus aureus* bacteraemia. *Lancet Infectious Diseases*, **11**(3): 208–22.

## Endocarditis

Gould, F. K., Denning, D. W., Elliott, T. S., Foweraker, J., Perry, J. D., Prendergast, B. D., Sandoe, J. A., Spry, M. J., and Watkin, R. W. (2012) Guidelines for the diagnosis and antibiotic treatment of endocarditis in adults: a report of the Working Party of the British Society for Antimicrobial Chemotherapy. *The Journal of Antimicrobial Chemotherapy*, **67**(2): 269–89.

# Chapter 27

# Bone and joint infections

## Septic arthritis

Bacteria can infect joints via the bloodstream (haematogenous septic arthritis) from a distant focus of infection such as a septic skin lesion, otitis media, pneumonia, meningitis, gonorrhoea, or an infection of the urinary tract. However, in adults, prosthetic joint infection is now by far the most common presentation. Rarely, bacteria may be introduced directly into the synovial space following a penetrating wound or an intra-articular injection. Also, the joint may become infected by direct spread from an adjacent area of osteomyelitis or cellulitis. Once established, septic arthritis can give rise to secondary bacteraemia.

### Aetiology

#### Haematogenous septic arthritis

*Staphylococcus aureus* accounts for most bacteriologically proven joint infections. Other bacteria are important in specific age groups. *Escherichia coli* and streptococci of Lancefield group B (*Streptococcus agalactiae*) occur in neonates. Pneumococci, *Str. pyogenes*, and coliform bacilli are found in elderly people. *Haemophilus influenzae* of serotype b cause septicaemia and pyogenic arthritis in children under the age of 6 but childhood immunization with the *H. influenzae* conjugate vaccine has markedly reduced the incidence of this infection. *Neisseria gonorrhoeae* occasionally causes septic arthritis in young adults. Patients with meningococcal infection may develop septic arthritis during the course of their illness. Other rare causes include *Mycobacterium tuberculosis*, opportunist mycobacteria, *Brucella* spp., fungi, and *Borrelia burgdorferi*, the spirochaete that causes Lyme disease.

#### Prosthetic joint infection

Acute infections (within one year of the primary operation) are often caused by *Staph. aureus* or *Str. pyogenes*. Infections occurring more than a year after surgery are caused by a much wider range of bacteria, including coagulase-negative staphylococci, enterococci, aerobic Gram-negative bacilli, and anaerobic bacteria.

### Management

#### Haematogenous septic arthritis

In 90 per cent of cases, a single joint is involved, most commonly the knee, followed by the hip. Typically, the patient is a child with a high temperature and a red, hot, swollen joint with restricted movement. However, septic arthritis is not uncommon in elderly and debilitated people, who may have non-specific symptoms. Patients with rheumatoid arthritis have an increased incidence of septic arthritis and a poorer prognosis, which may in part be attributable to delay in making the clinical diagnosis.

**Table 27.1** Initial antimicrobial therapy in septic arthritis when bacteria are seen in the Gram-film of the joint aspirate.

| Description of the Gram-film | Probable organism | Initial choice of antibiotic | Comments |
|---|---|---|---|
| Gram-positive cocci in clusters | Staphylococci | Flucloxacillin | Clindamycin if penicillin allergic |
| Gram-positive cocci in chains or pairs | Streptococci | Benzylpenicillin | Clindamycin if penicillin allergic |
| Gram-negative coccobacilli | *Haemophilus Influenzae* | Fluoroquinolone | May change to ampicillin if sensitive |
| Gram-negative large rods | Coliform bacilli or *Pseudomonas* | Fluoroquinolone | Modify according to culture results |
| Gram-negative diplococci | *Neisseria* spp. | Benzylpenicillin | Ciprofloxacin if penicillin allergic or resistant |

A presumptive diagnosis rests on the immediate examination of the joint fluid, because of the difficulty on clinical grounds in distinguishing other conditions with similar features, such as an exacerbation of rheumatoid arthritis, gout, acute rheumatic fever, or trauma to the joint. Typically, the fluid is cloudy or purulent with a marked excess of neutrophils. The Gram-film is of immediate help not only in confirming the diagnosis but also in the choice of the most appropriate antimicrobial therapy (Table 27.1). Despite the microscopic evidence of bacterial infection, culture of synovial fluid may sometimes fail to yield the pathogen, and blood cultures should always be taken at the same time. In suspected gonococcal arthritis, cervical, urethral, rectal, and throat swabs should also be taken for culture before starting antimicrobial therapy.

In young adults who present with acute mono-arthritis but do not have purulent joint fluid, a diagnosis of reactive arthritis secondary to sexually transmitted disease should be suspected (Chapter 24).

It is very important that a diagnosis is made rapidly and appropriate therapy started immediately, because permanent damage to the joint may occur and lead to long-term residual abnormalities. Most patients who are treated promptly recover completely. Infection of the hip joint is more difficult to treat since, in addition to antibiotics, open surgical drainage is needed because of the technical difficulty of needle aspiration. The key to success is a combination of antibiotics and drainage. In most cases this is achieved by multidisciplinary management, including input from orthopaedic surgeons, medical microbiologists, and physicians. Surgeons in particular should determine whether drainage of pus should be repeated needle aspiration or wash-out of the joint in an operating theatre.

The choice of initial antibiotic therapy depends on the age of the patient and the findings in the Gram-film. If organisms can be identified with reasonable confidence before culture, the appropriate antibiotic for that particular organism is the automatic choice, irrespective of the age (Table 27.1). If bacteria are not seen at this stage, the initial choice is influenced by the age of the patient or the underlying disease. Antibiotics are chosen to cover the most likely bacterial causes of the infection (Table 27.2) and can be modified subsequently if a pathogen is isolated.

**Table 27.2** Initial antimicrobial therapy in septic arthritis when no organisms are seen in the Gram-film of the joint aspirate.

| Type of patient | Most common organisms | Less common organisms | Initial choice of antibiotic |
|---|---|---|---|
| Neonate (0–2 months) | *Staphylococcus aureus*, group B streptococci, Gram-negative bacilli | | Flucloxacillin[c] +gentamicin or cefuroxime/cefotaxime |
| Infant (2 months–6 years) | *Staph. Aureus* | *Streptococcus pyogenes*, *Str. pneumoniae*, *Haemophilus influenzae*[a] | Flucloxacillin[c] +cefotaxime, or cefuroxime |
| Child (7–14 years) | *Staph. Aureus* | MRSA[b] | Flucloxacillin[c] |
| Adult (>15 years) | *Staph. Aureus* | *Neisseria gonorrhoeae*, MRSA | Flucloxacillin[c] |
| Elderly or debilitated | *Staph. Aureus* | *Str. pyogenes*, *Str. pneumoniae*, MRSA, Gram-negative bacilli | Flucloxacillin[c] +gentamicin |

[a] Now rare where vaccine has been introduced.

[b] MRSA, methicillin-resistant *Staphylococcus aureus*.

[c] Vancomycin if MRSA likely.

Most antimicrobial agents given parenterally achieve therapeutic levels in the infected joint, so intra-articular injection of antibiotics is not recommended, particularly as it may induce chemical synovitis. A sequential intravenous–oral regimen, carefully monitored at the time of oral therapy, is widely used. In all cases, the initial treatment must be with parenteral antibiotics until the condition of the patient has stabilized (usually seven to ten days) and the joint is reasonably dry. Switch to oral therapy is appropriate once the condition has stabilized, as all of the first-choice drugs are well absorbed after oral administration. The total duration of treatment is usually between 4 and 8 weeks. Close monitoring is required to ensure not only that signs of joint inflammation disappear but that inflammatory markers (white blood cell count and C-reactive protein or erythrocyte sedimentation rate) normalize.

## Prosthetic joint infection

Most patients with prosthetic joint infection (PJI) are not systemically unwell. Infection should be suspected in any patient who develops pain or signs of local inflammation in the joint, although it is impossible to distinguish between mechanical loosening of the joint and infection unless there are obvious signs of infection such as purulent discharge from a sinus. The chances of establishing a definitive microbiological diagnosis are greatly enhanced if empirical antibiotics are not given. Serious systemic illness, which is rare, is the only reason for giving empirical antibiotics, and it is extremely unlikely that PJI will resolve with antibiotic therapy alone.

Patients with suspected PJI should be referred urgently to an orthopaedic surgeon who specializes in revision surgery for prosthetic joints and who is likely to work closely with medical microbiologists and infectious diseases physicians. As coagulase-negative staphylococci are frequent causes of PJI and are also common contaminants, interpretation of results is not straightforward. It is of crucial importance that joint tissue specimens are carefully collected to minimize cross-contamination, and that all recovered microorganisms are considered as potential pathogens.

Treatment decisions are complex and, for more details, the reader is referred to recently published (2013) guidelines which include evidence- and opinion-based recommendations for the diagnosis and management of patients with PJI treated with debridement and retention of the prosthesis, resection arthroplasty with or without subsequent staged reimplantation, one-stage reimplantation, and amputation.

# Osteomyelitis

Osteomyelitis is infection of bone and is usually caused by bacteria. Unlike soft tissues, bone is a rigid structure and cannot swell. As infection proceeds and pus forms, there is a marked rise of pressure in the affected part of the bone; this pressure, if unchecked or unrelieved, may impair the blood supply to a wide area and result in areas of infected dead bone. Once this chronic phase of osteomyelitis is established, necrotic bone (sequestrum) must be removed surgically, in addition to the use of antibiotics, if the infection is to be eradicated.

## Pathogenesis and aetiology

Osteomyelitis may be haematogenous (infected through the bloodstream) or non-haematogenous (infected directly through a wound, including a fracture or an overlying chronic ulcer).

### Haematogenous osteomyelitis

This type of infection is most commonly caused by staphylococci that reach the site through the bloodstream, usually with no obvious primary focus of infection. Acute haematogenous osteomyelitis is principally a disease of children under 16 years, in whom more than 85 per cent of cases occur. The usual sites are the long bones (femur, tibia, humerus) near the metaphysis, where the blood supply to the bone is most dense. However, when the disease occurs in adults, the vertebrae are commonly affected.

*Staph. aureus* accounts for about half of all cases and for more than 90 per cent of cases in otherwise normal children. In the elderly with underlying malignancies and other diseases and in drug addicts, Gram-negative bacilli (coliform bacilli and *Pseudomonas aeruginosa*) are reported with increasing frequency. Coliforms are particularly likely to cause vertebral osteomyelitis, as it is associated with recurrent urinary tract infection. *H. influenzae* has become very rare since the introduction of the conjugate vaccine. Other rare causes of haematogenous osteomyelitis include *M. tuberculosis*, *Brucella abortus*, and, particularly in parts of the world where sickle-cell anaemia is prevalent, salmonellae.

### Non-haematogenous osteomyelitis

When bones are infected by the introduction of organisms through traumatic or post-operative wounds, *Staph. aureus* is still the commonest cause, although Gram-negative bacteria may also be found. *Ps. aeruginosa* may occasionally produce osteomyelitis of the metatarsals or calcaneum following a puncture wound of the sole of the foot and *Pasteurella multocida* infection may follow animal bites. Patients with infected pressure sores over a bone, or those with peripheral vascular disease or diabetes mellitus, may develop osteomyelitis with mixed aerobic and anaerobic organisms (coliforms and *Bacteroides* species), although *Staph. aureus* is an important cause of osteomyelitis by this route also.

## Clinical and diagnostic considerations

The typical manifestations of acute, haematogenous osteomyelitis include the abrupt onset of high fever and systemic toxicity, with marked redness, pain, and swelling over the bone involved. In vertebral osteomyelitis, there may be general malaise, with or without low-grade fever and low back pain. If the infection is not controlled, it may spread to produce a spinal epidural abscess, with consequent neurological symptoms.

The diagnosis of osteomyelitis is confirmed by bone biopsy. A bone scan may help to localize the site and extent of the infection. However, a positive bone scan is simply a demonstration of increased blood supply to the affected area and cannot distinguish between infection and other causes of inflammation. A positive bone scan should be a stimulus to further investigation, whereas a negative bone scan makes the diagnosis of osteomyelitis unlikely. Magnetic resonance imaging provides additional information about the presence and location of a sequestrum. Blood cultures should be taken in addition to bone biopsy. In patients with chronic osteomyelitis, it may be misleading to base antibiotic treatment on the results of cultures of pus obtained from a draining sinus, which will often yield organisms that are secondarily colonizing the sinus. For precise bacteriological diagnosis, material must be obtained during the surgical removal of dead bone and tissue.

## Guidelines for antibiotic therapy and management

It is generally agreed that acute haematogenous osteomyelitis can be cured without surgical intervention, provided antibiotics are given while the bone retains its blood supply and before extensive necrosis has occurred. In practice, this is within the first 72 hours of the development of symptoms. Antibiotic therapy must, therefore, start immediately after a bone biopsy and blood cultures have been obtained. Results from a Gram-film of aspirated material may help in the initial choice of antibiotic. If no organisms are seen, *Staph. aureus* is the prime suspect in any age group, and an antistaphylococcal agent should be used (flucloxacillin or clindamycin). If Gram-negative bacteria are isolated, a fluoroquinolone is the drug of choice.

To ensure adequate concentration at the site of infection, high doses of antibiotics should be given parenterally. If an abscess has already formed when the patient is first seen, or there is no significant clinical improvement within 24 hours of starting parenteral therapy, then surgical drainage of the abscess is essential. Combination antimicrobial therapy is often used in osteo-myelitis, especially for chronic infections and those cases caused by more resistant pathogens, for example, methicillin-resistant *Staphylococcus aureus* (MRSA). However, recent reviews have concluded that the evidence for combination therapy is inconsistent and is based primarily on in vitro and particularly animal experiments. Rifampicin may be beneficial, as part of combination treatment, in device or bone infections due to its activity against slow-growing staphylococcal cells that are found in biofilms. It should be noted that, for deep seated infections such as osteomyelitis, when using combination therapy, ideally the individual antibiotics should both achieve good penetration to the site of infection. If this does not happen, then the bacteria may in effect only be exposed to therapeutic concentrations of one drug. This scenario increases the risk of selecting resistant strains, especially during prolonged therapy and/or with some agents known to be associated with a high risk of resistance emergence (e.g. rifampicin and fusidic acid).

It is clear that the details of treatment, including duration of intravenous therapy and total duration of treatment, should be determined by specialists with experience in the management of these complex conditions.

## Key points

- *Staph. aureus* is the most important cause of septic arthritis and osteomyelitis and is particularly common in children.
- The management of PJI requires close liaison between a specialist orthopaedic surgeon and medical microbiologists/infectious diseases physicians.
- Coagulase-negative staphylococci are frequent causes of PJI but are also common contaminants, so interpretation of results is not straightforward.
- Chronic osteomyelitis is often treated with combination antibiotic therapy for prolonged periods and requires close monitoring of inflammatory markers.

## Further reading

Nguyen, H. M. and Graber, C. J. (2010) Limitations of antibiotic options for invasive infections caused by meticillin-resistant *Staphylococcus aureus*: is combination therapy the answer? *Journal of Antimicrobial Chemotherapy*, **65**(1): 24–36.

Osmon, D.R., Berbari, E.F., Berendt, A. R., Lew, D., Zimmerli, W., Steckelberg, J. M., Rao, N., Hanssen, A., and Wilson, W. R. (2013) Diagnosis and management of prosthetic joint infection: clinical practice guidelines. *Clinical Infectious Diseases*, **56**(1):e1–e25.

Rao, N., Ziran, B. H.,and Lipsky, B. A. (2011) Treating osteomyelitis: antibiotics and surgery. *Plastic Reconstructive Surgery*, **127**(Suppl 1): 177S–87S.

# Chapter 28

# Infections of the central nervous system

## Introduction to infections of the central nervous system

Infections of the central nervous system include meningitis, encephalitis, and brain abscess. These can be caused by viruses, bacteria, fungi, and protozoa; however, bacterial and viral causes predominate.

Bacterial infection is generally acquired from an exogenous source and spreads to the central nervous system via the bloodstream. Penetrating injuries and trauma, including neurological procedures, can be complicated by infection. In the case of brain abscess, bloodstream or spread from adjacent infected sites (middle ear, sinuses) are also important. All infections of the central nervous system are serious. Many infections, notably, meningitis, encephalitis, and brain abscess, will prove fatal unless diagnosed and treated promptly.

## Meningitis

Meningitis is an infection within the subarachnoid space resulting in inflammation of the membranes covering the brain and the spinal cord. Infection is usually caused by bacteria, viruses, and occasionally fungi (Table 28.1).

Viral meningitis is usually self-limiting, requiring no specific treatment; whereas bacterial meningitis is associated with a mortality of 10 to 30 per cent. Long-term neurological sequelae in survivors are common especially in neonates, infants, and those infected with *Streptococcus pneumoniae*.

### Bacterial meningitis

About 500 cases of bacterial meningitis are notified annually in the United Kingdom; most are caused by *Neisseria meningitidis* serogroup B and *Str. pneumoniae*. The introduction of a conjugate vaccine against *Haemophilus influenzae* type b in 1992 has now virtually eliminated infection with this organism. The introduction of a conjugate vaccine against *N. meningitidis* serogroup C in 1999 resulted in a dramatic reduction in meningitis caused by this organism. Recently, a vaccine against serogroup B has been shown to be safe and immunogenic; the results of trials confirming its effectiveness are awaited but this new vaccine is now recommended in the United Kingdom for patients at high risk of invasive meningococcal disease (e.g. splenic dysfunction or complement deficiency).

The incidence of the various forms of bacterial meningitis is age related. Enterobacteriacae and *Str. agalactiae* (group B streptococcus) cause most neonatal meningitis, with *Listeria monocytogenes* a rare but important agent. *N. meningitidis* and *Str. pneumoniae* cause the majority of meningitis in childhood and early adult life. After the age of 40, meningitis is most commonly caused by *Str. pneumoniae*. *L. monocytogenes* causes disease in the immunocompromised, be it through pregnancy, drugs, or old age.

**Table 28.1** Important infectious causes of meningitis.

| Bacteria | Viruses | Fungi |
|---|---|---|
| *Neisseria meningitidis* | Enteroviruses | *Cryptococcus neoformans* |
| *Streptococcus pneumoniae* | Mumps | |
| *Haemophilus influenzae* | Herpes simplex | |
| *Streptococcus agalactiae* (group B) | HIV | |
| Enterobacteriaceae e.g. *Escherichia coli* | | |
| *Staphylococcus aureus* | | |
| *Listeria monocytogenes* | | |
| *Mycobacterium tuberculosis* | | |
| *Treponema pallidum* | | |
| *Borrelia burgdorferi* (Lyme disease) | | |

Tuberculous meningitis, caused by *Mycobacterium tuberculosis*, is an extremely important cause of meningitis in tuberculosis endemic regions. It particularly affects young children and those infected with HIV.

## Pathogenesis and clinical features

*Str. pneumoniae* and *N. meningitidis* are found as normal upper respiratory tract commensals in 10–30 per cent of the population. Meningitis most commonly follows haematogenous spread of the microorganism from the nasopharynx. The sequence of events is believed to be mucosal colonization, passage through the mucosal epithelium, bacteraemia, penetration of the blood–brain barrier, and multiplication within the subarachnoid space. Occasionally, haematogenous spread from the middle ear, or other infected focus, may occur. Rarely, bacteria reach the cerebrospinal fluid (CSF) by direct extension from adjacent suppurative tissues or a ruptured intracranial abscess or may be directly implanted into the subarachnoid space from the nasopharynx through dural defects of congenital or traumatic origin. Once a pathogen is introduced into the subarachnoid space, bacteria multiply rapidly because of inadequate local defences. There follows an intense inflammatory process with marked congestion, oedema, outpouring of exudate, and raised intracranial pressure. Blood vessels and nerves may be involved in the inflammatory process leading to arteritis, infective thrombophlebitis, and cranial nerve palsies, and the thick exudate may interfere with CSF circulation and absorption leading to blockage and hydrocephalus.

Bacterial meningitis usually presents with a short history (hours, or 1–2 days) of headache, fever, and vomiting. In contrast, tuberculous meningitis typically presents with many days or weeks of symptoms. In each condition, however, the clinical picture reflects the signs and symptoms of systemic illness (e.g. general malaise, fever, toxicity, poor feeding, leucocytosis) increased intracranial pressure (e.g. headache, vomiting, irritability, disturbance of consciousness, seizures), and meningeal irritation (e.g. photophobia, neck pain, positive Kernig's sign). However, in a prospective nationwide cohort of 696 adults with culture–proven acute bacterial meningitis, the classic triad of fever, nuchal rigidity, and altered mental status was present in only 44 per cent of episodes; however, 95 per cent of episodes were characterized by at least two of the four symptoms of headache, fever, nuchal rigidity, and altered mental status. In neonates, infants, and old people the signs and symptoms may be non-specific and subtle. The presence of a petechial or purpuric rash, predominantly on the extremities, in a patient with meningeal signs almost always indicates meningococcal disease and requires immediate antibiotic therapy and admission to hospital.

## Laboratory diagnosis

**CSF examination** Examination of the CSF obtained by lumbar puncture is an essential investigation for the diagnosis of all suspected central nervous system infections. Other than in infants, it is safe to take at least 5 ml of CSF for cellular, biochemical, and microbiological analysis. The microbiological diagnostic yield increases with the volume of CSF examined. Paired blood and CSF samples for the estimation of glucose should always be sent for analysis.

Examination of the CSF should include total white and red blood cell counts (including white cell differential), and estimation of protein and glucose concentration. The deposit of centrifuged CSF should be Gram and Ziehl–Neelsen stained, followed by microscopy to look for bacteria.

Typical laboratory findings in bacterial and viral meningitis are shown in Table 28.2.

Lumbar puncture is an essential early investigation, although it is often delayed by requests for brain imaging. There is a common perception, especially among junior clinicians, that lumbar puncture cannot be performed safely without the prior exclusion of a space-occupying brain lesion and diffuse cerebral oedema, which may contraindicate the procedure by increasing the risk of 'coning' (brain stem herniation through the foramen magnum). Whether brain imaging should be mandatory for this purpose before all emergency lumbar punctures excites diverse opinion, but the following is widely recognized:

- brain imaging is not good at predicting those at risk of 'coning' following lumbar puncture;

- imaging should precede a lumbar puncture if the patient is immunocompromised, comatose, has had recent seizures, has papilloedema, or has focal neurological signs; and

- lumbar puncture can be performed safely without prior brain imaging in young, immune-competent, alert, and orientated individuals without focal neurological signs or coagulopathy.

**Table 28.2** Typical cerebrospinal fluid changes in bacterial, tuberculous, and viral meningitis.

| Property | Normal cerebrospinal fluid | Bacterial meningitis | Tuberculous meningitis | Viral meningitis |
|---|---|---|---|---|
| Appearance | Clear, colourless | Purulent or cloudy | Clear or slightly cloudy | Clear or slightly opalescent |
| Cell count (per μl) | 0–5 | 1,000–10,000 | 50–1,000 | 10–500 |
| Main cell type | Lymphocytes | Polymorphs[a] | Mix of polymorphs and lymphocytes | Lymphocytes[b] |
| Protein concentration | 0.1–0.4 g/l | 1.0–3.0 g/l | 1.0–5.0 g/l | 0.5–1.0 g/l |
| Glucose concentration | ≈60% blood glucose | <50% blood glucose | <50% blood glucose | >50% blood glucose |
| Gram stain | Negative | Positive (50%) | Negative | Negative |
| Ziehl–Neelsen stain | Negative | Negative | Positive (10–50%) | Negative |

[a] Exceptions: partially treated pyogenic meningitis; listerial, cryptococcal, or leptospiral meningitis, in which a lymphocytic response is common.

[b] In early cases an increased polymorph count may be seen.

**Blood cultures** Blood cultures (two sets) should be collected, ideally before antimicrobial therapy is begun, from patients with suspected meningitis, since bacteraemia is present in a high proportion of patients with meningococcal or pneumococcal disease.

## Therapeutic considerations

All patients with suspected bacterial meningitis should be treated immediately with broad-spectrum antibiotics (usually a third generation cephalosporin, like ceftriaxone or cefotaxime) without waiting for the results of investigations. In general, choice of antibiotic therapy is determined by the predicted in vitro drug susceptibility of the likely organism and the achievable concentrations of the drug within the central nervous system.

## Penetration of antibiotics into cerebrospinal fluid

Antibiotic penetration of the blood brain barrier into the CSF is important for the successful treatment of bacterial meningitis and depends upon antibiotic size, charge, lipophilicity, protein binding, efflux pumps, and the disruption of the barrier's integrity by inflammation.

Antimicrobial agents can be divided according to their ability to penetrate into CSF:

- those that penetrate inflamed and non-inflamed meninges in standard doses—chloramphenicol, sulphonamides, trimethoprim, metronidazole, isoniazid, pyrazinamide, and fluconazole;
- those that penetrate in the presence of inflamed meninges or when used in high doses—benzylpenicillin, ampicillin, flucloxacillin, cefotaxime, ceftriaxone, vancomycin, rifampicin, amphotericin, and flucytosine; and
- those that penetrate poorly even when the meninges are inflamed—aminoglycosides, erythromycin, tetracyclines, and fusidic acid.

## Choice of antimicrobial agent

In the United Kingdom, ceftriaxone and cefotaxime are currently active against all strains of *N. meningitidis*, *H. influenzae*, and nearly all *Str. pneumoniae*. Either of these drugs are the recommended front-line therapy. *Str. pneumoniae* strains resistant to ceftriaxone/cefotaxime are more common in the United States, Spain, and parts of southern Africa than in the United Kingdom; so, unless a patient has recently lived in one of these regions, the immediate empirical addition of vancomycin (to cover the possibility of cephalosporin resistance) is unnecessary.

*L. monocytogenes* is a rare cause of bacterial meningitis but has innate resistance to all cephalosporins. Ampicillin/ amoxicillin is effective and should be given to immune-suppressed patients with meningitis, including those in pregnancy and older age (>50 years). Alert the laboratory if you are considering listeria meningitis: *L. monocytogenes* is a Gram-positive rod, a characteristic shared by many benign skin bacteria; when isolated from blood and/or CSF, it may be wrongly ignored by the laboratory as a contaminant.

## Duration of therapy

Antibiotics need to be given long enough to kill all the bacteria and prevent disease recurrence but when this point is reached varies widely between patients, dependent on the causative bacteria, the disease severity, and the antibiotic used. A meta-analysis of five randomized controlled trials investigating short (4–7 days) versus longer (7–14 days) antibiotic therapy for all causes of bacterial meningitis found no difference in outcome between the two treatment groups. A recent randomized controlled trial in 1,027 African children with bacterial meningitis of all cause found no differences in treatment failure or relapse between those given 5 versus 10 days of ceftriaxone.

Nevertheless, many authorities in high-income countries recommend at least 7 days' treatment for haemophilus and meningococcal meningitis, and 10–14 days' treatment for pneumococcal meningitis. Listeria meningitis should be treated for at least 3 weeks.

## Adjunctive therapy

Whether dexamethasone improves outcome from bacterial meningitis remains uncertain and its administration is not mandatory. Dexamethasone may improve survival in HIV-uninfected adults with confirmed bacterial meningitis (positive CSF Gram stain or culture) and it probably should be given to patients who conform to these characteristics (0.15 mg/kg 6 hourly for 4 days).

# Meningococcal disease

Infections caused by *N. meningitidis* are both endemic and epidemic. Epidemics may occur in closed institutions, such as schools, halls of residence, and military barracks. In sub-Saharan Africa, epidemics occur every few years. *N. meningitidis* affects primarily infants, children, and young adults. The disease has a seasonal incidence, with most cases occurring in winter and spring. Coexisting or antecedent viral infection may play a part in invasive meningococcal disease. The following broad clinical groups can be recognized in patients with meningococcal disease according to the presenting clinical features.

## Sepsis syndrome with or without meningitis

About 15 to 20 per cent of cases of meningococcal disease are characterized by the rapid development over a period of 24 to 48 hours. The symptoms include fever, rigours, myalgias, and a petechial rash. In a few patients, headache, confusion, and neck stiffness may develop later, signifying the onset of meningitis. However, the onset of illness in those with fulminant meningococcal septicaemia is much more abrupt and dramatic. The duration of illness is often less than 24 hours, and, on admission, the patient is gravely ill, shocked, and covered with a rapidly spreading purpuric rash, which may coalesce, become ecchymotic, and even proceed to tissue necrosis. Disseminated intravascular coagulation may follow and death can occur within hours. Blood cultures are invariably positive. There may be no signs of meningism but it is not uncommon for *N. meningitidis* to be recovered from an otherwise normal CSF, implying the onset of early meningitis. Mortality is around 25 per cent in patients with meningococcal sepsis.

## Meningitis with or without the sepsis syndrome

This is the commonest presentation, with signs and symptoms of meningitis that may occur rapidly or evolve more gradually over several days. The CSF is typically cloudy with a high polymorphonuclear leucocyte count, raised protein, and low glucose concentration. A typical petechial or purpuric rash is present in about 60 per cent of patients; occasionally the rash may be initially maculopapular. Blood cultures are positive in about 40 per cent of cases. With appropriate treatment, mortality is around 5 per cent.

## Rarer forms of meningococcal disease

Occasionally *N. meningitidis* may localize in the joints or on heart valves producing acute septic arthritis or endocarditis. Chronic meningococcal septicaemia, although uncommon, is characterized by intermittent pyrexia, rash, and arthralgia. Occasionally a diagnosis is made retrospectively because of transient positive blood cultures in children with mild, self-limiting, febrile illness. They usually recover quickly and spontaneously without the use of antibiotics.

## Treatment and prophylaxis

Ceftriaxone is the drug of choice. Therapy should be started on first suspicion of meningococcal disease. Although most strains of *N. meningitidis* are highly sensitive to penicillin (minimum inhibitory concentration <0.16 mg/l), some strains of reduced sensitivity are occasionally encountered, which is why ceftriaxone is the preferred agent.

To prevent secondary cases of meningococcal disease, household and secretion (kissing) contacts are offered antibiotic prophylaxis. The standard agent for prophylaxis is oral rifampicin, twice daily for 2 days (adults 600 mg; children 10 mg/kg). Rifampicin-resistant strains occur but are presently uncommon. A single intramuscular injection of ceftriaxone (adults 250 mg; children 125 mg) or a single oral dose of ciprofloxacin (adults 500 mg) is an alternative prophylactic regimen. Pregnant women should be offered ceftriaxone rather than rifampicin.

## Pneumococcal meningitis

Meningitis caused by *Str. pneumoniae* may occur at any age. The mortality in children and adults is around 20 per cent and 30 per cent, respectively. The outlook is grave in those over the age of 60 years. There is often a pre-existing focus of infection elsewhere (e.g. pneumonia, acute otitis media, or acute sinusitis), predisposing risk factor (e.g. recent or remote head trauma, recent neurosurgical procedure, CSF leak, sickle cell anaemia, an immunodeficiency state, alcoholism, or an absent spleen). *Str. pneumoniae* is the commonest cause of recurrent or post-traumatic meningitis. Patients who have had a splenectomy are at particular risk of developing overwhelming pneumococcal infection. The onset of pneumococcal meningitis may be sudden, and the course rapid with death occurring within 12 hours. Alterations of consciousness and focal neurological defects may occur and survivors often suffer significant neurological deficits.

### Treatment

Ceftriaxone is the preferred agent to treat pneumococcal meningitis. The global spread of penicillin-resistant pneumococci has eroded the efficacy of benzylpenicillin, which was formerly the drug of choice. Strains of pneumococci that are resistant to expanded-spectrum cephalosporins such as ceftriaxone are being increasingly reported from around the world but are currently rare in the United Kingdom; rifampicin and/or vancomycin have been used in such cases.

## Haemophilus meningitis

Almost all cases of meningitis due to *H. influenzae* are caused by the capsulate type b strains. Before the introduction of the highly successful conjugate vaccine, *H. influenzae* meningitis affected children under 6 years of age. It is now a very rare cause of meningitis. Cefotaxime or ceftriaxone, both of which are active against β-lactamase-producing and non-β-lactamase-producing strains of *H. influenzae*, are the agents of choice for treatment. Rifampicin is used as prophylaxis for all household contacts when there is an unvaccinated sibling in the house aged 4 years or younger.

## Culture-negative pyogenic meningitis

About 40 per cent of patients presenting with meningitis will already have received antimicrobial therapy before lumbar puncture and this may lead to a change in the clinical presentation and failure to isolate an organism. The CSF white cell counts may be lower than expected, with a higher proportion of lymphocytes. Diagnostic confusion with tuberculous meningitis is common. Repeat the lumbar puncture if the diagnosis remains uncertain.

## Tuberculous meningitis

Tuberculous meningitis is hard to diagnose and treat. Death or severe neurological disability is strongly associated with treatment delay, yet there is no single laboratory test that will reliably make or exclude the diagnosis. In many cases treatment must be started and continued on the basis of compatible clinical features. Suspect tuberculous meningitis in any patient with more than 5 days of symptoms of meningitis and remember the following:

- The diagnostic yield of CSF Ziehl–Neelsen stain and culture for *Mycob. tuberculosis* increases with the volume of CSF submitted: take at least 8 ml for these tests alone and discuss your diagnostic requirements with the laboratory.
- Clinical or radiological evidence of extra-neural tuberculosis may allow further diagnostic specimens.
- Isolation of an organism is essential for determining bacterial drug susceptibility.

Treat tuberculous meningitis with four antituberculosis drugs and adjunctive dexamethasone: rifampicin, isoniazid, and pyrazinamide (see Chapter 30). The fourth drug—usually ethambutol—covers the possibility of isoniazid-resistant bacteria (around 5% in the United Kingdom); it adds little to the intracerebral activity of the other drugs in drug-susceptible disease. Six to eight weeks adjunctive dexamethasone (starting at 0.4 mg/kg/day and reducing gradually to stop over 8 weeks) improves survival from tuberculous meningitis. HIV-associated tuberculous meningitis should receive the same treatment regimen, although the benefit of corticosteroids is uncertain and there are important interactions between rifampicin and antiretroviral drugs.

Patients often get worse before they get better, commonly due to hydrocephalus, cerebral infarction, expanding tuberculoma, and hyponatraemia. Drug resistance should be suspected early in those previously treated for tuberculosis. Never change the antituberculosis regimen without consulting with tuberculosis experts.

## Neonatal meningitis

The highest risk of developing meningitis in the newborn is within the first 2 months of life, the incidence being about 0.3 per 1,000 live births. Neonatal meningitis carries a high mortality. The incidence of neurological deficits in those who survive is also high. Brain abscess is a rare complication.

Predisposing factors include prematurity, low birth weight, prolonged and difficult labour, prolonged rupture of membranes, and maternal perinatal infection. Some cases complicate congenital defects of the neuraxis.

Neonatal meningitis is usually the result of vertical transfer of pathogens from the mother in utero or during delivery, leading to early-onset (occurring within seven days of delivery) septicaemia or meningitis; less commonly, they are acquired from the environment, leading to late-onset meningitis (occurring after seven days and occasionally up to two months after delivery). Early-onset disease often presents as overwhelming sepsis syndrome with apnoea and shock. About 1 in 100 newborns colonized with group B streptococci develop early-onset disease. Late-onset disease usually presents as meningitis, and mortality is about 20 per cent.

The early signs and symptoms are often non-specific and include fever, lethargy, and refusal of feed. A bulging fontanelle, resulting from raised intracranial pressure, is a relatively late sign. A high degree of suspicion and prompt investigation with lumbar puncture is essential. Of those who survive, about half will have evidence of neurological damage.

## Treatment

Neonatal meningitis is difficult to treat. A wide variety of organisms may be involved and their susceptibility to antibiotics can be unpredictable. The chosen therapy should be supported by appropriate laboratory tests.

**Group B haemolytic streptococci** The treatment of choice is high-dose benzylpenicillin for at least 2 weeks. There may be enhanced bacterial killing when benzylpenicillin is combined with gentamicin, and many centres give this combination for the first 7–10 days.

*Escherichia coli* **and other enterobacteraciae** The most widely used antibiotic is high-dose cefotaxime, often in combination with gentamicin. Ceftazidime plus gentamicin, or a carbapenem, is used to treat *Pseudomonas aeruginosa* infections. The duration of treatment should be at least 3 weeks.

*L. monocytogenes* The organism is sensitive to a variety of agents, but the treatment of choice is high-dose ampicillin with or without gentamicin. The duration of therapy should be 3 weeks, since cerebritis may accompany the meningitis and requires more prolonged treatment.

A summary of current recommendations for the initial therapy of the commoner forms of bacterial meningitis is outlined in Table 28.3.

## Rarer forms of bacterial meningitis

### Staphylococcus aureus

Meningitis due to *Staph. aureus* may occur in patients with fulminating septicaemia secondary to pneumonia or endocarditis, or as a complication of penetrating head injury, recent neurosurgical procedures (including insertion of shunts), and ruptured cerebral or epidural abscess. Mortality is high, and neurological sequelae are common in survivors. See Table 28.4 for recommended treatment regimens. Treatment should be given for at least 4 weeks.

### Shunt-associated meningitis

In patients with hydrocephalus, the ventricular CSF is diverted to other compartments of the body (usually the peritoneal cavity) with a silastic catheter (shunt). Unfortunately, 15–25 per cent of these patients develop meningitis at some point in the life of the shunt. *Staph. epidermidis* accounts for about half, and *Staph. aureus* for about a quarter of shunt infections. Among many other microorganisms associated with such infections are *Propionibacterium acnes*, diphtheroids, enterococci, and Gram-negative bacilli. Most infections are believed to be due to colonization of the shunt at the time of surgery; occasionally, organisms may reach the CSF and shunt through the bloodstream or by retrograde spread. Examination of the CSF obtained by needle aspiration of the reservoir is essential and yields an organism in over 90 per cent of cases. It is not unusual to isolate bacteria from an otherwise normal CSF. Blood cultures are positive only if meningitis is associated with a ventriculo-atrial shunt.

Many infections will fail to be controlled unless there is complete removal of the shunt. Therapy should be commenced with parenteral vancomycin combined with oral rifampicin and daily intraventricular vancomycin. High-dose flucloxacillin should be substituted for parenteral vancomycin if the isolate proves sensitive. Treatment should be continued for 2–3 weeks before a new shunt is inserted.

**Table 28.3** Antibiotic treatment of the common types of bacterial meningitis.

| Age | Cerebrospinal fluid Gram-film findings | Presumptive organism | Treatment of choice | | Comments |
|---|---|---|---|---|---|
| | | | Antibiotic(s) | Minimum duration | |
| <2 months | Gram-positive cocci in chains | Group B streptococci | Benzyl penicillin+ gentamicin | 2 weeks | In selected patients, gentamicin may be discontinued after 7–10 days |
| | Gram-negative bacilli | 'Coliforms' (usually *Escherichia coli*) | Cefotaxime+gentamicin | 3 weeks | Change to ceftazidime if *Pseudomonas aeruginosa* |
| | Gram-positive bacilli | *Listeria monocytogenes* | Ampicillin+/–gentamicin | 3 weeks | Rare cause of neonatal meningitis |
| | No organisms seen | Any of the above | Cefotaxime+/–gentamicin +/–ampicillin | Variable[a] | Ampicillin added if *L. monocytogenes* strongly suspected |
| 2 months–6 years | Gram-negative diplococcic | *Neisseria meningitidis* | Cefotaxime or Ceftriaxone | 7 days | Can use benzylpenicillin if sensitivity confirmed |
| | Gram-positive diplococcic | *Streptococcus pneumonia* | Cefotaxime or ceftriaxone[b] | 10 days | Can use benzylpenicillin if sensitivity confirmed; in young infants and complicated cases treatment may be extended to 2 weeks |
| | Gram-negative coccobacilli | *Haemophilus influenza* | Cefotaxime or ceftriaxone | 10 days | Chloramphenicol in patients with severe cephalosporin allergy |
| | No organisms seen | Any of the above three | Cefotaxime or ceftriaxone | Variable[a] | Change as appropriate according to culture result |
| >6–40 years | Gram-negative diplococci | *N. meningitidis* | Cefotaxime or ceftriaxone | 7 days | As above |
| | Gram-positive diplococci | *Str. pneumonia* | Cefotaxime or ceftriaxone[b] | 10 days | As above |
| | No organisms seen | Either of the above two | Cefotaxime or ceftriaxone | Variable[a] | Change as appropriate according to culture result |

*(continued)*

**Table 28.3** (continued).

| Age | Cerebrospinal fluid Gram-film findings | Presumptive organism | Treatment of choice | | Minimum duration | Comments |
|---|---|---|---|---|---|---|
| | | | **Antibiotic(s)** | | | |
| >40 years | Gram-positive diplococci | *Str. pneumonia* | Cefotaxime or ceftriaxone[b] | | 10 days | As above |
| | Gram-positive bacilli | *L. monocytogenes* | Ampicillin+gentamicin | | 2–3 weeks | Co-trimoxazole if the patient is allergic to penicillin |
| | Gram-negative bacilli | 'Coliforms' (usually *E. coli*) | Cefotaxime or ceftriaxone+gentamicin | | 3 weeks | Change according to susceptibility results |
| | No organisms seen | Pneumococci or listeria | Cefotaxime or ceftriaxone+ampicillin | | Variable[b] | Add vancomycin for neurosurgical patients; change as appropriate according to culture result |
| Any age | Gram-positive cocci in clusters | Staphylococci (usually *Staphylococcus aureus*) | Flucloxacillin | | 3–4 weeks | If shunt-associated, removal of shunt usually necessary; vancomycin instead of flucloxacillin if patient is allergic to penicillin; MRSA[c] is present, or *Staph. epidermidis* is isolated |

[a] Duration will depend on the organism isolated or suspected.

[b] Add vancomycin and/or rifampicin if reduced susceptibility to ceftriaxone suspected or known.

[c] MRSA, methicillin-resistant *Staphylococcus aureus*.

**Table 28.4** Selected agents responsible for encephalitis.

| Viruses | Bacteria | Protozoa |
|---|---|---|
| Arboviruses[a] | Listeria monocytogenes | Toxoplasma gondii |
| Cytomegalovirus | Rickettsia spp. | Naegleria fowleri |
| Echoviruses | Treponema pallidum | Trypanosoma brucei |
| Enteroviruses | Tropheryma whipplei (Whipple's disease) | Trypanosoma rhodesiense |
| Epstein–Barr virus | | |
| Herpes simplex 1 and 2 | | |
| HIV | | |
| Influenza | | |
| Measles | | |
| Mumps | | |
| Rabies virus | | |
| Varicella-zoster | | |

[a] Includes Ross River, West Nile, Japanese encephalitis, and tick-borne encephalitis viruses.

## Cryptococcal meningitis

*Cryptococcus neoformans* is a yeast which causes subacute or chronic meningitis in patients with impaired cell-mediated immunity, most commonly through advanced HIV disease (blood CD4 count <100 cells/mm$^3$). Occasionally, it causes meningitis in immune-competent individuals; usually with a more virulent subspecies (*C. neoformans* var. gatti).

Clinically, the disease is indistinguishable from tuberculous meningitis. However, the yeast can be seen easily in CSF by India ink staining and can be cultured. There is also a highly sensitive and specific cryptococcal antigen (CrAg) test on blood and CSF.

Management revolves around killing the yeast, relieving any raised intracranial pressure and hydrocephalus, and addressing, if possible, the underlying immune suppression as follow:

- Kill the yeast with amphotericin B (the liposomal formulation is less nephrotoxic) and flucytosine (which enhances killing).
  - After 2 weeks, or once the CSF is sterile, treat with oral fluconazole for a further 8 weeks. If the patient remains severely immunosuppressed, lifelong low-dose fluconazole may be required.
- There is little evidence to determine optimal management of raised intracranial pressure. CSF manometry is essential at the start of treatment to determine whether repeated, sometimes daily, therapeutic lumbar punctures are required to lower pressure. Consider a lumbar drain or ventriculo-peritoneal shunt if the patient deteriorates despite these measures.

Without correction of the immune deficit, the outlook for many patients is bleak. However, current data from HIV-infected patients suggests outcomes are worse if antiretroviral therapy is started immediately. Delaying antiretroviral therapy by around two months may be a safer strategy.

### Lyme meningitis

Lyme disease is caused by *Borrelia burgdorferi*, a multisystem tick-borne disorder endemic in forested areas of North America, Europe, and Asia. A rash (erythema migrans) can occur at the site of inoculation, and the bacteria may disseminate to the central nervous system. Cranial nerve lesions (especially the VIIth nerve), lymphocytic meningitis, radiculitis, peripheral neuropathy, and rarely encephalitis may occur weeks to months after the initial infection. A later (but very rare) complication is chronic progressive encephalomyelitis, which mimics multiple sclerosis. Treat neurological Lyme disease with ceftriaxone/cefotaxime.

Overdiagnosis based on non-specific serological tests has been a problem. International guidelines now recommend positive screening tests must be confirmed by western blot.

### Viral meningitis

In the United Kingdom, viruses cause more acute meningitis than bacteria; predominantly enteroviruses, herpes simplex viruses (HSV) 1 and 2, and (in the unvaccinated) mumps. Antiviral treatment is not required as long as there is no evidence of encephalitis (see 'Encephalitis').

All the common viral causes of meningitis can be diagnosed by polymerase chain reaction (PCR) on CSF.

If the cause of meningitis remains elusive, revisit the history, re-examine the patient, and repeat the lumbar puncture; and consider rare causes of meningitis, or conditions with similar symptoms and signs. And remember, all patients with an unexplained neurological illness require an HIV test.

## Encephalitis

Encephalitis can be infectious, post-infectious, or immune mediated. In the majority (50–70%) no cause is found. However, the important infectious causes are as follows:

- ◆ HSV and varicella-zoster virus (VZV) are the commonest infectious causes in the United Kingdom, although cytomegalovirus (CMV), human herpesvirus type 6 (HHV-6), and *Toxoplasma gondii* cause encephalitis in immune-compromised patients.
- ◆ Worldwide, *AR*thropod-*BO*rne viruses (arboviruses) such as Japanese encephalitis and West Nile virus cause significant numbers of cases, and rabies (which is invariably fatal) remains endemic in many countries.
- ◆ Measles virus and *Mycoplasma pneumoniae* are the commonest causes of post-infectious encephalitis.

Other causes are listed in Table 28.4.

## Clinical features

Patients with acute encephalitis have fever, altered consciousness, and CSF pleocytosis, with or without seizures; although these findings are not universal. It can be difficult to distinguish acute encephalitis from septic encephalopathy. The latter is a syndrome of brain dysfunction associated with systemic sepsis. Its clinical features range from mild slowing of mentation and impairment of attention, to coma. Focal neurological signs, especially when lateralized, or seizures strongly suggest encephalitis. Neurological findings in septic encephalopathy are usually symmetrical, such as paratonic rigidity; asterixis, tremor, or myoclonus are uncommon. CSF abnormalities are unusual except for mildly raised protein. Septic encephalopathy is a diagnosis of exclusion.

## Treatment

Aciclovir reduces death and disability from HSV encephalitis (HSE) and should be prescribed empirically to all patients with suspected encephalitis as soon as is possible, until the cause has been determined (delay in treatment while awaiting diagnosis will lead to irreversible brain damage if the diagnosis does indeed turn out to be HSE). Diffusion-weighted magnetic resonance imaging (MRI) reveals early changes of HSE, which typically affects the fronto-temporal lobes. CSF HSV PCR early (<48 hours of symptoms) may be falsely negative; in this circumstance, aciclovir should be continued and CSF HSV PCR repeated. A negative HSV PCR after 72 hours of symptoms has a high negative predictive value. In proven cases, treat with 14–21 days aciclovir; beware aciclovir-induced renal toxicity. Adjunctive corticosteroids are not recommended.

## Brain abscess

*Staph. aureus*, many streptococci (e.g. *Str. pyogenes*, *Str. pneumoniae*, *Str. milleri*) and some anaerobic bacteria (e.g. *Bacteroides fragilis*) are associated with pus and abscess formation. They can infect the brain parenchyma (cerebral abscess) or occur between the dura and arachnoid mater (subdural empyema) through penetrating traumatic injuries, neurosurgery, haematogenous seeding (e.g. endocarditis), or contiguous spread (e.g. mastoiditis). Right-to-left circulatory shunts increase the risk of brain abscesses. *Mycob. tuberculosis* can mimic all the above infections.

Collections of pus cause swinging fevers; when involving the brain, they also cause headache and, depending on location, focal neurological deficits and seizures.

Abscess and empyema drainage is the key to rapid resolution; cure is affected more often by the surgeon's knife than the choice of antibiotic. Determining the cause of the infection is important; however, take pretreatment blood cultures and submit pus for staining and culture (including for *Mycob. tuberculosis*).

Community-acquired brain abscesses should be treated with a third generation cephalosporin and metronidazole. If a haematogenous infection source is suspected (e.g. *Staph. aureus* bacteraemia), arrange an echocardiogram and search for any foci of extracranial infection.

## Key points

- Viral meningitis is common and requires no treatment; bacterial meningitis is a life-threatening disease and requires rapid diagnosis and treatment.
- *Str. pneumoniae* and *N. meningitidis* are the lead causes of bacterial meningitis. In the neonate, *E. coli* and group B streptococci predominate.
- Treatment requires high-dose parenteral antibiotic such as penicillin or ceftriaxone that can penetrate the CSF; treatment is tailored to the particular pathogen.
- Herpes simplex encephalitis is a medical emergency; treatment with intravenous aciclovir MUST be given as soon as possible, before the diagnosis is proven or refuted.
- Abscesses of the brain vary by site; their microbiology is often mixed and reflects the predisposing condition. Their management requires coordination of radiological, neurosurgical and antibiotic expertise. Other causes of CNS infections include mycobacteria, viruses (meningitis and encephalitis), and rarely fungi and parasites.

## Further reading

Brouwer, M. C., McIntyre, P., Prasad, K., and van de Beek, D. (2013) Corticosteroids for acute bacterial meningitis. *Cochrane Database of Systematic Reviews*, **Issue 6**: Art. No. CD004405.

Brouwer, M. C., Thwaites, G. E., Tunkel, A. R., and van de Beek D. (2012) Dilemmas in the diagnosis of acute community-acquired bacterial meningitis. *Lancet*, **380**(9854):1684–92.

Kasanmoentalib, E. S., Brouwer, M. C., and van de Beek, D. (2013) Update on bacterial meningitis: epidemiology, trials and genetic association studies. *Current Opinion in Neurology*, **26**(3): 282–88.

Solomon, T., Michael, B. D., Smith, P. E., et al. (2012) Management of suspected viral encephalitis in adults—Association of British Neurologists and British Infection Association National Guidelines. *The Journal of Infection*, **64**(4):347–73.

Thwaites, G. E., van Toorn, R., and Schoeman, J. (2013) Tuberculous meningitis: more questions, still too few answers. *Lancet Neurology*, **12**(10): 999–1010.

van de Beek, D., Brouwer, M. C., Thwaites, G. E., and Tunkel, A. R. (2012) Advances in treatment of bacterial meningitis. *Lancet*, **380**(9854): 1693–1702.

# Chapter 29

# Skin and soft-tissue infections

## General considerations

At birth the skin of the baby rapidly becomes colonized with bacteria from the mother, other handlers, and the environment. Some of these essentially non-pathogenic microbes, including coryneforms, coagulase-negative staphylococci, micrococci, and propionibacteria, become established as the resident flora of the normal skin. In intact skin these microorganisms usually prevent potential pathogens such as *Staphylococcus aureus* and *Streptococcus pyogenes* (haemolytic streptococci of Lancefield group A) from becoming established. However, if the skin is broken by accidental or surgical trauma, burns, a foreign body, or a primary skin disease (psoriasis, atopic dermatitis), these pathogens may not only become established as resident organisms—they may also give rise to infection of the skin and subcutaneous tissue.

Many different microorganisms, including bacteria, fungi, and some viruses, may be involved in skin and soft-tissue infections. However, by far the commonest bacterial causes are *Staph. aureus* and *Str. pyogenes*. Thrush is usually caused by the yeast *Candida albicans*, and cold sores by the virus herpes simplex.

Skin and soft-tissue infections are common (Fig. 29.1) and frequently severe (Table 29.1). In European hospitals skin, soft-tissue, bone, and joint infections account for 19 per cent of all antibiotic treatments, second only to respiratory tract infections (Fig. 29.1) Nearly a quarter of hospital inpatients with skin and soft-tissue infection have sepsis, and a third of patients with severe sepsis die (Table 29.1).

## Common clinical presentations

### Impetigo

Impetigo consists of discrete purulent lesions on the exposed areas of the body, especially the face and extremities. It is nearly always caused by *Str. pyogenes* or *Staph. aureus*. Impetigo is most common in tropical countries but is also prevalent in more temperate zones, especially during the summer. It is most common in children aged 2–5 years but can occur in older children or adults. The prevalence is strongly related to personal hygiene, and impetigo is much commoner in socially deprived communities.

The lesions of impetigo start with papules that evolve into pustules and then form a characteristic thick crust over 4–7 days. The lesions are sometimes bullous. Antibacterial treatment can be either topical or systemic (Table 29.2).

### Pustular lesions

Such lesions of the skin are by far the commonest bacterial infection in man and include

- folliculitis (pimples), where the infection is confined to hair follicles and does not involve the surrounding skin or subcutaneous tissue—such infections are usually mild and self-limiting, and do not need medical attention;

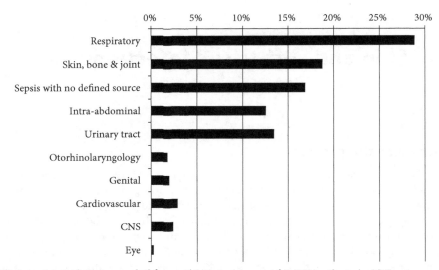

**Fig. 29.1** Anatomical sites recorded for antibiotic treatment of 2,760 patients in 20 European hospitals.

Source: data from of Ansari, F et al., The European surveillance of antimicrobial consumption (ESAC) point-prevalence survey of antibacterial use in 20 European hospitals in 2006, *Clinical Infectious Disease*, Volume 49, Issue 10, pp. 1496–1504, Copyright © 2010 British Society for Antimicrobial Chemotherapy.

- ◆ furuncles (boils), where the folliculitis has spread deeper and is surrounded by an area of cellulitis; and

- ◆ carbuncles, where several furuncles have coalesced and extended into subcutaneous fat to form a large, indurated, painful lesion that contains loculated pus with multiple drainage points.

Antibiotics are rarely required for these lesions unless they are recurrent (Table 29.2). Acne is discussed in Chapter 22.

**Table 29.1** Appropriateness of antibiotic treatment and mortality by severity of sepsis for 189 hospital inpatients with skin and soft-tissue infection.

| Severity of sepsis | Number (% total) | Treatment classification by comparison with UK guidance | | | Mortality |
|---|---|---|---|---|---|
| | | **Appropriate treatment** | **Over-treatment** | **Under-treatment** | |
| No sepsis | 144 (76%) | 27% | 63% | 24% | 6% |
| Sepsis without organ impairment | 33 (18%) | 30% | 30% | 39% | 18% |
| Severe sepsis | 12 (6%) | 8% | 0% | 92% | 33% |
| All | 189 | 26% | 43% | 31% | 10% |

Source: data from Marwick C et al., Severity assessment of skin and soft tissue infections: cohort study of management and outcomes for hospitalised patients, *Journal of Antimicrobial Chemotherapy*, Volume 66, Issue 2, pp. 387–397, Copyright © 2011 British Society for Antimicrobial Chemotherapy.

**Table 29.2** Most likely bacterial causes and antibacterial treatment for common skin infections.

| Clinical diagnosis | Most likely causes | Antibacterial treatment |
|---|---|---|
| Impetigo | *Streptococcus pyogenes*<br>Staphylococcus aureus | Topical: fusidic acid or mupirocin; reserve for patients with a limited number of lesions |
| | | Systemic: antistaphylococcal penicillin (e.g. flucloxacillin), clindamycin or a tetracycline |
| Pustules, furuncles and carbuncles | *Staph. aureus* | Small lesions: no treatment is required in most cases |
| | | Larger lesions: incision and drainage; antibiotics required only if there are signs of spreading cellulitis or systemic inflammation |
| | | Recurrent lesions: topical mupirocin to the nose for the first 5 days of each month; if this fails, try clindamycin 150 mg once daily dose for 3 months |
| Uncomplicated cellulitis and erysipelas | *Str. pyogenes*<br>*Staph. aureus* | Antistaphylococcal penicillin (e.g. flucloxacillin), clindamycin or a tetracycline;<br>see Fig. 29.2 for management of severe infections |
| Animal bites | Bacteria from the animal's normal mouth flora (e.g. *Pasteurella multocida*) | Co-amoxiclav; for penicillin-allergic patients, doxycycline plus metronidazole |
| Human bites | Mixed aerobic and anaerobic mouth flora | Co-amoxiclav; for penicillin-allergic patients, clindamycin plus a fluoroquinolone |
| Diabetic foot infections | *Str. pyogenes*<br>*Staph. aureus*<br>Gram-negative aerobic bacteria<br>Anaerobic bacteria | Co-amoxiclav; for penicillin-allergic patients, clindamycin+a fluoroquinolone unless at high risk of *Clostridium difficile* infection |

## Cellulitis and erysipelas

These are both diffuse, spreading skin lesions. Cellulitis, which is much more common, occurs in the deeper layers of the skin and subcutaneous tissues. The obviously affected area is red and hot but the demarcation between this and the normal skin is gradual and there is no palpable raised margin. It is more common if there is obstruction to venous or lymphatic drainage or gross obesity, which make the skin more fragile and local host defences less effective. In contrast, erysipelas occurs in the superficial layers of the skin and results in a very clear, abrupt line of demarcation between the affected and normal skin, with a palpable lesion that is raised above the level of the normal skin. Cellulitis may be caused by *Str. pyogenes* or *Staph. aureus*, whereas erysipelas is almost always caused by *Str. pyogenes*. Erysipelas usually occurs on the face or on the legs, whereas cellulitis can occur anywhere on the body, although it is commonest on the legs. Both types of lesion are usually preceded by a break in the skin. Methicillin-resistant *Staph. aureus* (MRSA) is increasingly incriminated in community-acquired cellulitis in some countries.

Signs of spreading infection include extension of the line of demarcation, lymphangitis (infection spreading up the lymph vessels with a characteristic thin streak of erythema running up to a lymph node), and painful tender lymph nodes distal to the lesion. Systemic inflammatory response means that the patient has sepsis and is at risk of progressing to severe sepsis or septic shock (see Chapter 26). Blood cultures should be taken from patients with sepsis arising from cellulitis, as about 50 per cent are positive.

Both cellulitis and erysipelas can be treated with an antistaphylococcal penicillin. In theory, erysipelas could be treated with penicillin V but it is not worth taking the risk that the cause may be *Staph. aureus*. There is a belief that an antistaphylococcal penicillin should be combined with benzylpenicillin or penicillin V, since the latter are much more active against *Str. pyogenes*. However, provided antistaphylococcal penicillins are given in adequate dosage, they are just as effective alone.

Prevention of recurrent cellulitis requires enhancement of host defences by preventing breaks in the skin (e.g. dry thoroughly between the toes after washing) or wearing compression stockings to reduce oedema. If these measures fail, then long-term prophylactic antibiotics are unfortunately not usually effective. It is preferable to give the patient a course of antibiotics to start as soon as symptoms begin.

## Cellulitis following animal or human bites

Infections following animal bites are polymicrobial, often including anaerobic bacteria and unusual organisms such as *Pasteurella multocida*, a human pathogen that is part of the normal oral flora of cats. Human bites are often associated with greater damage to the skin and soft tissues and are also polymicrobial, with aerobic and anaerobic bacteria. Co-amoxiclav is an effective treatment for all these infections (Table 29.2).

## Diabetic foot infections

Infections of the feet are particularly common in diabetics because several important host defences, including circulation and sensation, are compromised. This enables minor injuries to progress to advanced stages of infection rapidly and with very few symptoms. Consequently it is vital to educate patients with diabetes about how to avoid trauma to the feet and how to recognize infection early. Patients with diabetes also have impaired healing, so chronic ulcers are common.

Chronic ulcers without spreading cellulitis do not require antibiotic treatment, even if there is some purulence in the exudate, as this simply indicates bacterial colonization of the ulcer. If there is cellulitis spreading up to 2 cm from the margin of the ulcer, the infection is likely to respond to oral antibiotics but, if the infection spreads more widely or is associated with signs of sepsis, then referral to hospital for intravenous treatment should be considered. Taking swabs from chronic ulcers is not helpful because they will be colonized with possibly harmless bacteria; even if infection is present, the bacteria cultured are not always the ones that are responsible. Meaningful cultures can be obtained only by debriding the ulcer and then obtaining tissue specimens from the base of the lesion by curettage (scrapings with a sterile blade). Empirical treatment should cover both aerobic and anaerobic pathogens (Table 29.2).

Because of the combination of impaired circulation and sensation, diabetic foot infections are particularly likely to progress to osteomyelitis because they may be present for weeks before the patient seeks medical attention. Osteomyelitis should be considered as a potential complication of any deep or extensive ulcer, especially if it is overlying a bony prominence or contains visible bone particles. Management of osteomyelitis is considered in Chapter 27.

## Miscellaneous infections

Viral infections of the skin, such as herpes simplex and varicella zoster, are discussed in Chapter 32. Superficial fungal infections usually respond to topical therapy (Chapter 22), although dermatophyte infections of finger- or toenails may require oral treatment with terbinafine for up to 3 months or with griseofulvin for a year or more. These agents are deposited in newly formed keratin, and the prolonged treatment is needed to allow healthy nail to replace the diseased tissue. Even so, treatment of chronic infections of toenails may be unsuccessful, although terbinafine is more reliable in this respect than griseofulvin.

# Severe skin and soft-tissue infections

Necrotizing fasciitis and toxic shock syndrome have received considerable media attention. However both of these problems are rare in comparison with severe sepsis associated with cellulitis. In comparison with pneumonia, relatively little attention has been given to auditing and improving the management of severe skin and soft-tissue infection. The principles of treatment are not complex (Table 29.1 and Fig. 29.2):

1 Oral, narrow-spectrum therapy for uncomplicated cellulitis.

2 Intravenous narrow-spectrum therapy for sepsis without organ impairment.

3 Broad-spectrum intravenous therapy for patients with severe sepsis or evidence of necrotizing fasciitis. This should include clindamycin both for cover against anaerobic bacteria and because clindamycin reduces toxin production by bacteria.

However, studies of the management of skin and soft-tissue infection show that most antibiotic treatment is inappropriate, with under-treatment of severe infections as well as over-treatment of uncomplicated infections (Table 29.1). It is important to be aware that 20 per cent of patients with severe community-acquired cellulitis do not have signs of systemic inflammatory response on admission to hospital, so re-assessment within the first 24 hours of admission is essential. In this cohort study (Table 29.1), 35 different antibiotic regimens were used for initial treatment of skin and soft-tissue infections, whereas the protocol in Fig. 29.2 contains 6 regimens that should cover all eventualities. Hospitals need to audit and improve their management of these common infections.

## Necrotizing skin and soft-tissue infections

These are rapidly spreading and life-threatening forms of cellulitis that involve the deeper fascial and/or muscle compartments in addition to skin and subcutaneous tissue. Infection usually arises following a break in the skin after trauma or elective surgery. Most cases are caused by *Str. pyogenes* either alone or in combination with other bacteria, including *Staph. aureus*, coliform bacilli, and anaerobes. *Staph. aureus* strains that produce the PVL (Panton–Vallentine leukocidin) toxin are also associated with necrotizing infections. Many variations of necrotizing skin and soft-tissue infections have been described according to the tissues involved, the anatomical site of the infection, and the microbial causes but the basic principles of management are the same. The key is early distinction between a cellulitis that will respond to antibacterial treatment and a deeper necrotizing infection that is likely to require surgical debridement as well. The following clinical features indicate the possibility of necrotizing infection:

- severe, constant pain that is disproportionate to the visible inflammation in the skin;
- bullae on the skin, which occur because of occlusion of deep blood vessels that cross the fascia or muscle compartments;

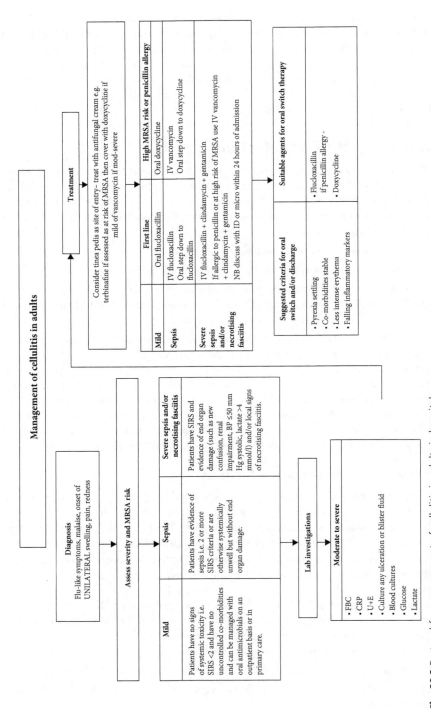

**Fig. 29.2** Protocol for management of cellulitis in adults in hospitals.

Adapted with permission from NHS Tayside Area Formulary, *Antibiotic Policy*, available from http://www.nhstaysideadtc.scot.nhs.uk/TAPG%20html/MAIN/front%20page.htm

- skin necrosis or bruising;
- gas in the soft tissues detected by palpation or imaging;
- oedema that extends beyond the margin of erythema;
- cutaneous anaesthesia;
- systemic toxicity, manifested by signs of severe sepsis (see Chapter 26); and
- rapid spread of infection despite appropriate antibiotic therapy.

Blood cultures are often positive, and streptococci can also be isolated from the bullous lesions. The management of these rare conditions is primarily surgical, with radical debridement of all necrotic tissue, intensive life-support therapy, and the treatment of shock. Antimicrobial therapy must be directed against aerobic Gram-positive and Gram-negative bacteria and against anaerobic bacteria until the results of cultures are available. Clindamycin is active against aerobic Gram-positive and anaerobic pathogens; it also suppresses toxin production by group A streptococci and may be superior to penicillins for these infections. Gentamicin should be added initially to treat Gram-negative aerobic pathogens.

## Gas gangrene

Gas gangrene (clostridial myositis) is a life-threatening, invasive infection that can be caused by several species of *Clostridium*, principally *Clo. perfringens*. These bacteria are part of the normal intestinal flora of man and animals, and clostridial spores are common in soil. Gas gangrene develops when impaired blood supply, tissue necrosis, or the presence of foreign bodies produce a low oxygen tension in the tissues and thus create conditions in which the spores can germinate. Extensive soft-tissue injury contaminated with soil or dirt carries an increased risk of gas gangrene. Gas gangrene may rarely complicate surgical wounds, particularly after intestinal or biliary surgery, or be a complication of septic abortion. Clostridial anaerobic cellulitis occurs under similar circumstances but exploration of the wound usually reveals that the muscle is spared.

A clinical diagnosis is made on the basis of palpable (crepitus) or radiological signs of a spreading, gas-producing infection in a toxic patient with the above risk factors. Immediate and extensive surgical excision of all involved tissues and the removal of any foreign body are essential and may mean hysterectomy (after septic abortion), excision of subcutaneous tissue and muscle of the abdominal wall, or even amputation of a limb. Parenteral benzylpenicillin should also be given promptly in high dosage. For patients allergic to penicillin, metronidazole may be used. Despite these desperate and mutilating measures, the mortality remains high.

## Toxic shock syndrome

Certain phage types of *Staph. aureus* and *Str. pyogenes* produce toxins that cause a multisystem disease characterized by the sudden onset of fever, myalgia, vomiting, diarrhoea, hypotension, and an erythematous rash: the toxic shock syndrome. Staphylococcal toxic shock syndrome was originally thought to affect only menstruating women who used a particular type of tampon; it is now known to be a rare sequel of any type of staphylococcal infection. An antistaphylococcal penicillin (e.g. flucloxacillin) or clindamycin should be given but antibiotic therapy is secondary to systemic support. Clinical results with intravenous immunoglobulin are inconsistent, probably because different batches of immunoglobulin contain variable quantities of neutralizing antibodies to some of these toxins.

# MRSA infections and PVL toxin

MRSA is most likely to cause skin and soft-tissue infections in hospital patients in Europe but in some settings (e.g. N. America) is a common community pathogen. In the United Kingdom, screening for MRSA is recommended for most hospital admissions. Screening requires swabs from two body sites, the nose and the perineum. If the latter is not clinically possible, then an alternative is throat swabbing; however, the diagnostic effectiveness of nasal and throat swabbing is significantly lower than nasal and perineal swabbing.

Patients may present from the community with MRSA infection despite having no contact with hospitals or health care. Strains of MRSA that cause community-acquired infection are genetically and phenotypically distinct from hospital-acquired MRSA and often produce PVL, a toxin that destroys white blood cells and is a staphylococcal virulence factor. PVL toxin related infection should be suspected in patients with recurrent boils or abscesses, with necrotizing skin infection, or with community-acquired necrotizing or haemorrhagic pneumonia.

## Key points

- Many different microorganisms, including bacteria, fungi, and some viruses, may be involved in skin and soft-tissue infections. However, by far the commonest bacterial causes are *Staph. aureus* and *Str. pyogenes*.
- Skin and soft-tissue infections are common and may be severe. In European hospitals, skin, soft-tissue, bone and joint infections account for 19 per cent of all antibiotic treatments, second only to respiratory tract infections. Nearly a quarter of hospital inpatients with skin and soft-tissue infection have sepsis, and a third of patients with severe sepsis die.
- Many skin infections are localized (impetigo, pustules, and abscesses). However, spreading cellulitis indicates invasive infection with risk of progression to sepsis.
- The principles of treatment are simple, and so it is disturbing that both over-treatment of mild cases and under-treatment of severe cases are common.

  1 Oral, narrow-spectrum therapy for uncomplicated cellulitis.

  2 Intravenous narrow-spectrum therapy for sepsis without organ impairment.

  3 Broad-spectrum intravenous therapy for patients with severe sepsis or evidence of necrotizing fasciitis. This should include clindamycin, both for cover against anaerobic bacteria and because clindamycin reduces toxin production by bacteria.

## Further reading

**Health Protection Agency.** Meticillin Resistant Staphylococcus aureus (MRSA) Screening and Suppression Quick Reference Guide for Primary Care—for consultation and local adaptation 2009 [Cited 9 February 2014] Available from: <https://www.gov.uk/government/uploads/system/uploads/attachment_data/file/330793/MRSA_screening_and_supression_primary_care_guidance.pdf>

**Health Protection Scotland.** (2014) *MRSA Screening Pathfinder Programme for Professionals.* <http://www.hps.scot.nhs.uk/haiic/sshaip/mrsascreeningpathfinderprofessionals.aspx>, accessed 3 December 2014.

**Leese, G., Nathwani, D., Young, M., Seaton, A., Kennon, B., Hopkinson, H., Stang, D., Lipsky, B., Jeffcoate, W., and Berendt, T.** (2009) Use of antibiotics in people with diabetic foot disease: a consensus statement. *The Diabetic Foot Journal*, **12**(2): 62–74.

Marwick, C, Rae, N., Irvine, N., and Davey, P. (2012) Prospective study of severity assessment and management of acute medical admissions with skin and soft tissue infection. *Journal of Antimicrobial Chemotherapy,* **67**(4): 1016–19.

Nathwani, D., Morgan, M., Masterton, R. G., Dryden, M., Cookson, B. D., French, G., and Lewis, D. (2008) Guidelines for UK practice for the diagnosis and management of methicillin-resistant *Staphylococcus aureus* (MRSA) infections presenting in the community. *Journal of Antimicrobial Chemotherapy,* **61**(5): 976–94.

Stevens, D. L., Bisno, A. L., Chambers, H. F., Everett, E. D., Dellinger, P., Goldstein, E. J., Gorbach, S.L., Hirschmann , J. V., Kaplan, E. L., Montoya, J. G., and Wade, J. C. (2005) Practice guidelines for the diagnosis and management of skin and soft-tissue infections. *Clinical Infectious Diseases,* **41**(10): 1373–1406.

# Chapter 30

# Tuberculosis and other mycobacterial diseases

## Tuberculosis

Tuberculosis is caused by *Mycobacterium tuberculosis*, a slow-growing bacillus with the important property of being able to resist decolourization with acidified alcohol following carbol fuchsin staining (the Ziehl–Neelsen stain). This property of 'acid fastness' is shared by all mycobacteria but the demonstration of 'acid-fast bacilli' in clinical specimens (e.g. sputum) has been the basis of the main diagnostic test for active tuberculosis for more than 100 years.

   *M. tuberculosis* is transmitted between humans by aerosol: people with pulmonary tuberculosis cough and expel bacteria into the surrounding air for them to be inhaled by others. The lungs are almost always the first organ infected. One of the most important characteristics of *M. tuberculosis* is its ability to cause prolonged, asymptomatic infection, commonly known as 'latent' infection. The World Health Organization (WHO) estimates that a third of the world's population is latently infected with *M. tuberculosis*; around 1 in 10 of these will develop clinical tuberculosis, falling to 1 in 3 if the individual is co-infected with HIV. Other risk factors for the development of active disease include tobacco smoking, diabetes, malnutrition, gastrectomy, and silicosis. Most recently, the antitumour necrosis factor biological agents (e.g. infliximab) for the treatment of autoimmune inflammatory conditions make patients uniquely susceptible to active tuberculosis.

   Clinical disease can take many forms, as almost any organ of the body can be affected but in around 70 per cent the primary focus of infection is the lungs (Table 30.1). Pulmonary tuberculosis is characterized by many weeks or months of symptoms, usually starting with weight loss, anorexia, fever, and a cough. As the cough progresses, sputum is produced, which may be bloody. Typically, the apices of the lungs are affected with infiltrates and cavitation. Associated mediastinal lymph node enlargement is common. Extrapulmonary disease is particularly common in untreated HIV infection and can take many forms. Prolonged bloodstream infection can lead to 'miliary' tuberculosis, with numerous foci of infection throughout the lung fields and other organs. Brain infection with meningitis is especially serious (see Chapter 28), as it is always fatal if left untreated.

   Drug resistance is one of the greatest challenges to physicians treating tuberculosis and those responsible for control programmes. Multidrug-resistant tuberculosis (MDR-TB)—defined as resistance to at least the two key drugs isoniazid and rifampicin—is becoming increasingly common and is very hard to treat. It takes 24 months to treat MDR-TB, rather than 6 months for sensitive disease, and the drugs are more toxic.

### Principles of management

Pulmonary tuberculosis is responsible for ongoing tuberculosis transmission and disease. Therefore, the effective management of pulmonary tuberculosis remains the greatest priority in disease control. The key components of management and tuberculosis control are

**Table 30.1** Tuberculosis: disease forms.

| Common | Less common | Uncommon |
|---|---|---|
| Pulmonary | Miliary | Pericardial |
| Lymph node | Meningitis | Skin |
| | Intra-abdominal | |
| | Pleural | |
| | Bone | |
| | Genito-urinary | |

- rapid and reliable microbiological detection of active disease;
- supervised treatment with combination chemotherapy;
- notification of cases and contact tracing;
- prevention of disease in contacts, either by vaccination or chemotherapy; and
- continuous reporting and surveillance, especially for drug resistance.

## Diagnosis

### Active tuberculosis

The diagnosis of active tuberculosis is dependent upon demonstrating the presence of *M. tuberculosis* in affected tissues. This is currently done in three main ways:

1 Finding 'acid-fast bacilli' in a clinical specimen, for example, sputum, cerebrospinal fluid (CSF), or tissue biopsy, by microscopy following Ziehl–Neelsen staining.

2 The demonstration of *M. tuberculosis* nucleic acid in a clinical specimen by nucleic acid amplification techniques, for example, polymerase chain reaction (PCR).

3 The culture of *M. tuberculosis* from a clinical specimen.

Microscopy is fast and cheap, but lacks sensitivity (around 50% on sputum for pulmonary tuberculosis diagnosis) and specificity. Mycobacteria other than *M. tuberculosis* are also 'acid fast' and may be either contaminating the specimen or causing disease (see 'Other forms of tuberculosis').

Nucleic acid amplification is rapid, more sensitive than microscopy, and some assays for example, the GeneXpert MTB/RIF test, can also detect the genetic mutations responsible for drug resistance. These assays are expensive and require specialized equipment but are becoming more widely available.

*M. tuberculosis* culture is too slow to aid clinical decision making. It takes at least 2 weeks to get a result, and sometimes up to 8 weeks. However, most drug susceptibility tests are dependent upon having a pure growth of the bacteria. Therefore, culture should always be attempted.

### Latent tuberculosis

In contrast, the diagnosis of latent tuberculosis is *not* dependent upon demonstrating the presence of *M. tuberculosis* within tissues but, instead, an immune response to the bacteria. There are two ways to diagnose latent tuberculosis:

1 Intradermal injection of purified protein derivative (PPD or 'tuberculin') of *M. tuberculosis* with measurement of the subsequent inflammatory induration after 48–72 hours. There are a

number of forms of these skin tests: for example, the Mantoux and Heaf tests. If the skin induration is greater than a defined threshold, latent infection is diagnosed.

2 More recently, blood tests have been devised to diagnose latent tuberculosis called the 'interferon-γ release assays' (IGRAs). The principle of these assays is to stimulate either whole blood or its mononuclear white cells with specific *M. tuberculosis* antigens and measure the expression of interferon-γ (an important cytokine in tuberculosis immunity). IGRAs are more specific than skin tests, and do not require recall of the patient to read the result. However, they are probably only marginally more sensitive than skin tests and are more expensive, requiring special laboratory equipment. IGRAs are not good at diagnosing active tuberculosis.

## Treatment

### Active tuberculosis

Tuberculosis became a treatable disease in the late 1940s with the discovery of streptomycin and *para*-aminosalicylic acid. The randomized comparison of streptomycin versus bed rest for pulmonary tuberculosis, published in the *BMJ* in 1948, was a landmark trial. It not only showed that streptomycin improved outcomes from tuberculosis but is widely credited as the first randomized controlled trial. Over the next 40 years, a series of randomized controlled trials were used to define the role of new antituberculosis agents as they became available (isoniazid, rifampicin, pyrazinamide, ethambutol) and the optimal treatment regimen.

The current standard first-line treatment for tuberculosis has not changed since the completion of these trials 30 years ago (see Table 30.2).

**Table 30.2** Recommended first-line treatment regimens for tuberculosis in adults.

| Drug | Initial phase (2 months) | Continuation phase (4 months) | Major side effects |
|---|---|---|---|
| **Standard regimen** | | | |
| Rifampicin | 10 mg/kg/day (450–600 mg/day) | 10 mg/kg/day (450–600 mg/day) | Hepatitis; gastrointestinal upsets |
| Isoniazid[a] | 5 mg/kg/day (300 mg/day) | 5 mg/kg/day (300 mg/day) | Peripheral neuropathy; hepatitis |
| Pyrazinamide | 30 mg/kg/day (1.5–2.0 g/day) | | Hepatitis; gout |
| Ethambutol | 15 mg/kg/day | | Retrobulbar optic neuritis |
| **Intermittent regimen (3 times weekly)** | | | |
| Rifampicin | 10 mg/kg | 10 mg/kg | As above |
| Isoniazid | 15 mg/kg | 15 mg/kg | |
| Pyrazinamide | 50 mg/kg | | |
| Ethambutol | 30 mg/kg | | |

[a] Or streptomycin (15 mg/kg/day or 0.75–1.00 g/day for 2 months if resistant to isoniazid). The rationale for this multidrug regimen is to provide the shortest possible, most effective therapy, while preventing the emergence of drug-resistant bacteria.

Treatment of tuberculosis requires expert supervision and should be under the direction of a specialist in respiratory medicine or infectious diseases and supporting staff. The key factors to a successful outcome are compliance with the regimen, an assured supply of medication, avoidance of interactions with any other concomitant medicines, early detection of drug toxicity, and dose adjustment for weight and renal function, since these may alter during the period of treatment.

Tuberculosis is a notifiable disease in many countries. This ensures that there is not only close supervision of the infected person but that household and other contacts can be assessed for evidence of infection (a positive tuberculin skin test) or active disease based on symptoms and a positive chest X-ray. Outbreaks continue to occur, emphasizing the importance of notification and contact tracing.

## Latent tuberculosis

The diagnosis and treatment of latent tuberculosis is a major part of many tuberculosis control programmes. There are two standard regimens:

1 Monotherapy with isoniazid, daily, for 6 months.
2 Rifampicin and isoniazid, daily, for 3 months.

Both regimens are probably equally effective; the rifampicin-containing regimen has the advantage of shorter duration but the rifampicin may interact with other drugs and may cause more hepatic toxicity. Isoniazid monotherapy is generally well tolerated (although hepatitis may occur) and there are no major interactions with other drugs.

# First-line antituberculosis drugs

## Isoniazid (isonicotinic acid hydrazide)

Isoniazid is a potent killer of *M. tuberculosis*, especially during the first few days of treatment. It penetrates rapidly into all tissues, including CSF. It is given as a single daily oral dose and metabolized mainly by acetylation in the liver, at a rate which is genetically determined. Patients can be divided into two groups—rapid and slow acetylators. This is probably of little clinical significance in patients treated daily but rapid acetylators given intermittent regimens may have worse treatment outcomes.

Primary resistance in *M. tuberculosis* in the United Kingdom is uncommon (<5%) but increasing. The impact of isoniazid resistance on clinical outcomes from lung tuberculosis is relatively modest, unless combined with rifampicin resistance (MDR-TB). However, isoniazid resistance causes substantially worse outcomes in patient with severe, disseminated tuberculosis with HIV co-infection, and alternative drugs should be used.

Adverse reactions are uncommon but include hypersensitivity rashes and hepatitis (0.1%). The latter is potentially serious and the risk increases with age. It can be easily managed by prompt withdrawal of treatment. A sharp rise in serum transaminases at the outset of treatment is relatively common and may be enhanced by the concomitant use of rifampicin but is usually of little significance. Liver function tests should be checked before starting treatment as a yardstick to measure any subsequent adverse reactions. Isoniazid interferes competitively with pyridoxine metabolism by inhibiting the formation of the active form of the vitamin and hence often results in peripheral neuropathy, which can be prevented by co-administration of pyridoxine. Rarely, isoniazid can cause a lupus-like syndrome and confusion and convulsions.

## Rifampicin and other rifamycins

Rifampicin is one of the most important of the antituberculosis drugs, as demonstrated by the major detrimental impact of resistance on treatment outcomes. Rifampicin may be given daily or as part of an intermittent, three-times-a-week regimen. Whenever possible, it should be used throughout treatment.

The important side effects of rifampicin are hepatitis, rash, and a flu-like illness when given as part of intermittent regimens. The drug also turns urine, sweat, and tears orange but this effect is harmless and stops once the drug is removed. Rifampicin also induces the hepatic metabolism of many drugs and this interaction must carefully be considered whenever prescribing rifampicin. The full and very extensive list of interactions can be found in the appendix of the *British National Formulary* but the most common, clinically important interactions are with warfarin, many anti-HIV drugs, and the combined oral contraceptive pill: the activity of all these agents are substantially reduced by co-administration with rifampicin.

Rifampicin is also key to the drug treatment of leprosy (see 'Leprosy') and is sometimes used in the treatment of life-threatening staphylococcal infections and in the prophylaxis of meningococcal and *Haemophilus influenzae* meningitis. There are a two other rifamycins in clinical usage: rifabutin and rifapentine. Both are active against *M. tuberculosis*. Rifabutin is a less potent inducer of hepatic metabolism than rifampicin and is therefore often used in combination with antiretroviral drugs in the treatment of tuberculosis in HIV co-infected patients. Rifapentine has a much longer half-life than rifampicin and can be given once or twice weekly, although these regimens have been associated with unacceptably high rates of tuberculosis recurrence in HIV-infected patients.

## Pyrazinamide

Pyrazinamide is used in the first 2 months of treatment and is an important 'sterilizing' agent, killing intracellular bacilli in acidic conditions that are relatively resistant to the activity of the other antituberculosis drugs. It reduces the duration of therapy required and the risk of relapse. It is given orally, produces high serum levels, and penetrates freely into CSF. Hepatitis, arthralgia, gout, anorexia, nausea, and rash are well-reported side effects. Hypersensitivity reactions and photosensitivity of the skin also occur.

## Ethambutol

Ethambutol is active against *M. tuberculosis* and many non-tuberculous mycobacteria. It is rapidly absorbed after oral administration and high serum levels are found after 2 hours.

The most important side effect is dose-dependent optic (retrobulbar) neuritis, which can result in impairment of visual acuity and colour vision. Early changes are usually reversible but blindness can occur if treatment is not discontinued promptly. It is unusual (<1%) at currently recommended doses but it is recommended that the patient's visual acuity and colour vision (Ishihara chart) be tested before ethambutol is first prescribed and monitored during treatment. The risk of optic neuritis increases substantially in those with renal impairment, and the drug should be used cautiously in such patients, with dose adjustments and regular visual assessments.

## Streptomycin

Streptomycin is an aminoglycoside and is not absorbed when given orally. It must be administered as a deep intramuscular injection, which is painful and must be administered daily for up to 2 months. This requirement, combined with relatively high prevalence of streptomycin resistance worldwide, has meant that ethambutol is generally preferred to streptomycin as the fourth drug in standard antituberculosis regimens. Furthermore, streptomycin is oto- and nephrotoxic. Vestibular damage occurs in about 30 per cent of cases; deafness is less common. Serum levels need to be monitored in those with renal impairment.

## Second-line drugs

### Fluoroquinolones

The fluoroquinolones have become essential agents in the treatment of MDR-TB. Most of the fluoroquinolones are active against *M. tuberculosis* but moxifloxacin, levofloxacin, and gatifloxacin are the most active. Ciprofloxacin is least active and should not be used in tuberculosis treatment whenever possible. Fluoroquinolones are well absorbed orally and achieve adequate concentrations in the CSF. There are generally very well tolerated but important side effects include prolongation of the QTc interval on echocardiograms; dysglycaemia; confusion; tendon rupture; and, rarely, hepatitis.

### Amikacin, kanamycin, and capreomycin

All these agents must be given by parenteral injection, and at least one should be used in the initial treatment of MDR-TB. Amikacin is most often used in this role and can be given either by daily or intermittent injection. Plasma drug concentrations should be measured to reduce the risk of nephrotoxicity and ototoxicity. Patients expected to have more than 2 weeks of amikacin should also have regular audiology to detect early subclinical hearing loss. Similar precautions are required for long-term kanamycin treatment.

Capreomycin is a cyclic peptide antibiotic but, like the above aminoglycosides, it can cause nephro- and ototoxicity. It must be given by deep intramuscular injection, and doses should be adjusted in renal impairment.

Bacteria resistant to fluoroquinolones and the injectable agents are termed extensively drug resistant (XDR) and are extremely hard to treat.

### Thiacetazone

Thiacetazone is one of the earliest antituberculosis drugs, and is cheap to manufacture. However, it is rarely used now because of rare but serious side effects of fatal exfoliative dermatitis and acute liver failure. It is well absorbed from the gastrointestinal tract, and plasma levels are sustained for long periods of time. Other side effects include nausea, vomiting, diarrhoea, and bone marrow depression.

### Ethionamide and protionamide

Ethionamide and protionamide have been used increasingly over the last few years in the treatment of MDR-TB. They are also used by some physicians (notably in South Africa) as the fourth drug in the first-line treatment of drug-susceptible tuberculous meningitis because they achieve high CSF concentrations. Their commonest side effect is nausea, sometimes with abdominal pain and diarrhoea. Hypothyroidism also occurs, especially when the drug is used in combination with *para*-aminosalicylic acid (PAS).

### Cycloserine

Cycloserine inhibits cell-wall biosynthesis in a range of Gram-positive and Gram-negative bacteria but its use is restricted to the treatment of MDR-TB. The drug is rapidly and almost completely absorbed following oral administration and has the important property of achieving high concentrations in the central nervous system. This accounts for its important neurological side effects of convulsions, confusion, depression, psychosis, and suicidal ideation; but it also means the drug is useful in the treatment of MDR-TB meningitis. Other reported side effects include allergy, rash, megaloblastic anaemia, and elevated serum aminotransferases, especially in patients with pre-existing liver disease.

### PAS

PAS was discovered at almost exactly the same time as streptomycin and was used in early treatment regimens to prevent the emergence of resistance. Up to 10–12 g a day were given orally, in two or three doses. The drug tastes most unpleasant, and gastrointestinal intolerance was common. The drug fell out of use for many years until the rise of MDR-TB; its use is increasing again as resistance increases to other agents.

## Short-course and intermittent therapy

Short-course antituberculosis chemotherapy is not well named. It describes the regimen defined by a remarkable series of clinical trials performed between 1960 and 1985 but its duration is still 6 months (Table 30.2). Nevertheless, 6 months was a major advance on the 18–24 month regimens used before the trials but it is still too long. Adherence to 6 months of multidrug treatment presents major challenges, both to the individuals taking the drugs and the institutions responsible for delivering the treatment. Until much shorter regimens are devised, tuberculosis will remain a global problem.

Intermittent regimens have become popular in developing countries for ease of administration and are probably as effective as daily regimens for the treatment of uncomplicated disease. Rifampicin in standard dose, together with isoniazid and pyrazinamide at doses higher than the standard regimen, are given on 3 days of the week, again for a total of 6 months (Table 30.2). However, most authorities recommend daily medication for the treatment of severe, disseminated tuberculosis, particularly if it involves the brain.

The treatment of MDR-TB is much less straightforward than that of drug-susceptible disease. Second-line agents for treating MDR-TB (Table 30.3) are not only less active but often more toxic than first-line drugs and must be given for 18–24 months.

## Directly observed therapy

To ensure compliance with medication and to avoid the risk of relapsing disease and the development of drug-resistant bacteria, directly observed therapy has been employed. A healthcare provider or other responsible person observes the ingestion of antituberculosis drugs by the patient. This practice is one of the fundamental tenets of tuberculosis control espoused by the WHO.

Use of fixed drug combinations (e.g. Rifinah: rifampicin + isoniazid; Rifater: rifampicin + isoniazid + pyrazinamide) may also help adherence to treatment, although care must be taken to prescribe the right number of tablets to ensure the doses of the individual drugs are correct.

## Non-antimicrobial treatment

Adjunctive corticosteroids have a limited place in the routine management of tuberculosis but have been shown to improve survival from tuberculous pericarditis and meningitis. They may also have a role in the management of severe miliary tuberculosis with respiratory distress, and when tuberculous lymph nodes enlarge and cause worsening symptoms and signs of disease after the start of antituberculosis treatment.

**Table 30.3** Second-line drugs for the treatment of tuberculosis in adults.

| Drug | Usual adult dose | Toxicity |
|---|---|---|
| Amikacin | 7.5 mg/kg every 12 h[a] | Nephrotoxicity, ototoxicity, rash, neuromuscular blockade, eosinophilia |
| Capreomycin | 1 g/day | Nephrotoxicity, ototoxicity, hypersensitivity |
| Moxifloxacin[b] | 400 mg every 24 h | Gastrointestinal intolerance, convulsions, rash, hepatitis, dysglycaemia, prolonged QTc interval on an echocardiogram |
| Cycloserine | 250 mg every 12 h or every 8 h | Seizures, psychoses, various central nervous system effects |
| Ethionamide (protionamide) | 0.5–1.0 g/day (divided dose) | Gastrointestinal intolerance, hepatitis, hypersensitivity, convulsions, depression, alopecia |
| Kanamycin | 15 mg every 12 h[a] | Nephrotoxicity, ototoxicity, hypersensitivity |
| *para*-Aminosalicylic acid | 12 g/day (divided doses) | Gastrointestinal intolerance, hypersensitivity, hypothyroidism, crystaluria |
| Thiacetazone | 150 mg daily | Gastrointestinal intolerance, Stevens–Johnson syndrome, bone marrow depression, ototoxicity, hepatitis |

[a] Peak drug levels should be less than 3 mg/dl (30 mg/l) and troughs less than 1 mg/dl (10 mg/l).

[b] Levofloxacin is an alternative.

Surgical resection is rarely necessary except for rare situations such as severe repeated haemoptysis or resection of extensive disease of a lobe or lung in those with multidrug-resistant or poorly responsive tuberculosis.

## Monitoring the therapeutic response

Inadequate adherence to treatment is the most important cause of therapeutic failure. Most cases of chronic or relapsing tuberculosis are the result of irregular, inadequate administration of prescribed drugs or the use of less potent regimens, and often result in the selection of resistant strains. The clinical response to treatment requires monitoring weight changes, fever, and symptoms of cough and shortness of breath. Where resources permit, cultures and smears can be examined for acid-fast bacilli. Fixed-dose combinations that include rifampicin can be detected by observing the red-orange discoloration of urine.

## Pregnancy and lactation

Treatment should not be interrupted or postponed if tuberculosis is diagnosed during pregnancy; indeed, treatment is essential to prevent harm to both mother and baby. Congenital tuberculosis is a rare but very serious condition with a high mortality. Rifampicin, isoniazid, and pyrazinamide are safe in pregnancy. Aminoglycosides, such as streptomycin and amikacin, and the fluoroquinolones should be avoided, when possible. Patients can breastfeed normally while taking antituberculosis drugs.

## Tuberculosis and HIV infection

HIV infection results in progressive depletion and dysfunction of CD4 lymphocytes and impaired macrophage and monocyte function. Because CD4 cells and macrophages are essential to the host response to tuberculosis, advanced untreated HIV infection results in exquisite susceptibility to *M. tuberculosis* infection. Higher rates of reactivation disease occur (7–10% per year, compared with 5–8% per lifetime for HIV-negative patients). There are also much higher rates of acute disease (with extrapulmonary dissemination), and possible malabsorption of antituberculosis drugs owing to enteropathy. The presenting features of pulmonary tuberculosis also differ according to the stage of HIV infection. In early disease, conventional presentations with lung cavitation occur. However, in advanced disease, chest X-ray changes may be atypical or absent. Serious drug–drug interactions can occur, especially between rifamycins, protease inhibitors, and non-nucleoside reverse transcriptase inhibitors used to treat HIV.

The treatment of tuberculosis in HIV-positive patients is therefore challenging and requires expert knowledge of both antituberculosis and antiretroviral drugs. The microbiological diagnosis of tuberculosis in HIV-positive individuals may also be difficult, owing to concurrent infection with *Pneumocystis jiroveci* (*P. carinii*), cytomegalovirus, or fungi. Non-tuberculous mycobacterial infections (see 'Non-tuberculous (atypical) mycobacteria') are also more frequent in these patients.

## Prevention of tuberculosis in the community

There are a number of strategies used to prevent tuberculosis. These include the following:

1 Vaccination with BCG (primarily given to neonates to prevent disseminated tuberculosis in childhood).

2 Rapid identification and treatment of infectious cases.

3 Case-contact tracing with either vaccination or chemoprophylaxis (see regimens above) of contacts.

4 'Find and treat' screening programmes of high-risk patients (e.g. homeless).

5 Screening and treatment of latent infection in important/high-risk groups (e.g. health-care workers, HIV infection, those about to receive antitumour necrosis factor treatment).

No one strategy is universally successful, and different countries have different approaches. For example, the United States uses case-contact tracing and chemoprophylaxis rather than BCG in tuberculosis control programmes, whereas the United Kingdom has a hybrid approach of BCG-vaccinating all high-risk neonates (parents from regions with a high prevalence of tuberculosis) and the identification and treatment of latently infected people. In resource-poor settings with a high burden of disease, BCG may be given to all at birth but efforts are primarily focused on the rapid identification and successful treatment of infectious cases.

## Prevention of tuberculosis transmission in hospitals

Health-care workers and other patients are at risk of acquiring tuberculosis from patients with infectious pulmonary tuberculosis. Patients with unsuspected, untreated disease pose the greatest risk, especially if they have drug-resistant disease.

Infection control measures require the early detection and isolation of patients with smear-positive lung tuberculosis, especially if multidrug-resistant *M. tuberculosis* is suspected. Ideally, these patients should be cared for in negative-pressure isolation rooms, although these facilities are often limited, even in well-resourced hospitals. Filter masks should be worn by the patient if they leave the room (e.g. for investigations) and by medical staff anticipating exposure to respiratory secretions. Masks should be worn all time by patient, staff, and visitors, if MDR-TB is suspected or proven. Fully drug-susceptible pulmonary tuberculosis can assumed to be non-infectious once 2 weeks of standard four-drug therapy has been given.

## Extrapulmonary tuberculosis

### Tuberculous meningitis

Tuberculous meningitis is the most lethal form of tuberculosis. It is universally fatal if left untreated, and death or severe neurological disability occurs in a high proportion if treatment is delayed. The management of tuberculous meningitis is discussed in Chapter 28.

### Other forms of tuberculosis

*M. tuberculosis* can affect any system in the body including, in decreasing order of frequency, superficial lymph nodes, bone and joints, the genito-urinary tract, the abdomen, the breast, and skin. Patients with non-respiratory tuberculosis are not infectious, unless they have concurrent pulmonary disease. Generally, the chemotherapeutic principles described for the treatment of pulmonary tuberculosis apply to all forms of tuberculosis. Six months of treatment is adequate, unless the patient is infected with drug-resistant bacteria or they cannot tolerate the first-line drugs.

## Non-tuberculous (atypical) mycobacteria

A number of non-tuberculous or 'atypical' mycobacteria can cause human disease. They include *M. kansasii*, *M. marinum*, *M. avium*, *M. intracellulare*, *M. fortuitum*, and several others. The isolation of one of these mycobacteria does not prove that disease is present unless the organism is isolated repeatedly in the context of compatible pathology or is from a normally sterile body site (e.g. blood). Mucosal surface colonization with these organisms, especially in those with abnormal lungs (e.g. cystic fibrosis, chronic obstructive pulmonary disease (COPD), bronchiectasis), is not uncommon. Nevertheless, disease, when it occurs, may be indistinguishable clinically from tuberculosis.

Treatment is organism specific and highly variable and it not within the scope of this textbook to provide all the details. However, in general, non-tuberculous mycobacteria do not respond to conventional antituberculosis regimens. All are resistant to pyrazinamide and most are not susceptible to isoniazid. Rifampicin, ethambutol, and the macrolides are more commonly effective, although some mycobacteria (e.g. *M. abscessus*) are resistant to all conventional antituberculosis drugs and respond to some cephalosporins, carbapenems, and aminoglycosides.

Patients with advanced HIV infection with CD4 counts <100 cells/mm$^3$ are especially prone to disseminated infection with *M. avium intracellulare* complex but this has become much less common following the advent of highly active retroviral therapy. Treatment is with a rifamycin (often rifabutin to reduce interactions with the anti-HIV drugs) and a macrolide (usually azithromycin), although macrolide resistance occurs.

## Leprosy

This is a chronic communicable tropical disease caused by infection with *M. leprae*, which mainly affects the skin and peripheral nerves, causing anaesthesia, muscle weakness, paralysis, and consequent injury and deformity. Currently, the disease is restricted to six countries as a result of a WHO eradication programme. Over the centuries, those with leprosy have often been ostracized and excluded from society, despite the fact that it is not very contagious. Transmission is caused by respiratory droplet spread from close contact. There is a spectrum of disease determined by the extent of cell-mediated immune response by the host. This not only distinguishes the major types of the disease but also has implications for treatment (Fig. 30.1).

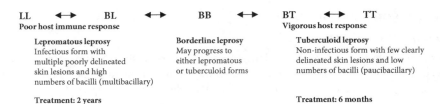

**Fig. 30.1** The spectrum of leprosy as determined by host response and bacillary load and its implications for treatment. LL, lepromatous leprosy; BL, borderline lepromatous; BB, borderline leprosy; BT, borderline tuberculoid; TT, tuberculoid leprosy.

Two major types are described: lepromatous and tuberculoid leprosy. In lepromatous leprosy there is diffuse involvement of skin and mucous membranes, with ulceration, iritis, and keratitis; scrapings of skin or mucous membranes contain numerous acid-fast bacilli. The tuberculoid form is more localized but nerve involvement occurs early; only scanty bacilli are present. In both forms, progress of the disease is slow. The tuberculoid form may heal spontaneously in a few years. Death is usually due to other causes.

The approach to leprosy control includes early case detection, adequate treatment with a combination of dapsone, rifampicin, and clofazimine, and the prevention of disabilities and rehabilitation of sufferers. Paucibacillary (tuberculoid) disease is cured in 6 months with dapsone and rifampicin, while multibacillary (lepromatous) disease requires at least 2 years' treatment with dapsone, clofazimine, and rifampicin. Dapsone (diaminodiphenylsulphone) resistance is avoided by the use of triple therapy. Rifampicin is more rapidly bactericidal than dapsone but resistance may arise if it is used alone. Clofazimine is effective but some patients develop discoloration of the skin that may prove unacceptable. The treatment of leprosy requires specialist expertise.

With such long and complicated regimens, patient compliance is naturally a problem, particularly in areas of the world where leprosy is most prevalent. Second-line agents include minocycline, ofloxacin, and clarithromycin. Furthermore, a single-dose triple combination of rifampicin, ofloxacin, and minocycline has been successful in lepromatous leprosy and provides a further alternative.

## Key points

- Tuberculosis is caused by *M. tuberculosis*, an acid-fast bacillus.

- *M. tuberculosis* can cause asymptomatic latent infection, or active disease.

- *M. tuberculosis* is transmitted by aerosol droplet spread from coughing patients with pulmonary tuberculosis.

- Active tuberculosis is diagnosed by demonstrating the bacilli in affected tissues, either by microscopy, culture, or nucleic acid amplification (e.g. PCR).

- Treatment is 6 months of multiple drugs: four drugs for 2 months; two drugs for 4 months.

- Drug resistance is increasing and complicates treatment substantially: multidrug-resistant tuberculosis takes 18–24 months to treat.

- BCG vaccination prevents severe disease in childhood but only has a modest protective effect in adults against pulmonary disease.

- Tuberculosis control has many facets, including rapid identification and treatment of infectious cases, case-contact tracing, and the treatment of latent infection.

## Further reading

Abubakar, I., Dara, M., Manissero, D., and Zumla, A. (2012) Tackling the spread of drug-resistant tuberculosis in Europe. *Lancet*, **379**(9813): e21–e23.

Grant, A., Gothard, P., and Thwaites, G. (2008) Managing drug resistant tuberculosis. *BMJ*, **337**: a1110.

Harrop, T., Aird, J., and Thwaites, G. (2011) How to minimise risk of acquiring tuberculosis when working in a high prevalence setting: a guide for healthcare workers. *BMJ*, **342**: d1544.

Lawn, S. D. and Zumla, A. I. (2011) Tuberculosis. *Lancet*, **378**(9785): 57–72.

Maartens, G. and Wilkinson, R. J. (2007) Tuberculosis. *Lancet*, **370**(9604): 2030–43.

Zenner, D., Zumla, A., Gill, P., Cosford, P., and Abubakar, I. (2013) Reversing the tide of the UK tuberculosis epidemic. *Lancet*, **382**(9901): 1311–12.

Zumla, A., George, A., Sharma, V., Herbert, N., and Baroness Masham of Illton. (2013) WHO's 2013 global report on tuberculosis: successes, threats, and opportunities. *Lancet*, **382**(9907): 1765–7.

# Chapter 31

# Infections in immunocompromised patients, including HIV/AIDS

## Introduction to infections in immunocompromised patients

The care of the immunocompromised patient is an increasingly important and challenging aspect of medicine that encompasses individuals suffering from a variety of underlying disease states which render them especially vulnerable to microbial challenge. The term immunocompromised describes patients who have immunodeficiency states or those who are immunosuppressed, for example, following the administration of drugs.

## Immunodeficiency

Immunodeficiency may be congenital or acquired and can affect humoral (antibody or complement) or cell-mediated immunity, or both. In general, the nature of the deficiency predicts the types of infections suffered (see Table 31.1). Worldwide, the most important cause of acquired immune-deficiency is HIV infection. HIV infection causes an inexorable decline in cell-mediated immune function as a result of the virus targeting and killing CD4-positive T lymphocytes, which have a central role in orchestrating the immune system and cells of the monocyte/macrophage series. However, iatrogenic immune compromise is becoming increasing important, especially in resource-rich parts of the world where the use of targeted biological agents (e.g. against specific cells or cytokines/chemokines of the immune system) are becoming increasingly important in the treatment of autoimmune diseases and some cancers. These agents can produce highly selective immune deficiencies with susceptibility to very specific infections (see Table 31.1).

## Immunosuppression

In contrast to immunodeficiency states, immunosuppression affects patients whose immune defences are impaired, either as a result of an underlying disease or its management by cytotoxic, immunosuppressive, or radiation therapy. The commonest immunosuppressive state is diabetes mellitus, with nearly 300 million sufferers worldwide. Diabetes predisposes to a range of bacterial infections, especially those involving the skin and soft tissue; it is also a major risk factor for tuberculosis.

The hospitalized immunosuppressed patient often has an underlying malignant disease or has undergone organ or bone marrow transplantation. In both situations, part of the therapeutic strategy involves temporary suppression or ablation of host immune functions. The vulnerability of the patient to infection may be compounded by the use of intravascular catheters, bladder catheters, and in the case of ventilated patients, endotracheal tubes. These either interfere with pharyngeotracheal clearance mechanisms (respiratory tract) or connect a normally sterile body site (bladder, vascular compartment) with the external environment.

**Table 31.1** Examples of immunodeficiency states associated with an increased frequency of severity of infection.

| Congenital immunodeficiencies | Common associated infections* |
|---|---|
| B-cell deficiencies | |
| Selective IgA deficiency | Usually healthy (can predispose to coeliac disease and other autoimmune conditions) |
| X-linked hypogammaglobulinaemia | Encapsulated bacterial infections, gastrointestinal bacterial infections, giardiasis, chronic mycoplasma and ureaplasma infections, enteroviral infections |
| Common variable immunodeficiency | As for X-linked hypogammaglobulinaemia, depending on severity |
| IgG subclass deficiency | As for X-linked hypogammaglobulinaemia, depending on severity |
| T-cell deficiencies | |
| DiGeorge anomaly | Recurrent and severe childhood infections with encapsulated bacteria, herpesvirus infections (CMV, EBV, HSV, VZV), candida, *Pneumocystis jiroveci*, atypical mycobacteria |
| Wiskott–Aldrich syndrome | |
| Ataxia telangiectasia | |
| X-linked hyper-IgM syndrome | Recurrent respiratory, sinus, ear, and gastrointestinal bacterial infections |
| Combined T- and B-cell defects | |
| Severe combined immunodeficiency | Recurrent and severe childhood infections with encapsulated bacteria, herpesvirus infections (CMV, EBV, HSV, VZV), candida, *Pneumocystis jiroveci*, atypical mycobacteria |
| Congenital deficiency of phagocytosis | |
| Congenital neutropenia | Recurrent pneumonia, lymphadenitis, abscesses, osteomyelitis, and septicaemia with *Staphylococcus aureus*, *Aspergillus* spp., and Gram-negative bacteria such *Serratia* spp. and *Burkholderia cepacia* |
| Chronic granulomatous disease | |
| Leucocyte adhesion deficiency | |
| *Congenital complement deficiencies* | |
| C1–4 deficiencies | Variable; C3 deficiency most marked, with susceptibility to encapsulated bacteria (especially *Streptococcus pneumoniae*) |
| C5–9 (terminal attack complex) deficiencies | *Neisseria meningitidis* and *N. gonorrhoeae* infections |
| **Acquired immunodeficiencies** | |
| HIV infection/AIDS | Bacterial infections (*Str. pneumoniae*), Mycobacterial infections (especially tuberculosis), fungal infections (*Pne. jiroveci*, *Candida* spp., cryptococcosis, histoplasmosis), herpesvirus infections (CMV, HSV, VZV), parasitic infections (toxoplasmosis, other gastrointestinal protozoa) |
| Cytotoxic antineoplastic therapy | Depends on duration of neutropenia/lymphopaenia but initially severe invasive bacterial and fungal infections (*Aspergillus* spp. and other moulds); if prolonged T-lymphocyte depletion, as for HIV/AIDS |

(continued)

**Table 31.1** (continued).

| Congenital immunodeficiencies | Common associated infections* |
|---|---|
| Lymphoproliferative and myeloproliferative disorders | Encapsulated bacteria, especially *Str. pneumoniae*; lymphomas, dependent on their type, can predispose to *Pne. jiroveci* and other infections associated with T-cell depletion; recurrent herpesvirus infections |
| Hyposplenism/asplenism | Encapsulated bacteria, *Salmonella* spp., malaria |
| Autoimmune neutropenia | As for congenital neutropenia |
| New 'biological therapies' | Specific infections dependent upon agent: |
| e.g. | ♦ mycobacterial infections, listeriosis |
| ♦ antitumour necrosis factor | ♦ upper respiratory tract infections/sinusitis |
| ♦ anti-interleukin-1β | ♦ viral infections, reactivation of hepatitis B |
| ♦ anti-B-cell | |

* CMV, cytomegalovirus; EBV, Epstein–Barr virus; HSV, herpes simplex virus; VZV, varicella-zoster virus.

**Table 31.2** Examples of immunosuppressive states associated with an increased frequency or severity of infection according to altered host defences.*

| Disease | Mucosal surfaces | Phagocytosis | Humoral immunity | CMI |
|---|---|---|---|---|
| Acute lymphoblastic leukaemia | + | ++ | − | + |
| Acute myeloblastic leukaemia | + | ++ | − | + |
| Chronic lymphocytic leukaemia | − | − | ++ | + |
| Hodgkin, non-Hodgkin lymphoma | − | − | − | + |
| Solid tumours | ++ | − | − | + |
| Multiple myeloma | − | − | ++ | − |

* CMI, cell-mediated immunity; −, association absent; +, definite association; ++, marked association.

The major features of immunosuppression associated with various malignant conditions are summarized in Table 31.2. Such patients are often cared for in high dependency or intensive care facilities that provide opportunities for cross-infection and the acquisition of hospital-associated, and therefore frequently antibiotic-resistant, pathogens.

## Microbial complications in the immunocompromised host

A wide variety of infections may occur in immunocompromised patients, dependent on the nature of compromise (see Table 31.1). The encapsulated bacteria—*Streptococcus pneumoniae*, *Haemophilus influenzae*, and *Neisseria meningitidis*—are the commonest organisms responsible for infections in those with impaired humoral responses. *Str. pneumoniae* is also an important pathogen in those with impaired cell-mediated responses, for example, HIV infection. However, prolonged hospitalization for any reason comes with the increased risk of acquiring a range of bacterial infections, many of which are now resistant to first-line antibiotic therapy, for example, methicillin-resistant *Staphylococcus aureus* (MRSA), vancomycin-resistant enterococcal (VRE) species, and multidrug-resistant Gram-negative bacteria.

The herpesvirus group—cytomegalovirus (CMV), Epstein–Barr virus (EBV), herpes simplex virus (HSV), and varicella-zoster virus (VZV)—are the predominant opportunistic viral pathogens in those with impaired cell-mediated immunity. Disease may represent primary infection or reactivation of latent virus, and these infections are often more severe than those in the immunocompetent host and can cause multi-organ involvement. Severe adenovirus and para-influenza virus infections of the lung are also observed in profoundly neutropenic patients.

Fungal infections can be particularly severe, especially in those with protracted neutropenia or severe T-cell-mediated deficiency. Candidiasis of the mouth and upper gastrointestinal tract is particularly common in those with untreated HIV and can result in bloodstream spread to other organs. *Cryptococcus neoformans* is an important cause of indolent meningitis in those with advanced HIV infection but it occasionally complicates organ transplantation and malignant lymphoma.

Among the filamentous fungi, *Aspergillus* spp. are the most common pathogens. Their ubiquitous spores are normally harmless to the immunocompetent but, in the immunocompromised patient, they can cause serious lung infection that may disseminate throughout the body. This risk is greatest in patients with profound neutropenia. Aspergillosis is not only difficult to treat but also difficult to diagnose, especially in the early stages of infection.

*Pneumocystis jiroveci* (previously 'carinii') is an important opportunistic fungal infection complicating HIV infection. It primarily affects the lung, where it produces a severe progressive pneumonia, which may be fatal unless treated early. Pneumocystosis may also occur in patients undergoing organ transplantation and in those with lymphoblastic leukaemia or malignant lymphoma; profound impairment of cell-mediated immunity characterizes all these conditions. *Pne. jiroveci*, although a fungus, has a pattern of susceptibility to chemotherapeutic agents that is more in keeping with a protozoon. Other parasitic infections in the immunocompromised host include toxoplasmosis and in endemic regions, leishmaniasis. There are also a variety of gut infections such as giardiasis, cryptosporidiosis, microsporidiosis, and strongyloidiasis. The latter can progress to a state of hyperinfection with extensive larval invasion of the body.

## Chemoprophylaxis

The seriousness of infections in the severely immunosuppressed patient has led to the use of chemoprophylactic drug regimens, particularly in patients with advanced HIV infection, in those undergoing cytotoxic chemotherapy for haematological malignancies, and in bone marrow transplant recipients. Regimens are directed at the microorganisms most likely to result in disease (see Chapter 18).

In advanced HIV infection, there is a substantial body of evidence to indicate prophylaxis against *Pne. jiroveci* pneumonia and toxoplasmosis with trimethoprim–sulphamethoxazole (Septrin) is highly effective, and azithromycin or clarithromycin prevents *Mycobacterium avium* complex infections in those with CD4 T-cell counts <50 cells/µl. Identification and treatment of latent *M. tuberculosis* infections also prevents tuberculosis, although the effect is not long lasting if the patient is in a region with high tuberculosis transmission.

Prophylaxis against bacterial infection in neutropenic patients is more controversial. Studies have suggested prophylactic fluoroquinolones may reduce infections and reduce their associated mortality but there are major concerns regarding the development of resistance and the increasing the risk of *Clostridium difficile*-associated diarrhoea. Therefore, this approach is not widely recommended. In patients at high risk of invasive fungal infections, including those following haematopoietic stem cell transplantation, voriconazole is used as prophylaxis.

Antiviral prophylaxis with aciclovir (and derivatives) or ganciclovir/valganciclovir, mostly to prevent serious CMV infection, is well established practice for patients undergoing solid organ or bone marrow transplantation.

## Principles of chemotherapeutic control

The vulnerability of the immunocompromised patient to infection has been emphasized. Not only is the range of possible infections broad but, because of the state of immunosuppression, the presentation may be atypical and the course fulminant. A specific clinical and microbiological diagnosis can be difficult to establish; the therapeutic management of such patients is consequently based on a set of principles that has evolved to meet their particular needs.

It is essential that the patient is thoroughly examined at the earliest suspicion of infection. Particular attention should be paid to the skin, perineum, entry sites for catheters, the mouth, lungs, and abdomen. Appropriate microbiological samples should be collected and necessary radiographic investigations obtained. Timely biopsy of lymph nodes, bone marrow, cutaneous, or intrapulmonary lesions is essential in selective cases. The approach to the chemotherapeutic management of the immunocompromised patient is particularly well demonstrated in

- patients with haematological malignancies undergoing cytotoxic chemotherapy or bone marrow transplantation, especially during episodes of profound neutropenia;
- patients with HIV/AIDS; and
- those with specific immunological defects such as hyposplenism.

### Neutropenic patients

Infection in the neutropenic patient can develop rapidly over a matter of hours and, if untreated, can prove fatal. If fever above 38°C persists for 2 hours or more, blood cultures should be taken and broad-spectrum antibiotic therapy should be administered promptly by the intravenous route. However, documentation of infection can be difficult: about 15 per cent of infections will be documented by blood culture, a further 20 per cent by other microbiological investigations, and a further 20 per cent by clinical criteria. In the remainder, infection may only be strongly suspected without supporting clinical or laboratory evidence; non-microbial causes such as drug reactions, blood or platelet transfusions, or the underlying disease state may be responsible for the febrile episode.

The variety and relative frequency of bloodstream pathogens in the neutropenic patient are summarized in Table 31.3. There has been an increase in Gram-positive infections in recent years, which in part relates to the widespread use of vascular catheters for drug administration, as well as the selective pressure arising from the use of broad-spectrum antibiotics, notably β-lactam and quinolone agents.

The empirical treatment of 'neutropenic sepsis' has evolved over the last decade in response to increasing Gram-positive infections and drug resistance. Most centres recommend a combination of a β-lactam antibiotic and an aminoglycoside, which together are active against most of the likely pathogens. Among the β-lactam agents, those with antipseudomonal activity have been favoured: ceftazidime, piperacillin in combination with tazobactam ('Tazocin'), or meropenem. The latter is being increasingly used as resistance to the other two agents steadily increases among Gram-negative bacteria. An aminoglycoside such as gentamicin or amikacin is administered

**Table 31.3** Distribution of the more common bloodstream isolates complicating neutropenic states.

| Microorganism | Approximate percentage |
|---|---|
| **Gram-positive bacteria** | |
| *Staphylococcus epidermidis* | 28 |
| *Staph. Aureus* | 10 |
| *Corynebacterium* spp. | 5 |
| Streptococci | 12 |
| **Gram-negative bacteria** | |
| Gram-negative enteric bacilli | 28 |
| *Pseudomonas aeruginosa* | 7 |
| Others | 7 |
| **Fungi** | |
| *Candida* spp. | 3 |

simultaneously since both are active against Gram-negative bacilli, including *Pseudomonas aeruginosa*.

The increase in Gram-positive infections caused by staphylococci, enterococci, and streptococci is also complicated by an increase in resistance among these organisms, especially to β-lactams. Glycopeptides, such as vancomycin or teicoplanin, may be needed, especially if MRSA is suspected. However, increased use of glycopeptides is being accompanied by infections caused by glycopeptide-resistant enterococci (GRE). Glycopeptide-resistant bacterial infections can be treated with linezolid or daptomycin.

Candida infection is best treated with either an echinocandin (e.g. caspofungin) or intravenous amphotericin, with the azoles as reserve agents (see Chapter 8). Amphotericin is a toxic drug, and careful dosaging and monitoring of renal function is essential to avoid serious nephrotoxicity. Lipid formulations of amphotericin are less nephrotoxic and increasingly used but much more expensive.

Cryptococcal yeast infections are managed with a combination of amphotericin and flucytosine (see 'Polyenes' in Chapter 8 and 'Cryptococcal meningitis' in Chapter 28). Filamentous fungal infections, notably *Aspergillus* infection, are best treated with intravenous voriconazole. Amphotericin provides an alternative choice. For unresponsive disease, caspofungin is used as salvage therapy.

# HIV/AIDS

The clinical impact of HIV infection lies in its persistent nature and the accompanying progressive immunodeficiency which gives rise to a range of complicating infections and malignancies. These target many organs as well as producing systemic illness. Table 31.4 summarizes the more important complicating infections.

In contrast to their effects in the immunocompetent host, these infections often present atypically and with heightened severity. Furthermore, many of the infections recur after treatment in those with advanced HIV disease. Thus, in the HIV-infected patient the initial course of treatment must be more intensive than in the immunocompetent host and, for many conditions, long-term

**Table 31.4** Common opportunist pathogens complicating HIV disease.

| Site | Microorganism |
|---|---|
| Gastrointestinal tract | *Cryptosporidium parvum* |
| | *Salmonella enterica* serotypes |
| | *Mycobacterium avium* complex |
| | Cytomegalovirus |
| | Herpes simplex virus |
| | *Candida* spp. |
| Respiratory tract | *Pneumocystis jiroveci (carinii)* |
| | *Streptococcus pneumonia* |
| | *M. tuberculosis* |
| | Cytomegalovirus |
| Central nervous system | *M. tuberculosis* |
| | *Toxoplasma gondii* |
| | *Cryptococcus neoformans* |
| | Cytomegalovirus |
| | Herpes simplex virus |
| | Varicella-zoster virus |
| | JC polyoma virus |

suppressive therapy is needed to prevent relapse. In addition, by controlling the underlying HIV infection, the frequency and severity of opportunistic infections can be reduced, as well as the risk of recurrent opportunistic infection.

The introduction of combination antiretroviral therapy (cART; sometimes referred to as highly active antiretroviral therapy (HAART)), in which three-drug regimens of two nucleoside analogues with a protease inhibitor, a non-nucleoside reverse transcriptase inhibitor, or an integrase inhibitor results in an increase in functional CD4 cells, thereby obviating the need for primary prophylaxis against *Pne. jiroveci* in selected patients. These regimens are discussed in Chapter 34. They are generally well tolerated and, provided the patient is compliant with the medication, have a major impact on the quality of life. Although they all act in a suppressive manner to delay disease progression, none is curative.

The chemotherapeutic approach to selected opportunistic infections is discussed in order to emphasize the principles and associated problems that arise.

## Pne. jiroveci pneumonia

*Pne. jiroveci* is a common cause of severe pneumonia is those with a CD4 count <200 cells/μl. The primary site of infection is the lung. Clinical disease represents reactivation of endogenous infection usually acquired in childhood. Typical symptoms include progressive shortness of breath with or without a relatively unproductive cough, progressive hypoxaemia, and diffuse bilateral chest radiograph infiltrates. The diagnosis has been greatly facilitated by the availability of a fluorescent antibody to *Pne. jiroveci*, as this antibody can be applied to expectorated sputum or to a saline lavage obtained by bronchoscopy.

The treatment of choice is high-dose trimethoprim-sulphamethoxazole (Septrin) by mouth or intravenously for 3 weeks. The risk of hypersensitivity to the sulphonamide component is greatly increased in HIV disease, and alternative regimens such as intravenous pentamidine, oral atovaquone, or a combination of clindamycin and primaquine may be necessary.

Once the patient has recovered, it is necessary to continue with secondary prophylaxis with low-dose Septrin for as long as CD4 counts remain below 200 cells/μl. Alternative agents that can be used in those intolerant of the standard regimens include dapsone and atovaquone. Nebulized pentamidine given once monthly as an aerosol inhalation provides another choice. In view of the seriousness of *Pne. jiroveci* pneumonia, patients with HIV infection are now offered primary prophylaxis when their CD4 lymphocyte counts fall below 200 cells/μl, in order to prevent infection. The choice of agent and frequency of administration is the same as for secondary prophylaxis.

## Toxoplasmosis

The protozoon *Toxoplasma gondii* can cause serious disease in people with HIV infection and a CD4 count <100 cells/μl. This may occur as a primary infection, although it more usually represents reactivation of dormant parasites. The disease presents most frequently as a space-occupying lesion of the brain with focal neurological features. The diagnosis is based on clinical suspicion and computed tomography scan. Serological tests can confirm past infection but cannot be used to diagnose reactivation. The presence of tachyzoites in brain biopsy is confirmatory. However, it is more usual to carry out a trial of chemotherapy in the first instance, since this can avoid potentially dangerous neurosurgery.

Toxoplasmosis is treated with pyrimethamine and sulphadiazine in high dosage for 6 weeks before reducing to a maintenance dose. This regimen often results in bone marrow suppression or is complicated by an allergic skin eruption. Alternative drugs include high-dose clindamycin or the azalide azithromycin in combination with pyrimethamine, which also exhibits useful activity. Atovaquone plus pyrimethamine provides a further option. The principles of treatment are similar to those for controlling *Pne. jiroveci* pneumonia in that initial control is followed by continuous maintenance therapy, until immune system function is restored following antiretroviral therapy.

## Cytomegalovirus infection

Cytomegalovirus infection is common in patients with advanced untreated HIV. In those with HIV infection, reactivation is associated with a range of manifestations, which may involve the gastrointestinal tract, lung, liver, and in particular the eye, where a progressive retinopathy may lead to loss of vision or total blindness. Treatment with ganciclovir, valganciclovir, foscarnet, or cidofovir is suppressive but not curative (see Chapter 32).

## Mycobacterial infections

Patients with HIV infection are at increased risk of all mycobacterial infections. These infections may be newly acquired or represent endogenous reactivation of latent infection as cell-mediated immunity steadily declines. *M. tuberculosis* is the commonest infecting organism but disease may present atypically owing to altered host immunity. In many parts of the world, drug-resistant tuberculosis has emerged as an important problem and there have been instances of spread within prisons and hospitals (see 'Tuberculosis' in Chapter 30). Antituberculosis treatment regimens are the same for HIV uninfected patients (see Chapter 30), although there is probably a higher risk of relapse and recurrent tuberculosis in those infected with HIV. Treatment is often complicated by interactions with the antiretroviral drugs.

Infection with organisms of the *M. avium* complex is a common problem in patients with very low CD4 counts (<50 cells/µl). Disease presents with fever, sweats, weight loss, and diarrhoea. Patients are frequently bacillaemic and have high bacterial loads within the gut and bone marrow. The organisms are resistant to conventional antituberculosis regimens, and a combination of clarithromycin with rifabutin and ethambutol is recommended. Response to treatment may, unfortunately, be short-lived. Attempts have therefore been directed at preventing disease with azithromycin or clarithromycin.

## Hyposplenism

The spleen is an important site of host defences, rich in lymphoid follicles and phagocytic cells. In its absence the patient is at increased risk of infection, including fulminating bacteraemia. Apart from splenectomy, a variety of medical conditions can cause hyposplenism. These include hereditary conditions such as sickle cell anaemia and hereditary spherocytosis. The risk of serious infections is greatest in early childhood but declines with age, although the risk remains throughout life. Among the fulminant infections are those caused by *Str. pneumoniae*, *H. influenzae*, *Escherichia coli*, *N. meningitidis*, and a rare pathogen of man, *Capnocytophaga canimorsus*. Hyposplenic or asplenic patients should be alerted to their increased risk and recommended to seek early medical attention in the presence of symptoms suggestive of severe infection. Immunization against pneumococcal infections is possible in those over 2 years of age and is the best form of prevention. Likewise, children should be immunized against *H. influenzae* and group C meningococcal infection. Long-term chemoprophylaxis with phenoxymethylpenicillin (penicillin V) is of proven benefit in children with sickle cell disease. However, the additional benefit of lifelong prophylaxis in those who have been actively immunized is marginal. Compliance with lifelong penicillin V prophylaxis is a further problem, as is the steady increase in resistance to penicillin among pneumococci, especially in parts of Europe and North America.

## Key points

- Patients with impaired immunity are an important and increasingly common part of modern medical practice.

- The nature and extent of the immune compromise must be understood to predict the likely infectious risks and provide the best management.

- Infection prevention strategies—vaccination and chemoprophylaxis, for example—are essential components in the management of immunocompromised patients.

## Further reading

Nelson, M., Dockrell, D. H., Edwards, S. and on behalf of the BHIVA Guidelines Subcommittee. (2011) Treatment of opportunistic infections in HIV-seropositive individuals. *HIV Medicine*, **12**(Suppl 2): 1–140.

Webster, A. D. B. (2013) The immunocompromised patient: primary immunodeficiencies. *Medicine*, **41**(11): 619–23.

# Chapter 32

# Viral infections

## Introduction to viral infections

Diseases caused by viruses are extremely common and range from trivial coughs and colds to life-threatening infections. Most viral infections are self-limiting, although some that normally cause relatively minor problems can be serious in immunosuppressed patients or neonates. Some viruses nearly always cause severe disease regardless of the initial status of the host. Rabies, human immunodeficiency virus (HIV), and several of the viruses causing haemorrhagic fevers fall into this category. Furthermore, long-term complications may arise from viral infections of the central nervous system (Chapter 28) or liver (Chapter 34).

Most success in the control of serious virus infections has been achieved by immunoprophylaxis, and to a lesser extent immunotherapy, notably to manage rabies and hepatitis B virus infections, rather than by the use of specific antiviral chemotherapy. However, there is an ever-increasing list of useful antiviral drugs (see Chapters 5 to 7) and, as knowledge of the molecular biology of viral replication increases, more potential targets are being identified. In general, the most widely treated virus infections comprise herpes viruses, respiratory tract infections (both dealt with in this chapter), HIV infection (see Chapter 33), and viral hepatitis (Chapter 34).

## Herpesvirus infections

All eight herpesviruses known to infect man (Table 32.1) exhibit the phenomenon of latency. Following acute infection, virus is not eliminated from the body but viral DNA remains quiescent without causing any apparent damage to the latently infected cells. Later, virus may be reactivated; the virus replicates, and disease may re-emerge. Herpesvirus infections can therefore be classified as primary, the host's first encounter with the virus, or secondary, due to reactivation of latent virus. Alternatively, secondary infection may arise from exogenous reinfection with a distinct strain of virus. The clinical features of primary and secondary herpesvirus infections are often very different.

Aciclovir is very active against certain herpesviruses and was the first truly selective antiviral agent. Two more oral anti-herpetic drugs have subsequently been developed: valaciclovir (an oral prodrug of aciclovir) and famciclovir (a prodrug of penciclovir) (see 'Properties of antiviral agents' in Chapter 5). These newer agents exhibit greater oral bioavailability than aciclovir, which allows an easier dosing schedule.

Herpesviruses differ in their sensitivity to aciclovir and penciclovir (Table 32.1). Cytomegalovirus (CMV) and human herpesvirus type 6 do not possess thymidine kinase and cannot activate the drugs efficiently. In practice, these drugs are useful only in the treatment of herpes simplex virus (HSV), in varicella-zoster virus (VZV) infection, and in certain unusual manifestations of Epstein–Barr virus infection. Clinical trials in various manifestations of herpes simplex and varicella-zoster infection have shown the two compounds to be equipotent. Aciclovir is the only agent licensed for intravenous use and thus must be used in life-threatening diseases necessitating

**Table 32.1** Human herpesviruses.

| Name | Usual abbreviation | Sensitivity to aciclovir |
| --- | --- | --- |
| Herpes simplex type 1 | HSV1 | Very sensitive |
| Herpes simplex type 2 | HSV2 | Very sensitive |
| Varicella-zoster virus | VZV | Fairly sensitive |
| Epstein–Barr virus | EBV | Poorly sensitive |
| Cytomegalovirus | CMV | Insensitive |
| Human herpes virus type 6 | HHV6 | Insensitive |
| Human herpes virus type 7 | HHV7 | Not known |
| Human herpes virus type 8 | HHV8 | Insensitive |

intravenous therapy. For oral therapy, the choice between aciclovir, valaciclovir, and famciclovir may depend on considerations of relative costs and convenience of dosing.

## HSV infections

Although most HSV infections are asymptomatic, there can be a wide range of clinical manifestations.

### Primary orolabial infection

Symptomatic primary infection, which usually occurs in children, presents with extensive painful blistering and ulceration of the lips, tongue, and mucous membranes of the mouth, sometimes with marked cervical lymphadenopathy and fever. Left untreated, the infection is self-limiting with complete healing in 2–3 weeks. Oral anti-herpes therapy reduces the manifestations of systemic disease, the formation of new lesions, the period of virus excretion, and the time to healing; it is of unquestioned therapeutic benefit.

### Recurrent orolabial infection

Resolution of primary disease is followed by the establishment of latency of HSV within the trigeminal nerve ganglion. This virus can be reactivated in later life and track back down the nerve to reach the mouth. The manifestations of reactivated disease in an immunocompetent host are much milder: there is no systemic upset, only a few lesions (cold sores), localized to a small area on the lips; the inflammatory response is less, with less pain and swelling, and the lesions heal in about 5–6 days. Aciclovir therapy enhances resolution of lesions by about 24 hours. Given the mild nature of recurrent disease (as compared with primary infection), and the marginal benefit of aciclovir, routine systemic treatment of cold sores is not recommended.

### Eczema herpeticum

Intact skin is a very efficient barrier to the spread of viruses. However, in patients with chronic dermatitis or eczema, this barrier is not intact, and virus can spread freely. Eczema herpeticum is a severe complication of primary or secondary orolabial HSV infection in patients with eczema. Lesions extend to large areas on the face, neck, and upper chest. Virus may also gain access to the bloodstream through cracks in the skin, putting the patient at risk of death from disseminated

HSV infection. Antiviral therapy is mandatory. Patients should be given supplies of valaciclovir or famciclovir so that they can self-medicate in the early stages of recurrent disease.

## Ocular HSV infection

HSV is the commonest infectious cause of blindness in the United Kingdom. Children are particularly prone to self-inoculating the eye with virus-infected oral secretions. Spread of virus to the cornea results in keratitis and may lead to severe inflammation and repeated reactivations predispose to chronic ulceration. Management should include systemic and topical aciclovir (together with consideration of the use of steroids to damp down the damaging host inflammatory response) and prompt referral for specialist ophthalmological assessment.

## Genital herpes

The clinical manifestations and management of primary and secondary genital herpes are analogous to those of orolabial disease. Thus primary infection may result in extensive bilateral, painful ulceration with spread to adjacent skin, inguinal adenopathy, and fever, lasting 2–3 weeks. Lesions close to the urethral meatus may give rise to pain when passing urine. Cervicitis with profuse discharge is common in women. Oral anti-herpes therapy is of proven benefit. Recurrent disease is much more localized, with no systemic upset, and shorter lasting; oral antiviral therapy is of marginal value.

Some unfortunate individuals may suffer severe recurrent attacks of genital herpes as frequently as once a month. The immunological basis for this debilitating and depressing condition is not understood. One approach to the management of these patients is to give them continuous prophylactic anti-herpes therapy. Patients are advised to titrate the dose down to that which keeps them free of recurrence. Therapy can be interrupted every 6–12 months to reassess recurrence frequency but otherwise can be continued for years and rarely gives rise to significant side effects.

## Neonatal herpes

Pregnant women with genital herpes are at risk of passing on the infection during childbirth. Neonatal HSV infection is a potentially devastating disease, as virus readily disseminates to internal organs, and such babies may die of HSV hepatitis, pneumonitis, or encephalitis. Survivors are almost invariably left with severe neurological sequelae. Although mortality from neonatal herpes has improved with the use of intravenous aciclovir, overall morbidity has scarcely been affected, presumably because by the time the diagnosis is made, and therapy initiated, the damage has already been done.

## Herpes simplex encephalitis

Herpes simplex encephalitis is the commonest form of sporadic viral encephalitis (Chapter 28), with an annual incidence of about one case per million population. Most cases occur in individuals with evidence of prior infection with HSV. Thus the disease is usually a manifestation of secondary infection, although the route by which virus gains access to the brain is not clear. Untreated, mortality is high, and survivors suffer severe long-term damage. Diagnosis is difficult but should be suspected in all patients with features of acute encephalitis with focal signs, especially when confirmed by computed tomography scans or magnetic resonance imaging of the brain. The cerebrospinal fluid usually shows a pleocytosis but it is very rare to succeed in isolating the virus from cerebrospinal fluid. HSV DNA can be detected in cerebrospinal fluid during the acute stage by genome amplification (e.g. the polymerase chain reaction). Intravenous aciclovir, in high dosage, improves the prognosis dramatically, provided therapy is started as soon as the diagnosis is suspected, without waiting for laboratory confirmation.

## Immunocompromised patients

Patients who are immunocompromised for whatever reason are at risk of severe primary or secondary HSV disease. All HSV infections in this group of patients should be treated promptly with aciclovir, if necessary by the intravenous route. In bone marrow transplant recipients, prophylactic aciclovir is recommended because of the potentially severe and life-threatening nature of such infections.

# VZV

## Chickenpox

The primary manifestation of infection with VZV is chickenpox. This is usually a trivial disease of children, despite the dramatic rash. The most important complication is varicella pneumonia, which can be life threatening. This is considerably more common in adults than in children, and is more common in smokers and pregnant women. Adults with chickenpox are thus at risk of severe pneumonitis and should be referred promptly to hospital for intravenous aciclovir therapy if evidence of respiratory involvement occurs.

It has been suggested that all children with chickenpox should be given aciclovir. The arguments in favour of this blanket approach are economic rather than medical. Aciclovir allows resolution of the disease earlier than would otherwise be the case, enabling adults, or carers of sick children to return to work that much sooner. Primary infection in adults is usually a more disabling disease than in children, and consideration of aciclovir therapy in this instance is reasonable.

## Neonatal chickenpox

Pregnant women who develop chickenpox in late pregnancy may pass this infection on to their baby if the child is born within a week of onset of the maternal rash (or the maternal rash arises within the first few days of giving birth) since there is insufficient time to allow the mother to generate protective antibodies that can be transferred across the placenta. Neonatal chickenpox is a feared disease, and babies at risk should be given passive immunization with varicella-zoster hyperimmune globulin. It is also reasonable to give such babies prophylactic aciclovir by mouth, although some withhold the drug until the baby develops signs of disease.

## Immunocompromised patients

Chickenpox in a patient who is immunocompromised may be life-threatening, especially if the immunodeficiency is in cell-mediated immunity (e.g. HIV-positive patients, transplant recipients on immunosuppressive drugs, patients on high-dose steroids). Such individuals should be tested for their immune status with regard to VZV and, if susceptible, should report all contacts with either chickenpox or herpes zoster, so that varicella-zoster immunoglobulin can be administered. Treatment of the disease itself in such individuals should be with high-dose intravenous aciclovir, no matter how trivial the disease appears to be when first seen.

## Herpes zoster

The site of latency of VZV is the dorsal root ganglion. The systemic nature of varicella infection means that dorsal root ganglia up and down the spinal cord become latently infected.

Reactivation of infection results in virus travelling down the dorsal nerve route in question, to reach the dermatome supplied by that nerve. This accounts for the characteristic dermatomal rash of shingles, or herpes zoster, the clinical manifestation of reactivated VZV infection. The onset of rash is often preceded by pain or abnormal sensation in the distribution of the dermatome. The rash usually heals uneventfully but pain in the area of the rash, known as post-herpetic neuralgia, may persist long after the rash itself has resolved and can be extremely debilitating. Risk factors for post-herpetic neuralgia include age (more likely in elderly patients), and severity of the initial zoster rash, as judged by the number and coverage of lesions.

Other complications of secondary VZV infection occasionally occur: reactivation of virus in the ophthalmic branch of the trigeminal nerve may result in keratitis and damage to the cornea; facial nerve involvement may cause a form of Bell's palsy; motor nerve damage may also be evident in zoster affecting the limbs; and involvement of sacral ganglia may result in urinary and anal retention.

A prolonged or atypical attack of herpes zoster may be the presenting feature of a number of diseases in which host immune responses are impaired. These include malignancy of the reticulo-endothelial system and HIV infection. In any immunocompromised patient with zoster, dissemination of the virus in the bloodstream may occur, with the appearance of lesions beyond the initial dermatome. This spread of virus also puts the patient at risk of life-threatening internal organ infection.

The aims of antiviral therapy include alleviation of the pain and discomfort of the rash, and the prevention of complications, including post-herpetic neuralgia and dissemination. Antiviral therapy given early in the course of zoster reduces the incidence of post-herpetic neuralgia and accelerates the resolution of pain. It is therefore logical to use antiviral therapy (aciclovir or its congeners) in the following types of zoster, provided this is started within 72 hours of onset of the rash (or longer for immunocompromised patients):

- any form of zoster in an immunocompromised patient, no matter how mild the attack appears to be on first presentation;
- ophthalmic zoster;
- zoster involving motor nerves, including the facial nerve;
- sacral zoster;
- zoster occurring in patients at 50 years of age or above who are therefore at increased risk of post-herpetic neuralgia.

## Epstein–Barr virus

Considerably larger doses of aciclovir are necessary to inhibit Epstein–Barr virus replication than HSV or VZV in vitro. This presumably reflects the differing efficiency of the phosphorylation of the drug by these viruses. The results of clinical trials of aciclovir in patients with infectious mononucleosis have been disappointing. The only manifestation of Epstein–Barr virus infection in which aciclovir is useful is oral hairy leukoplakia. This unusual disease arises only in immunocompromised patients, most commonly those with HIV infection. It presents as a whitish coating on the tongue or buccal mucosa, which may resemble candidiasis. The lesions are packed with replicating virus. The lesions may respond to aciclovir therapy but reappear when treatment is stopped, so that long-term use of the drug may be necessary.

# CMV

## Primary infections

Primary CMV infections of immunocompetent individuals are usually asymptomatic, although a small minority result in the infectious mononucleosis syndrome (glandular fever). Reactivation of latent virus fails to induce any recognizable disease in the individual concerned. There are two groups of patients, however, in whom the virus is a significant pathogen: babies infected in utero, and immunocompromised patients.

## Congenital infection

Transfer of CMV across the placenta may arise from both primary and reactivated maternal infection. Congenital infection affects about 1 in 300 live births in the United Kingdom. Most of these babies develop normally, but about 5 to 10 per cent are born with so-called cytomegalic inclusion disease, which has a poor prognosis. A further 5 to 10 per cent are normal at birth but later develop abnormalities such as deafness, impaired neurodevelopment, or learning difficulties. Controlled clinical trials of twice daily intravenous ganciclovir for 6 weeks in congenitally infected neonates with symptoms related to the central nervous system have shown significant benefit in terms of hearing outcome, and this has therefore become the standard of care for such neonates. Trials of oral valganciclovir for either 6 weeks or 6 months, and in neonates with manifestations other than those restricted to the central nervous system, are now in progress. There is currently no effective strategy for the prevention of congenital infection, although experimental vaccines have shown some promise in protecting susceptible individuals from infection. It may therefore be possible to protect women who reach child-bearing age without having had CMV infection from acquiring it during pregnancy.

## Immunocompromised patients

Symptomatic CMV disease may arise from primary or secondary infection in immunocompromised patients, including transplant recipients and those infected with HIV. In these patients, active CMV infection is a multisystem disease. In transplant recipients, it often presents with fever and leucopenia; other complications include hepatitis, myositis, and pneumonitis. In HIV-infected patients, retinitis is the commonest manifestation, accounting for 85 per cent of all CMV disease in patients with AIDS, but infection may also involve any part of the gastrointestinal tract, the brain, lungs, liver, adrenals, and peripheral nerves. Diagnosis is dependent upon clinical suspicion, demonstration of virus in normally sterile body samples, biopsy, and quantitative measurements of CMV viraemia. As management of HIV infection itself has improved significantly over the years, manifestations of CMV disease in HIV-infected patients have become less common.

## Treatment

Although several drugs are now available, the goal of a safe, easily administered, and effective therapy for CMV infection has yet to be attained. Ganciclovir, foscarnet, and cidofovir must all be given by intravenous infusion but fomivirsen is administered by intraocular injection. Side effects may be serious: bone marrow suppression (ganciclovir), nephrotoxicity (foscarnet and cidofovir), and painful penile ulceration (foscarnet) are the most notable. Further clinical trial data relating to brincidofovir, a lipid-bound version of cidofovir which is orally bioavailable, free of nephrotoxicity, and of enhanced antiviral potency compared to the parent compound, are awaited with interest.

Ganciclovir or valganciclovir (administered orally) are the drugs of first choice, with foscarnet as an alternative. Experience with cidofovir and fomivirsen is so far restricted to the management of CMV retinitis. Not all complications of CMV infection respond equally well to therapy. Drugs can save the sight of patients with retinitis, and infections of the bowel and liver also respond well but treatment of CMV pneumonitis in bone marrow transplant recipients is often unsuccessful because immune responses to the virus may also contribute to the disease process.

Therapy does not eliminate the virus, and in patients who remain immunosuppressed, CMV disease often recurs when therapy is stopped.

## Prophylaxis

Avoiding transplantation of material from latently infected donors to uninfected recipients can significantly reduce serious CMV disease in solid-organ transplant recipients. In contrast, bone marrow recipients most at risk of life-threatening CMV disease are those who are seropositive themselves but receive marrow from a seronegative donor. However, matching of CMV serostatus between donor and recipient in order to prevent the risk of disease is not a practicable solution to the problem. If recipients are deemed to be at risk, administration of CMV prophylaxis is appropriate. The exact regimen is a matter of debate but trials in different transplant settings have demonstrated the benefit of CMV immunoglobulin, oral valganciclovir, and, surprisingly, oral aciclovir or valaciclovir. Serum levels of aciclovir in these patients are well below the concentrations necessary to inhibit CMV replication but sufficiently high levels may be achieved inside infected cells.

# Human herpesviruses 6, 7, and 8

Human herpesvirus type 6 is the causative agent of roseola infantum, one of the many rashes of childhood. Occasional cases are associated with hepatitis or encephalitis, the latter being especially a problem in bone marrow transplant recipients. The virus is sensitive in vitro to ganciclovir but not aciclovir; however, the value of treatment is unknown. No disease has yet been associated with either primary or secondary infection with human herpesvirus type 7.

Human herpesvirus type 8, also known as Kaposi's sarcoma-associated herpesvirus, is the causative agent of all forms of Kaposi's sarcoma. Management of this malignant disease involves chemotherapy, and a role for antiviral drugs remains to be defined.

# Respiratory tract infections

## Upper respiratory tract infections

Infections of the upper respiratory tract with rhinoviruses (of which there are over 100 serotypes), corona-, entero-, adeno-, respiratory syncytial, and para-influenza viruses are extremely common but, fortunately, result in very little serious morbidity or mortality. Despite considerable effort, no specific antiviral therapy has been successfully developed for treatment or prevention of these infections. Intranasal interferon spray is effective in the treatment and prophylaxis of common colds that are caused by rhinoviruses but patients experience nasal stuffiness, irritation, and bleeding, which negates any possible therapeutic benefit. This approach to the management of the common cold has now been abandoned.

## Lower respiratory tract infections

Viral infection of the lower respiratory tract is potentially much more dangerous. The commonest viral infections giving rise to bronchiolitis and pneumonia are those due to respiratory syncytial and influenza viruses. Varicella pneumonia and CMV pneumonitis have been referred to above. In addition, giant cell pneumonia is a rare and fatal complication of measles, usually in leukaemic children who escaped vaccination. In the past decade, zoonotic transmissions of, first, severe acute respiratory syndrome and then Middle East respiratory syndrome coronaviruses (SARS-CoV and MERS-CoV, respectively) have resulted in diseases with significant mortality rates.

## Respiratory syncytial virus infection of infants

Bronchiolitis and pneumonia due to respiratory syncytial virus infection are relatively common in infants under 1 year of age. Ribavirin reduces viral shedding, hastens resolution of fever, improves respiration, and shortens stay in hospital. The main difficulty is that the drug needs to be administered by use of a small-particle aerosol generator. Moreover, for maximum benefit, the infant must breathe nebulized drug for at least 12 hours each day. Thus, ribavirin is not usually used in otherwise uncomplicated infection in an immunocompetent host. In babies with congenital immunodeficiency or heart or lung defects, where mortality from acute respiratory syncytial virus (RSV) infection may exceed 50 per cent, ribavirin can be lifesaving.

# Influenza

The preferred drugs for the management of influenza virus infections are the neuraminidase inhibitors (e.g. zanamivir, oseltamivir). Controlled trials have shown a shorter time to the resolution of symptoms and lower usage of antibiotics among patients treated with these drugs. However, they must be given within 48 hours of onset of symptoms for maximum benefit—a timeframe not often met by patients suffering influenzal symptoms. Zanamivir has poor oral bioavailability, is not licensed for children under 5 years of age, and has to be given by oral or nasal inhalation. Oseltamivir, in contrast, can be administered by mouth in capsules and a 5-day course is standard. Currently in the United Kingdom, it is recommended that neuraminidase inhibitors be used for the treatment of an influenza-like illness in an 'at-risk' individual when influenza is circulating in the community. 'At-risk' individuals comprise those with chronic respiratory, heart, renal, liver, or neurological disease, or diabetes mellitus, together with the immunocompromised and those aged 65 years or older.

These drugs can also be used, in the same target population groups, for post-exposure prophylaxis (PEP), assuming those individuals are not effectively protected by prior influenza vaccination. Such PEP is appropriate following exposure to someone suffering from an influenza-like illness in the same household or residential setting, when influenza is known to be circulating in the community.

The influenza pandemic of 2009 was the first in history to occur at a time when effective anti-influenza drugs were available. Most governments had stockpiled millions of doses of neuraminidase inhibitors (mostly oseltamivir) for just such an eventuality. When the pandemic first emerged, most use of the drugs was as prophylaxis for close contacts of laboratory-proven cases, in order to try and reduce the spread of disease (the containment phase). Once the infection was widespread in the community, the strategy switched to a treatment phase, where the drugs were used primarily as therapy for those with proven infection. It is difficult to assess how successful these tactics were as, fortunately, the causative pandemic virus was of relatively low virulence. Stockpiling as part of pandemic preparedness plans will continue and may prove to be of great benefit should a highly pathogenic virus such as avian influenza A H5N1 virus, which has been circulating at low levels in humans since 1997, adapt to become a human pandemic strain in the future.

Extensive use of the neuraminidase inhibitors, as treatment for both influenza A H5N1 and for pandemic influenza A H1N1 has, perhaps inevitably, been associated with the emergence of resistant variants. A single point mutation (H275Y) in the neuraminidase gene induces considerable resistance to oseltamivir. Resistance to zanamivir is less common and, indeed, oseltamivir-resistant strains may still be sensitive to zanamivir. For severely ill patients with oseltamivir resistance, zanamivir can be administered intravenously. There are also new neuraminidase inhibitors in the pipeline, such as peramivir, which can be administered via this route.

Some influenza A viruses are susceptible to the uncoating blockers amantadine and rimantadine. Clinical trials in boarding schools and other places in which large numbers of individuals are crowded together have shown that amantadine is effective in the treatment and prophylaxis of influenza A. Those treated with the drug have a milder, shorter-lasting infection. About 70 per cent of contacts given the drug are protected from infection. However, amantadine is unpopular in the elderly, who suffer the brunt of serious influenza, because of its stimulatory actions on the central nervous system. Patients become confused and agitated and may be unable to sleep. Rimantadine, a derivative of amantadine, is said to be equipotent in its anti-influenzal properties but less prone to side effects. However, it is not currently licensed in the United Kingdom. Viral resistance emerges rapidly in patients treated with either of these drugs and they are not currently recommended for the treatment or prophylaxis of influenza.

## Other infections

### Warts

Papillomavirus infections (warts) are amenable to physical (cryotherapy, surgery) and chemical (podophyllin and derivatives, salicylic acid) therapies. Interferons may have a place in the management of recalcitrant warts. About 50 per cent of warts disappear following intralesional or intramuscular interferon but they often recur. Topical application of imiquimod, a new imidazoquinoline that stimulates interferon and other cytokines, appears to be modestly effective.

More serious consequences of human papillomavirus (HPV) infection include cancer of the uterine cervix. New vaccines, containing the surface proteins of the commonest high-risk HPV types (16 and 18), and the commonest types associated with genital warts (6 and 11) are now licensed for the prevention of infection. Most countries have adopted a policy of targeting the vaccine at teenage girls.

### Polyomavirus infections

Progressive multifocal leukoencephalopathy, a disease that occurs almost exclusively in HIV-positive and other immunosuppressed patients, is a manifestation of reactivation of a polyomavirus in the brain. Treatment is difficult but there are reports that cidofovir (see 'Cidofovir' in Chapter 5) may be useful.

### Lassa fever

Ribavirin, taken orally, is very effective in the treatment and prophylaxis of Lassa fever, a haemorrhagic virus infection with a high mortality rate encountered in certain parts of West Africa.

### Diarrhoea

The treatment of viral gastroenteritis is considered in Chapter 25.

## Key points

- Aciclovir and derivatives (valaciclovir, famciclovir) are effective against infections with HSV-1, HSV-2 and VZV.

- Antiviral therapy is therefore recommended for all primary HSV infections (oropharyngeal or genital); eczema herpeticum; herpetic keratitis (primary or secondary); suspected herpes simplex encephalitis; and neonatal HSV infection. It may also be useful as prophylaxis against recurrent herpetic disease in heavily immunocompromised individuals or those who suffer frequent recurrent genital infection.

- Antiviral therapy is also recommended for primary VZV infection (chickenpox) in adults (including pregnant women if required); in any immunocompromised individual; and in neonatal varicella. In reactivated infection (herpes zoster or shingles), therapy is recommended for ophthalmic zoster; zoster involving motor nerves (e.g. facial palsy); any zoster in an immunocompromised patient; and zoster in anyone over the age of 50.

- Treatment of CMV infection with (val)ganciclovir, cidofovir, or foscarnet is less satisfactory owing to drug toxicities but may be life- or sightsaving in immunocompromised patients (e.g. HIV infection, solid-organ or bone marrow transplant recipients).

- Influenza virus infections can be treated with neuraminidase inhibitors. Ideally, therapy should be initiated within 72 hours of onset of symptoms. These drugs are targeted at those individuals at high risk of serious complications should they acquire influenza virus infection, although in the setting of an emerging pandemic, they may be offered universally either for prophylaxis or therapy.

## Further reading

Cohen, J. I. (2013) Clinical practice: herpes zoster. *New England Journal of Medicine*, **369**(3): 255–63.

Field, H. J. and Vere Hodge, R. A. (2013) Recent developments in anti-herpesvirus drugs. *British Medical Bulletin*, **106**: 213–49.

Yin, M. T., Brust, J. C. M., Tieu, H. V., and Hammer, S. M. (2009) Antiherpesvirus, anti-hepatitis virus, and anti-respiratory virus agents', in D. D. Richman, R. J. Whitely, and F. G. Hayden, eds, *Clinical Virology* (3rd edn). Washington, DC: ASM Press, pp. 217–64.

# Chapter 33

# Management of HIV infection

## Introduction to the management of HIV infection

There have been many significant advances in our understanding and management of HIV infection within the 30 years or so since the first appearance of patients with the acquired immunodeficiency syndrome (AIDS). Improvements in drug design and in understanding the replication cycle of HIV have led to the development of an increasing number of antiretroviral agents (see Table 6.1). Moreover, application of molecular biological techniques allows accurate monitoring of the amount of HIV RNA in peripheral blood (viral load) in individual patients. Treatment regimens and management protocols are becoming ever more complex. In order to achieve optimization and standardization of clinical practice, bodies such as the British HIV Association publish consensus guidelines for antiretroviral treatment of HIV-seropositive individuals. Such is the pace of change that these guidelines need regular revision. It is nevertheless possible to discern some important underlying principles governing the appropriate use of antiretroviral therapy, although their detailed application may vary from place to place and over time.

## Natural history of HIV infection

The natural history of HIV infection is relatively straightforward. The virus infects CD4-positive T cells and cells of the monocyte/macrophage series. Infection results in cell death. Initially, dying cells can be replenished but, over a prolonged period of time, there is an inexorable decline in the circulating CD4 T cell count. These cells play an integral role in the orchestration of adaptive immune responses, and their loss is accompanied by ever-increasing clinically evident immunodeficiency, culminating in AIDS. While there are differences in the rate of progression of disease between individuals, nevertheless, the vast majority of untreated patients will eventually die from the disease.

Following initial infection, which may or may not be associated with a 'seroconversion illness' about 4–6 weeks after infection, patients enter an asymptomatic phase. During this period, the viral load is a relatively stable marker within an individual patient—this is referred to as the viral load 'set-point'. This is a reflection of the turnover of virus replicating within cells, which in turn will reflect the rate of CD4 cell death, and it is therefore not surprising that the viral load set-point is the strongest predictor of how long it will take an individual patient to reach the clinical end point of AIDS. Disease progression can therefore be monitored by regular measurement of both the circulating CD4 T cell count, and the viral load.

## Treatment goals

The primary aim of therapy is to prevent the morbidity and mortality associated with the infection, while minimizing drug toxicity. This is achieved by suppressing viral replication, and thereby viral load, to as low as possible—preferably to levels which are undetectable using modern ultra-sensitive assays, which can detect down to around 40 copies of viral RNA per millilitre of blood. Suppression of viral replication will not only halt the decline of the CD4 T cell count, but will usually lead to an increase in CD4 T cell numbers. The returning CD4 T cells are functional and thus there is, to a greater or lesser extent, a reconstitution of the damaged host immune system. Indeed, this improvement in immune function may result in a profound inflammatory reaction against residual opportunistic or prior infecting organisms, resulting in the so-called immune reconstitution inflammatory syndrome (IRIS). Management may require administration of appropriate antibiotic or antiviral drugs. In particularly severe cases it may be necessary to use corticosteroids to dampen the immune response until the offending infection has been eliminated. As the immunodeficiency recedes, then the risk of those complications of HIV infection that define AIDS also recede. As a consequence, it is possible to discontinue prophylaxis against infections such as pneumocystis, toxoplasmosis, and cryptococcosis in patients responding successfully to therapy.

## When to treat?

Given that there are now drugs available that can substantially decrease the viral load within an individual patient, and that this can be monitored, the question arises as to when antiretroviral therapy should be started in an individual patient. This decision is an important one. It requires commitment from the patient to take the medication with strict adherence for a prolonged period, usually for life. This may incur both physical and psychological morbidity, disadvantages that have to be weighed against the potential therapeutic benefits to be gained. At present, UK guidelines recommend starting therapy in any patient with symptomatic HIV infection or AIDS regardless of their viral load or CD4 count. In those who are asymptomatic, the CD4 count is the major determinant for starting therapy. All those with counts ≤350 cells/μl should be offered therapy (Table 33.1). Those with counts between 350 and 500 cells/μl are evaluated further for viral load, rate of CD4 decline, evidence of coexisting conditions, and patient preference. Currently, treatment is deferred for those with CD4 counts above 500 cells/μl, although such patients could be enrolled into ongoing 'when to start' clinical trials. Current recommendations for treatment of primary infection are if there is neurological involvement, if the presentation is with an AIDS-defining illness, or if the CD4 count is <350 cells/μl. Otherwise, evidence for long-term survival benefit of early treatment of primary HIV infection is currently lacking, and this should only be considered as part of a clinical trial to address this question. Management of HIV infection in pregnancy is a further specialist issue (see 'Pregnancy').

**Table 33.1** When should combination antiretroviral therapy be initiated?

| |
|---|
| CD4 T cell count ≤350 cells/μl |
| History of an AIDS-defining illness |
| HIV-related co-morbidity e.g. nephropathy, HIV-associated neurocognitive disorders |
| Pregnancy |
| Co-infection with hepatitis B virus/hepatitis C virus |
| Non-AIDS-defining malignancies requiring immunosuppressive therapy |

# What to treat with?

The history of drug development in HIV infection demonstrates very clearly that successful therapy must consist of multiple drugs given in combination. Initially zidovudine (AZT) was the only option available. However, monotherapy with AZT invariably led to the selection of mutations in the error-prone reverse transcriptase gene, rendering the virus resistant to the drug after around 6 months. Thus, it is essential to model the treatment of HIV infection on that used for the treatment of tuberculosis: use of multiple agents to reduce the chances that the virus will become resistant to all of the drugs simultaneously. This principle has now been validated for a variety of combination therapies and has become the standard of care.

Triple drug combinations are highly effective in reducing viral load, both in degree and in duration of the effect. With the choice of agents including nucleoside and non-nucleoside inhibitors of reverse transcriptase, inhibitors of the viral protease and integrase enzymes, and entry and fusion inhibitors (Table 6.1), there are numerous possible triple drug combinations. The continuing emergence of new agents will complicate this even further. It is clearly not possible to test each one of these combinations in full-scale clinical trials but several regimens have proved to be highly effective. Such combination therapies are now collectively referred to as 'combination antiretroviral therapy' (cART), having formerly been known as 'highly active antiretroviral therapy' (HAART).

It is recommended in the United Kingdom that regimens for previously treatment naive patients consist of a backbone of two nucleos(t)ide reverse transcriptase inhibitors plus one of a non-nucleos(t)ide reverse transcriptase inhibitor, a ritonavir-boosted protease inhibitor, or an integrase inhibitor (Table 33.2). The reason for not selecting one drug of each category, which might appear intuitively to be the best idea, is to reserve some classes of drugs for the time when (if) initial therapy begins to fail. At this time, the virus present within the patient may have acquired a number of mutations conferring resistance to the drugs contained within his/her regimen but the virus should remain fully sensitive to drugs in the unused classes. In the absence of such 'class-sparing', the options for salvage therapy in the event of treatment failure are much reduced, as cross-resistance between drugs of the same class is common.

**Table 33.2** Recommended initial combination antiretroviral therapy regimens.[a]

|  | **First choice** | **Alternatives** |
| --- | --- | --- |
| NRTI backbone | Tenofovir+emtricitabine | Abacavir[b]+lamivudine |
| Third agent: |  |  |
| NNRTI | Efavirenz | Rilpivirine; nevirapine[c] |
| Protease inhibitors | Darunavir/ritonavir | Lopinavir/ritonavir |
|  | Atazanavir/ritonavir | Fosamprenavir/ritonavir |
| Integrase inhibitors | Raltegravir |  |
|  | Elvitegravir/cobicistat |  |

[a] NRTI, nucleos(t)ide analogue reverse transcriptase inhibitor; NNRTI, non-nucleos(t)ide analogue reverse transcriptase inhibitor.

[b] Must ensure patient is HLA-B*5701 negative.

[c] Contraindicated if baseline CD4 count is >250/400 cells/ μl in women/men.

The exact choice of drugs for an individual patient depends on a number of variables. It cannot be assumed that virus in a patient who has received no previous antiretroviral therapy will be sensitive to all drugs, as the patient may have been infected with a resistant strain. Such primary drug resistance now affects more than 10 per cent of newly diagnosed patients in the UK. Thus, virus from newly diagnosed patients should be sent for resistance testing prior to initiation of therapy. Moreover, adverse events are often unpredictable, and regimens may need tailoring to individual patients. Clearly, the more drugs a patient takes, the greater the risk of adverse reactions. For example, there is particular concern about the long-term safety of protease inhibitors,

**Table 33.3** Major adverse events associated with antiretroviral agents.

| Drug class | Drugs | Main adverse effects |
|---|---|---|
| Reverse transcriptase inhibitors: nucleos(t)ide analogues | Abacavir (ABC) | Hypersensitivity reactions in HLA B5701-positive patients |
| | Didanosine (ddI) | Peripheral neuropathy, pancreatitis |
| | Emtricitabine | Pruritus |
| | Lamivudine (3TC) | |
| | Stavudine (d4T) | Fat redistribution, peripheral neuropathy |
| | Tenofovir (TDF) | Increased serum phosphate, renal dysfunction |
| | Zidovudine (AZT) | Macrocytic anaemia, fat redistribution |
| Reverse transcriptase inhibitors: non-nucleoside analogues | Efavirenz | CNS toxicity, teratogenic— avoid in pregnancy |
| | Etravirine | Rash |
| | Nevirapine | Rash; may cause severe hepatotoxicity |
| Protease inhibitors | Atazanavir | Most are metabolized by the P450 CYP3A system and may cause drug–drug interactions; most are associated with hyperlipidaemia and possibly insulin resistance; many are associated with gastrointestinal disturbance (e.g. diarrhoea) |
| | Darunavir | |
| | Fosamprenavir | |
| | Indinavir | |
| | Lopinavir | |
| | Ritonavir | |
| | Saquinavir | |
| | Tipranavir | |
| Fusion inhibitors | Enfuvirtide | Must be given by subcutaneous injection; very expensive |
| CCR5 inhibitors | Maraviroc | |
| Integrase inhibitors | Raltegravir, elvitegravir, dolutegravir | Gastrointestinal upset, rash |

owing to their effect on lipid metabolism. Adverse events associated with the antiretroviral drugs are discussed in Chapter 6, and the more common/important ones are listed in Table 33.3.

As outlined earlier, antiretroviral therapy is monitored by serial viral load measurements. Viral load should decline significantly, and usually to undetectable levels, within 3 months of onset of cART. Regular monitoring at three monthly intervals thereafter is standard, as failure of treatment, for whatever reason, will first become apparent due to a rise in viral titres. Patients stabilized on cART are also reviewed frequently for CD4 T cell count, clinical assessment, lipid analysis, and evidence of organ or bone marrow toxicity arising from treatment or complications of their HIV infection.

## Treatment failure: non-compliance and resistance

Should viral load start to rise, then consideration must be given to understanding the reasons for treatment failure. The two most important are non-compliance with therapy, and emergence of drug resistance.

Drugs are only effective for as long as their concentration in the tissues is high enough. Failure to take the requisite regular doses of an antiviral drug leads to a fall in tissue levels, with a consequent risk of escape of the virus from inhibition of replication, and an increased likelihood of mutation to resistance. It is important, therefore, that patients adhere to the prescribed regimens. The more doses that are missed, the faster resistant virus will emerge.

Compliance is a significant problem, especially with multidrug regimens, in which some tablets should be taken with food and others on an empty stomach; some twice a day, others three or four times a day. By combining drugs in fixed dose formulations, compliance can be increased and this is now the preferred treatment approach, with the aim being 'one tablet, once a day'. Patients may also be on a variety of other agents (e.g. for prophylaxis against pneumocystis pneumonia or recurrent herpes simplex disease). Moreover, in any disease, and HIV infection is no exception, adherence to treatment is poorer in patients with symptom-free disease. Failure to take the tablets must always be considered as an explanation for a sudden rise in viral titre.

If non-compliance is ruled out, then the possible emergence of drug-resistant virus must be assessed. Resistance testing is performed in reference laboratories and is mostly based around sequencing of the target viral genes and comparison of those sequences against an extensive database of possible resistance mutations. Identification of which mutations are present in which viral genes will allow determination of which drugs within the cART regimen are failing, and therefore rational decision making about how to change the cART regimen. This may involve replacing one, two, or even all three of the drugs. Drug-resistance genotyping is expensive but has become integral to defining initial therapy and for identifying resistance arising during treatment. Comparative trials have shown that genotypic resistance testing confers a significant benefit on the virological response when choosing therapeutic alternatives.

## Pregnancy

A special consideration is the use of antiretroviral drugs in pregnancy. In the absence of any interventions, around 25 per cent of babies of infected mothers will acquire HIV infection themselves. However, mother-to-baby transmission of HIV is almost entirely preventable with appropriate interventions. As such interventions can only be applied to pregnant women who are known to be infected with HIV, it is imperative that HIV testing is routinely instituted for all pregnant women.

Such a policy of universal screening for HIV infection in pregnancy was introduced in the United Kingdom some years ago.

There is compelling evidence that the risk of vertical transmission of HIV from mother to baby is proportional to the maternal viral load during pregnancy. Reduction of maternal viral load by use of antiretroviral agents significantly reduces the risk of transmission. Thus, viral load should be determined in all HIV-infected pregnant women, and appropriate regimens of antiretroviral therapy offered dependent on the starting viral load, the patient's past history of antiretroviral usage, and the fact that some antiretroviral agents are contraindicated in pregnancy due to their potential teratogenicity, for example, efavirenz. Delivery by caesarean section may also reduce the risk of transmission, especially if the maternal viral load is above 50 copies/ml, although the benefit in women with undetectable viral load is minimal. Post-exposure prophylaxis should be given to the neonate—the precise regimen is dependent on maternal therapy and viral load at delivery. Breastfeeding is not advised, as this doubles the risk of transmission.

## Co-infection with hepatitis B or C viruses

Hepatitis B virus (HBV) and hepatitis C virus (HCV) share routes of transmission with HIV, and therefore co-infection is not unusual. As management of HIV infection has improved, co-infected patients have started to survive long enough to develop life-threatening liver disease arising from their chronic viral hepatitis. It is therefore important that all HIV-infected patients be tested to determine if they are co-infected with HBV or HCV. If they are, then appropriate management of both their HIV and HBV/HCV infections must be instituted. Treatment of HBV infection is complicated by the fact that most anti-HBV drugs (including tenofovir and entecavir) have anti-HIV activity as well (although entecavir is not used as an anti-HIV drug). Thus, while monotherapy for HBV infection may be the norm in non-HIV-infected patients, this is not acceptable in co-infection, as it may encourage the emergence of drug-resistant HIV. Anti-HBV therapy therefore needs to be performed with a combination of drugs effective against both viruses (e.g. tenofovir plus emtricitabine), or it must be in the setting of an effective cART regimen, even if cART is otherwise not indicated. In addition, in HCV co-infection, it may be necessary to treat the HIV infection in a patient who would not otherwise be offered it (e.g. a patient with a CD4 count between 350 and 500), purely for the purposes of enhancing the chances of successful anti-HCV therapy. Care must be exercised if the HCV infection is to be treated with directly acting agents emerging as optimal therapy against HCV (see Chapter 7), as there is considerable potential for drug–drug interactions between the anti-HCV and anti-HIV drugs.

## Conclusions

The complexity of HIV disease and its attendant complications, most notably of opportunistic infections (Chapter 31), requires specialist management over many years. The use of cART has substantially improved the survival and quality of life of those affected by HIV/AIDS—recent UK data indicate that the life expectancy of an HIV-infected patient has improved significantly in recent years. The disease remains incurable. New therapeutic approaches are needed, with novel modes of action, ideally including elimination of long-lived reservoirs of infected cells, and fewer side effects. This will remain the situation until an effective vaccine is developed, which despite an enormous research effort, remains an elusive goal.

HIV-positive patients are at risk of a wide range of serious infections. These are discussed in Chapter 31.

## Key points

- The aim of antiretroviral therapy is to prevent (or halt or reverse) immunological damage arising from HIV infection and so avert the associated risks of opportunistic infections and other morbidities associated with AIDS.

- HIV management is best delivered by a multidisciplinary team with appropriate experience. In addition, cART is essential in order to avoid the emergence of drug resistance.

- The use of cART should be considered for patients displaying symptomatic disease, having an AIDS-defining illness, or having a CD4 count lower than 350 cells/µl. Additional considerations are pregnancy, and co-infection with HBV or HCV.

- Drug-resistance testing should be performed prior to the initiation of therapy, as patients may be infected de novo with resistant strains.

- Recommended initial cART regimens include two nucleos(t)ide analogue reverse transcriptase inhibitors (NRTIs) plus one of a non-nucleos(t)ide analogue reverse transcriptase inhibitor (NNRTI), a protease inhibitor (PI), or an integrase inhibitor (INI). Response should be monitored by regular viral load testing.

- Compliance is essential but may be difficult to obtain. All antiretrovirals may give rise to adverse events, both short and long term. It may be necessary to try different regimens to find one that an individual patient can tolerate.

## Further reading

The BHIVA Treatment Guidelines Writing Group. (2013) British HIV association guidelines for the management of hepatitis viruses in adults infected with HIV 2013. *HIV Medicine*, **14**(Suppl 4): 1–71.

The BHIVA Treatment Guidelines Writing Group. (2014) British HIV association guidelines for the treatment of HIV-1 positive adults with antiretroviral therapy 2012. *HIV Medicine*, **15**(Suppl 1): 1–85.

The British HIV Association website contains a number of authoritative guidelines for the management of HIV infection, available at: <http://www.bhiva.org/guidelines.aspx>.

Maartens G, Celum C, Lewin SR. HIV infection: epidemiology, pathogenesis, treatment and prevention. *Lancet*, **384** (39): 258–381.

# Chapter 34

# Treatment of chronic viral hepatitis

## Introduction to the treatment of chronic viral hepatitis

With over 500 million individuals chronically infected with either hepatitis B virus (HBV) or hepatitis C virus (HCV) and thus at risk of developing end-stage liver disease or hepatocellular carcinoma, chronic viral hepatitis creates a huge health and economic burden worldwide. The outlook for such patients has dramatically improved in the last 10–15 years, with a number of antiviral therapies being shown in appropriately controlled clinical trials to be effective (see Chapter 7).

## Hepatitis B

### Natural history of chronic HBV infection

Chronic infection with HBV is defined as the persistence of hepatitis B surface antigen (HBsAg) in the peripheral blood for more than 6 months. However, HBsAg-positive individuals can be subdivided further into those in whom HBeAg (a breakdown product of the viral core antigen) can be detected, and those with antibodies to this antigen (anti-HBe). HBeAg is a surrogate marker of active viral replication in hepatocytes. HBe antigen seroconversion is therefore associated with a significant decline in the viral load detectable in peripheral blood.

HBV itself is not cytopathic—it is the immune response (especially that mediated by cytotoxic T cells) to infected hepatocytes which induces liver cell death. The intrahepatic response to liver cell injury is the laying down of fibrous tissue. Thus, the end result of the inflammatory hepatitis induced by chronic HBV infection is cirrhosis of the liver. However, liver disease progression is not linear over time, and a number of pathologically distinct phases of chronic infection are now recognized (see Table 34.1). Soon after the establishment of chronic infection, there is extensive virus replication within hepatocytes, with no apparent immune response. This is the immunotolerant phase. The patient will be HBeAg positive (a marker of active virus replication), the peripheral blood viral load will exceed $10^6$ IU/ml, but the serum level of alanine aminotransferase (ALT; a marker of liver cell death) will be normal. When, eventually, an immune response is mounted to the virus, there may be extensive hepatocyte death and an intense intrahepatic inflammation which may result in severe liver damage. This phase is referred to as immune clearance or 'e' seroconversion. During this phase, the ALT levels will be raised, indicating ongoing inflammation. Eventually, as the bulk of infected cells are killed, resulting in loss of replicating virus, HBeAg is lost from peripheral blood, the viral load declines to levels below $10^3$ IU/ml, and eventually anti-HBe is detectable in the peripheral blood. The patient then enters a quiescent phase of low or non-detectable virus replication. The intrahepatic inflammation has died down and therefore ALT levels return to normal. This has previously been referred to as an inactive carrier state but this terminology is perhaps slightly misleading, as virus is still present within the liver, and replication may recommence as the patient enters the reactivation phase. Reactivation occurs due to the emergence of virus that has acquired mutations in the pre-core region of its genome so that it

**Table 34.1** Natural history of chronic hepatitis B virus infection.*

| Phase | Intrahepatic viral replication | Viral load (IU/ml) in peripheral blood | HBeAg/anti-HBe status | Serum ALT | Active liver damage |
|---|---|---|---|---|---|
| Immunotolerant | High | >10$^6$ | HBeAg +ve | Normal | No |
| Immune clearance | Declining | Declining | Seroconverting | High | Yes |
| Low/non-replicative | Low | <10$^3$ | Anti-HBe +ve | Normal | No |
| Reactivation | Flares of high activity | >10$^4$ | Anti-HBe +ve | High | Yes |

* +ve, positive; ALT, alanine aminotransferase; note that patients remain HBsAg positive throughout all phases of infection.

is no longer able to synthesize HBeAg—these are so-called pre-core mutants. Virus reactivation is associated with increased viral loads and inflammatory responses despite the patient being anti-HBe positive, resulting in raised ALT and the propensity to cause progressive liver damage.

Progression through these phases of chronic infection is dependent on a number of factors including the following:

♦ Age at infection. Neonates who acquire infection at birth from their carrier mothers enter a prolonged immunotolerant phase which may last up to 30 years. In those who acquire infection as adults, this phase may only last for a year or two.

♦ Immune function, for obvious reasons.

♦ HBV genotype. The ease with which the virus can acquire the key pre-core mutations resulting in a replication competent strain which cannot synthesize HBeAg is dependent on the starting wild-type sequence, which differs between viral genotypes.

## Which patients should be treated?

Therapy should be directed at those patients most at risk of progressive liver disease. Several learned societies (e.g. the European Association for the Study of the Liver (EASL) or the American Association for the Study of Liver Disease (AASLD)) have issued extensive guidance on selection of patients for therapy. The fundamental principles are that the risk of progressive liver disease is highest in the immunoclearance and reactivation phases of infection and that high viral loads are an important prognostic indicator of long-term development of liver disease. Assessment of an individual patient for therapy therefore requires knowledge of

♦ their HBeAg/anti-HBe status;

♦ the viral load; and

♦ the ALT level (a marker of liver cell death/inflammation).

If in doubt, it may also be helpful to perform a liver biopsy and thereby obtain a histological assessment of disease activity. Patients most likely to warrant therapy will therefore be those who are

♦ HBeAg positive with high viral loads (HBV DNA >2,000 IU/ml), high ALT (above the upper limit of normal), and/or histological evidence of active liver disease (immunoclearance phase); or

♦ anti-HBe positive with high viral loads (as above), high ALT (again), and/or histological evidence of active liver disease.

## What should patients be treated with?

As outlined in Chapter 7, there are two strategies for the treatment of chronic HBV infection—immunomodulation with pegylated interferon-α, and viral suppressive therapy with nucleos(t)ide analogue polymerase inhibitors. Both modalities have their advantages and disadvantages.

Interferon enhances the expression of human leucocyte antigen (HLA) class I molecules on the surface of infected hepatocytes, thus resulting in the efficient elimination of these cells by circulating cytotoxic T lymphocytes. This in turn reduces the amount of virus in the liver, and the production of infectious virions, with a consequent reduction in viral load.

In a patient who is HBeAg positive, a typical response to interferon is shown in Fig. 34.1. At the onset of therapy, the patient is HBsAg and HBeAg positive and has a raised ALT level, which indicates an active inflammatory response as part of the immune clearance phase. Some weeks after the initiation of interferon therapy, there is a marked rise in ALT. Paradoxically, this indicates a good therapeutic response, since it shows that hepatocytes now express sufficient HLA class I molecules to allow recognition and destruction by cytotoxic T lymphocytes. At the end of therapy, liver function returns to normal and the patient is now anti-HBe positive. Note that the patient remains HBsAg positive. Thus virus has not been completely eliminated but passage through the period of immune clearance has been speeded up and the subsequent risk of ongoing liver damage is much reduced. The patient is also much less of an infection risk to sexual partners and family members. After a number of years, some patients do in fact eventually lose HBsAg.

Pegylated interferon-α is administered via weekly intramuscular injections for a standard period of 48 weeks. Some patients may find the side effects of myalgia, headache, and fever difficult to tolerate at first. Not all infected individuals will respond. Predictors of response include both host and viral factors. Thus, immunodeficient patients respond less well than

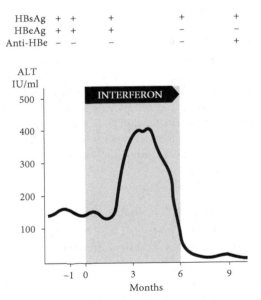

**Fig. 34.1** Treatment of chronic hepatitis B infection with interferon showing the change in ALT levels, loss of hepatitis B e antigen (HBeAg), and the appearance of antibody to HBe (anti-HBe). HBsAg is not eliminated.

immunocompetent ones, while HBV genotypes A and B respond better than genotypes C and D. In HBeAg-positive patients, anti-HBe seroconversion rates are of the order of 30 per cent. In anti-HBe positive patients in the reactivation phase, interferon may also be useful in guiding patients back into a non-replicative phase. Therapy in these patients can only be monitored by viral load and ALT measurement, as the patients are already anti-HBe positive.

Nucleos(t)ide analogue therapy has become more widely adopted in the last 5 years or so. First-line therapy should be with a highly potent drug with a high barrier to resistance (i.e. tenofovir or entecavir), although lamivudine is still widely used in many countries because it is cheaper. These drugs suppress viral replication, and monitoring should therefore be via viral load measurement. In HBeAg-positive patients, suppression of HBV DNA to undetectable levels after 12 months of therapy is achieved in around 70 per cent of patients with the more potent antivirals; this figure is even higher (90% plus) in anti-HBe positive patients. Around 30 per cent of HBeAg-positive patients will seroconvert to anti-HBe positivity on such therapy. Cessation of therapy may lead to recurrence of viral replication, and HBeAg sero-reversion in those who lost HBeAg on therapy, so knowing when to stop therapy is difficult. For HBeAg-positive patients, a rule of thumb is to consider stopping 6 months after anti-HBe seroconversion. For patients who are already anti-HBe positive, therapy may have to be very prolonged, which carries an increased risk of the emergence of resistant virus. There are also concerns about possible long-term adverse events, such as nephrotoxicity and reduced bone density associated with tenofovir. However, it is becoming apparent that the longer therapy is continued, the greater the chances of the patient losing HBsAg, and even converting to anti-HBs positivity, at which point it may be safe to discontinue therapy.

The success of therapy can be judged by monitoring HBeAg/anti-HBe status and by measurement of HBV DNA viral load. There is considerable interest in identifying laboratory markers which are predictive of response to therapy. The most promising of these is quantitative assessment of HBsAg levels. This allows generation of 'stopping rules'. The most robust of these is for patients being treated with interferon. If HBsAg levels have not declined by month 3 of therapy, the chances of a successful outcome are so small that it is not worth continuing the treatment. It is hoped that further development of such markers will inform clinical decision making about which treatment, and for how long, will provide most benefit to individual patients. Co-infection with HIV and HBV is increasingly recognized and requires specialist management. The danger here is that monotherapy for HBV infection with a drug also active against HIV will generate HIV resistance to the drug. Thus, the management of HBV should be undertaken either with adefovir, which has no anti-HIV activity, or only as part of combination antiretroviral therapy potent enough to bring HIV replication under control.

Another area in which these newer agents have shown promise is in the prophylaxis and treatment of hepatitis B-positive patients undergoing liver transplantation, or immunosuppressive therapy (e.g. treatment with rituximab), which may result in flares of HBV replication with consequent liver damage. There is a reduction in risk of infection of the transplanted liver, of severe disease if the grafted liver becomes infected, and a reduced rate of virus reactivation associated with immunosuppressive therapy.

# Hepatitis C

## Which patients should be treated?

The primary diagnostic test to determine if a patient has been infected with HCV is to look for anti-HCV antibodies in serum. Anti-HCV positivity, however, is only a marker of past infection, and a further test, looking for the presence of HCV RNA in serum, should then be performed to determine if the patient is still infected with the virus. Around 25 per cent of infected patients will clear their infection spontaneously (i.e. without intervention). The remaining 75 per cent become chronically infected and are at risk of progressive liver disease. Factors which increase that risk include older age at the time of infection, being male, drinking alcohol (which acts synergistically with HCV in inducing liver damage), and underlying immunodeficiency, including HIV co-infection. EASL and AASLD guidelines recommend that any patient with chronic HCV infection be considered for therapy, regardless of the degree of underlying liver damage at the time of diagnosis, and this is reflected in the National Institute for Health and Clinical Excellence (NICE) guidelines in the United Kingdom. Possible contra-indications to therapy include active injecting drug use (although most clinicians will treat active injectors), heavy alcohol intake, and chaotic lifestyle—all of which might militate against adherence to therapy over a prolonged period of time.

## Monitoring of therapy

Response to therapy is best monitored by measurement of the circulating HCV RNA load using quantitative real-time polymerase chain reaction (PCR) assays. Viral load may be assessed at different times after initiation of therapy, with several definitions of response:

◆ Rapid virological response (RVR). Assessed at 4 weeks of therapy. Must be HCV RNA-negative in an assay capable of detecting down to 30 IU/ml.

◆ Early virological response (EVR). Assessed at 12 weeks of therapy. Complete EVR (cEVR) means viral RNA is undetectable. Partial EVR (pEVR) means there has been at least a 2-log drop in viral load but not to negativity.

◆ End of treatment response (EoTR).

◆ Sustained virological response (SVR). Defined as HCV RNA negativity at particular time points after the end of treatment (EoT). SVR12 is the SVR determined at 12 weeks after EoT; SVR24 is the SVR determined at 24 weeks.

Overall treatment responses are classified (Fig. 34.2) as the following:

◆ SVR. This equates to cure—almost 100 per cent of individuals who reach SVR remain virus free when tested 5 years later.

◆ Non-response (NR)—viral RNA remains detectable throughout therapy.

◆ Relapser-responder (RR)—viral RNA becomes undetectable during therapy but reappears within 6 months of cessation of therapy.

| | | ANTI VIRAL THERAPY | | | | |
|---|---|---|---|---|---|---|
| | Pretreatment | 12 weeks | 24 weeks | 48 weeks | 72 weeks | |
| HCV RNA | + | + | + | + | + | Non-responder |
| | + | − | − | − | + | Responder-relapser |
| | + | − | − | − | − | Sustained virological responder |

**Fig. 34.2** Patterns of response to 48 weeks of PEG/RV therapy in chronic HCV infection.

Achievement of RVR is the best predictor that an SVR will be attained (see 'Likelihood of response to therapy'). Patients who have detectable viraemia after 4 weeks of therapy should be retested at 12 weeks. If an EVR has not been achieved, then there is very little chance that an SVR will eventuate, and there is little point in continuing therapy beyond this point. Such patients are non-responders.

Most patients do achieve an EVR and continue through to EoT. However, patients may relapse in the subsequent 6 months (almost always within 3 months) with reappearance of viraemia (RRs).

## Which drugs should be used?

Therapy for chronic HCV infection is undergoing a major revolution, with a number of directly acting antiviral agents (DAAs; see Chapter 7) successfully completing late stage clinical trials and achieving licensure for clinical use.

Pegylated interferon-α (PEG) and ribavirin (RV) combination therapy was the standard of care for many years and is still widely used. The mechanism of action of interferon in hepatitis C infection appears to be different from that in hepatitis B, as response is not usually accompanied by a rise in ALT levels. For patients infected with genotype 1 (or 4) virus, the recommended course is for 48 weeks and, even then, SVR rates are only of the order of 50 per cent. For those with genotype 2 or 3 infection, only 6 months therapy is required, and SVR rates are in excess of 70 per cent. The molecular basis for the differing sensitivities of the different viral genotypes to therapy is unknown. PEG/RV therapy gives rise to a number of adverse effects (see Chapter 7) and is not easy to tolerate. Patients require extensive support to get them through a tough regimen, which is usually provided by specialist hepatitis nurses. Even so, a significant number of patients may not be able to complete their allocated therapy—most clinical trials have dropout rates of the order of 10–15 per cent. Some of this is due to patient intolerance but also some patients develop adverse reactions, such as neutropaenia, thrombocytopaenia, suicidal ideation (all due to PEG), or haemolytic anaemia (due to RV) which make it dangerous to continue.

The NS3 protease inhibitors telaprevir and boceprevir were the first DAAs to be licensed in 2011, for use in genotype 1 infection only. When these are added to a PEG/RV backbone, SVR rates for genotype 1 infected patients increase to 65–75 per cent, and for those patients who lose detectable virus early on in therapy, duration of therapy can be shortened to 6 months ('response-guided therapy'; see 'Likelihood of response to therapy'). Moreover, this triple therapy regimen is also valuable in patients who have previously failed PEG/RV therapy. The SVR rate in previous RRs may be as high as 75 per cent; this figure is lower for previous partial responders (60%) or non-responders (30%). Such improvements in SVR rates do, however, come at a cost—quite literally, in the sense that a course of triple therapy may be as much as £30,000, meaning that it may not be possible to treat all patients in this way. There are also additional side effects such as anaemia, rash, and dysgeusia, which make a difficult regimen of PEG/RV even more stressful for the patient.

In the coming months and years, the situation will no doubt change again. Second-wave protease inhibitors (e.g. simeprevir, asunaprevir) are more potent and are better tolerated than the first generation ones but are still essentially restricted to the treatment of genotype 1 or 4 infection. Second-generation protease inhibitors (PIs; e.g. MK-5172) are expected to be more pangenotypic. Sofosbuvir is the most advanced nucleoside NS5b polymerase inhibitor, and trial data show this to be enormously promising. In combination with PEG/RV, SVR rates in genotype 1 patients are in excess of 90 per cent, and similarly high rates are reported in genotype 3 infection. For genotype 2 infection, it is likely that sofosbuvir plus ribavirin alone will be sufficient to generate similarly high SVR rates. The drug is well tolerated, with no significant serious adverse effects reported, and there is also an extremely high barrier to resistance, with the key resistance mutation (S282T) giving rise to significant fitness costs for the virus and therefore impaired virus replication and has only been reported in in vitro studies.

The development of yet another class of DAAs, the NS5a inhibitors (e.g. daclatasvir), which are very potent but have moderate barriers to resistance, has brought the concept of combination DAA therapy in the absence of an interferon backbone close to reality. Sofosbuvir plus daclatasvir therapy has achieved high SVR rates (although in relatively small numbers of patients). As more drugs come through trials, the number of possible combinations will increase, for example, protease inhibitor plus nucleoside NS5b inhibitor, or NS5a inhibitor plus nucleoside NS5b inhibitor. Non-nucleoside NS5b inhibitors have a much lower barrier to resistance and therefore are likely to be used only in triple regimens with both a PI and an NS5a inhibitor. One example of such a regimen is dasabuvir (targets NS5b) plus ombitasvir (NS5a) plus ritonavir-boosted paritaprevir (NS3). It is not possible at this stage to determine precisely what the most cost-effective combinations will be. Suffice it to say that, by the next edition of this text, all oral interferon- (and possibly ribavirin-) free regimens with minimal side effects taken for 12 weeks (perhaps even shorter) with SVR rates above 95 per cent across all genotypes will be the norm. Table 34.2 lists some of the more promising drugs in current trials.

## Likelihood of response to therapy

Several factors influence the likelihood of patients achieving viral clearance with PEG/RV therapy (see Table 34.3). The genotype of the infecting virus is the dominant viral factor—cure rates for patients with genotype 1 infection are around 45 per cent, whereas for genotype 2 infection, this approaches 90 per cent. The molecular basis for the differing sensitivities of the different viral genotypes to therapy is unknown. However, this fundamental property is reflected in the different treatment regimens recommended for each genotype (see above). Response rates are also related to pretreatment viral load. With regard to host factors, much interest has been generated by recent genome-wide association studies which have identified a cluster of single nucleotide

**Table 34.2** Directly acting antivirals in current trials for the treatment of hepatitis C infection.

| NS3 protease inhibitors | NS5a inhibitors | Nucelos(t)ide NS5b inhibitors | Non-nucleoside NS5b inhibitors |
| --- | --- | --- | --- |
| Telaprevir | Daclatasvir | Sofosbuvir | Dasabuvir |
| Boceprevir | Ledipasvir | Mericitabine | Deleobuvir |
| Simeprevir | Ombitasvir | | |
| Asunaprevir | Elbasvir | | |
| Paritaprevir* | | | |
| Grazoprevir | | | |

*Contains a boosting dose of ritonavir

**Table 34.3** Factors which influence the response to pegylated interferon/ribavirin therapy in chronic hepatitis C infection.*

| Factor | Good prognostic indicator | Poor prognostic indicator |
|---|---|---|
| Viral genotype | 2, 3 | 1, 4 |
| Pretreatment viral load | Low (<800,000 iµ/ml) | High (>800,000 iµ/ml) |
| Gender | Female | Male |
| Age at onset of therapy | Younger | Older |
| Liver disease severity | No or mild fibrosis | Significant fibrosis |
| Interleukin-28B genotype | Responder allele homozygosity | Non-responder homozygosity or responder/non-responder heterozygosity |
| Kinetics of viral loss | Achievement of RVR | Failure to achieve RVR |

* RVR, rapid virological response.

polymorphisms on chromosome 19; these polymorphisms are near *IL-28B*, the gene encoding interleukin-28B (IL-28B; also known as interferon-λ3), and segregate with response/non-response to therapy (see Chapter 7). Again, the molecular basis for these observations is not clear but it raises the possibility that particular therapeutic regimens may be selected for individual patients based on their *IL-28B* genotype. Severity of underlying liver disease is also an important factor in determining outcome – patients with established cirrhosis clearly respond less well to all treatment regimens.

However, the single most important predictor of treatment outcome is the kinetics of viral loss after the initiation of therapy. Achievement of an RVR (see 'Monitoring of therapy') means the patient is much more likely to achieve an SVR, regardless of the various other factors outlined above. Indeed, if patients with genotype 1 infection and a low pretreatment viral load (defined as less than 800,000 IU/ml) achieve RVR, then PEG/RV therapy can be shortened to just 6 months (as opposed to 12 months) without reducing their chances of an SVR. Similarly, a shortened course of therapy (e.g. to 16 weeks) is possible for genotype 2 and 3 patients with a low pretreatment viral load who achieve RVR. This concept of response-guided therapy (i.e. the regimen is adjusted to take into account the initial response) has also been adopted in the early triple therapy regimens of PEG/RV plus telaprevir or boceprevir, where therapy can be as short as 6 months, provided virus is not detectable after 4 weeks of therapy.

HCV infection is an important co-morbidity in patients with HIV infection. As management of the immunodeficiency has improved (see Chapter 33) and therefore infected patients are surviving longer, it has become apparent that development of end-stage liver disease is a real threat in co-infected patients. Treatment of chronic HCV infection in co-infected patients requires specialist selection and supervision. The timing of treatment of hepatitis C in relation to the stage of HIV infection is crucial. Overall, SVR rates in response to PEG/RV therapy in co-infected individuals are less than in immunocompetent patients. However, there are encouraging data suggesting that response rates to DAA-containing regimens may be as good as in mono-infected patients. There is considerable potential for drug–drug interactions between the anti-HCV DAAs and antiretroviral drugs, so it is important that co-infected patients are managed by suitably experienced clinical teams.

## Key points

- Chronic hepatitis B infection proceeds through a number of distinct phases. Liver damage is most likely to occur during the immunoclearance and reactivation phases.
- The need for therapy in chronic HBV is determined by measurement of HBeAg/anti-HBe status, HBV DNA, ALT, and, if necessary, histological assessment of liver biopsy.
- Therapeutic options comprise a time-limited course of pegylated interferon (acting as an immunomodulatory agent), or long-term nucleos(t)ide inhibitors of the viral polymerase. Tenofovir and entecavir are the first choice agents in this category, due to their high potency and high genetic barrier to resistance.
- Therapy should be monitored by viral load assessment, and HBeAg to anti-HBe seroconversion where appropriate.
- All patients with chronic HCV infection are eligible for therapy. Standard of care regimens are rapidly changing from dual therapy with pegylated interferon and ribavirin to triple therapy with PEG/RV plus a DAA and will soon become combination therapy with multiple DAAs (and possibly RV) in interferon-free regimens.
- Likelihood of response is dependent on viral genotype, viral load, age, gender, pre-existing liver disease, and host *IL-28B* genotype.
- Duration of therapy depends on viral genotype, pretreatment viral load, and the rate of on-treatment response to therapy. Overall cure rates for PEG/RV dual therapy are around 50 per cent (45% for genotype 1, 70–80% for genotypes 2 or 3) but are considerably higher (e.g. >90%) in trials of PEG/RV plus a DAA, and of multiple DAAs in interferon-free regimens, across all genotypes.

## Further reading

Cooke, G. S., Main, J., and Thursz, M. R. (2010) Treatment for hepatitis B. *BMJ*, **340**: 87–91.

Dusheiko, G. and Wedemeyer, H. (2012) New protease inhibitors and direct-acting antivirals for hepatitis C: interferon's long goodbye. *Gut*, **61**(12): 1647–52.

EASL Clinical Practice Guidelines. (2012) Management of chronic hepatitis B virus infection. *Journal of Hepatology*, **57**(1): 167–85.

EASL Clinical Practice Guidelines. (2014) Management of hepatitis C virus infection. *Journal of Hepatology*, **60**(1): 392–420.

# Chapter 35

# Parasitic disease

## Introduction to parasitic disease

The dictionary definition of a parasite is an organism which lives off or on another, without benefit to its host and often causing it harm. By this definition, almost all pathogenic agents are parasites but the word has a different meaning when applied to human infectious diseases. Classical human parasitic diseases are those caused by eukaryotic organisms; some are unicellular (e.g. protozoa), many are multi-cellular (e.g. helminths; see Fig. 35.1 for classification), and some are complex free-living organisms (e.g. arthropods). Parasitic infections are more common in tropical regions, and many are strongly associated with poverty, poor hygiene, and unclean water. Parasitic diseases are, however, far from being restricted to the tropics. Some parasites, such as *Trichomonas vaginalis* and threadworm (caused by *Enterobius vermicularis*), are at least as common in developed countries. Moreover, the speed and extent of international travel ensures that parasitic infections acquired in the tropics may present therapeutic challenges to medical practitioners everywhere.

## Protozoa infections

### Malaria

Malaria is the most important parasitic disease of man. Around 5 per cent of the world's population is infected and it causes approximately one million deaths each year. It is caused by four plasmodium species: *Plasmodium falciparum*, *Pla. vivax*, *Pla. malariae*, and *Pla. ovale*; and is transmitted by the bite of female anopheline mosquitoes. Infections are diagnosed through examination of thick and thin blood films for parasites within red cells; speciation depends on their morphology and requires a skilled microscopist. More recently, point-of-care malaria antigen detection 'dipsticks' have been developed, which provide rapid and highly sensitive and specific diagnosis of falciparum and non-falciparum malaria. *Pla. falciparum* causes the most severe infection and is a common cause of death among young children in endemic regions; the other species cause 'benign' malaria, although *Pla. vivax* has recently been associated with more severe disease, especially in parts of South East Asia.

Although indigenous malaria is now virtually restricted to the tropics and subtropics, it is commonly imported into many temperate countries because of the rapid increase in international travel. About 2,000 cases of imported malaria are recorded in the UK each year—a figure likely to be an underestimate because of considerable under-reporting.

### Falciparum malaria

Falciparum malaria is divided into uncomplicated or severe disease. Uncomplicated malaria is defined as symptomatic malaria without evidence of vital organ dysfunction. It can be treated

**Helminths**

**Protozoa**

**Namatodes (roundworms)**
**Intestinal:**
- Ascaris lumbricoides
- Enterobius vermicularis
- Trichuris trichuria
- Strongyloides stercoralis
- Ancylostoma duodenale
- Necator americanis

**Filarial/tissue:**
- Wunchereria bancrofti
- Brugia sp.
- Onchocerca volvulus
- Trichinella sp.
- Dracunculus sp. (guinea worm)

**Trematodes (flukes)**
- Schistosoma sp.
- Pargonimus sp.
- Fasciolopsis buski
- Fasciola hepatica
- Opisthorchis sinensis

**Cestodes (tapeworms)**
- Taenia sp.
- Echinococcus sp.
- Diphylobotrum latum

**Amoebae**
- Entamoeba histolytica
- Acanthamoeba sp.
- Naegleria sp.

**Flagellates**
- Giardia lamblia
- Trichomonas vaginalis
- Trypanosoma sp.
- Leishmania sp.

**Sporozoa**
**Intestinal:**
- Isospora belli
- Cryptosporidium parvum
- Cyclospora sp.

**Blood/tissue:**
- Plasmodium sp.
- Toxoplasma gondii

**Others**
*Microsporidia*
- Enterocytozoon
- Encephalocytozoon
*Ciliates*
Balantidium coli
*Babesia*

**Fig. 35.1** Classification of medically important parasites.

with orally delivered medication. The presence of one or more of the following variables defines severe malaria:

- Clinical features
  - Impaired consciousness or unrousable coma
  - Prostration, that is, generalized weakness so that the patient is unable walk or sit up without assistance
  - Failure to feed
  - Multiple convulsions—more than two episodes in 24 hours
  - Deep breathing, respiratory distress (acidotic breathing)
  - Circulatory collapse or shock; systolic blood pressure <70 mm Hg in adults and <50 mm Hg in children
  - Clinical jaundice plus evidence of other vital organ dysfunction
  - Haemoglobinuria
  - Abnormal spontaneous bleeding
  - Pulmonary oedema (radiological)
- Laboratory findings
  - Hypoglycaemia (blood glucose <2.2 mmol/l or <40 mg/dl)

- Metabolic acidosis (plasma bicarbonate <15 mmol/l)
- Severe normocytic anaemia (haemoglobin <5 g/dl, packed cell volume <15%)
- Haemoglobinuria
- Hyperparasitaemia (>2%/100,000/µl in low intensity transmission areas or >5% or 250,000/µl in areas of high stable malaria transmission intensity)
- Hyperlactataemia (lactate >5 mmol/l)
- Renal impairment (serum creatinine >265 µmol/l)

After the Second World War, chloroquine replaced the traditional remedy quinine as the drug of choice for the treatment of falciparum malaria. These agents are active against the blood forms of the parasite, which is important in the symptomatic stage of the disease when rapidly dividing schizonts cause red cell lysis. In its time, chloroquine revolutionized the treatment and prophylaxis of malaria, but extensive use led to the global spread of resistant strains of *Pla. falciparum*. Surprisingly for such an ancient remedy, resistance to quinine remains quite rare and the drug returned to favour for severe falciparum malaria, but has now replaced by the artemisinin derivatives because of their greater effectiveness.

Derivatives of a Chinese herbal remedy, qinghaosu (artemisinin), have become the major drugs in the treatment of *Pla. falciparum* infections. In April 2011, the WHO recommended artesunate as the first-line treatment of severe malaria (Table 35.1) in children and adults on the basis that large, international, multicentre clinical trials have shown it reduces mortality compared to quinine. Although animal experiments revealed a potential for neurotoxicity at very high dose, extensive trials, and increasing clinical experience have shown these compounds are safe. Various formulations, including artesunic acid (artesunate), artemotil (β-arteether), and artemether have been deployed for intravenous or intramuscular administration but artesunate is most widely used. Artesunate can also be given by mouth or rectal suppository, which is particularly useful in children. Artemisinin derivatives are now also recommended by the WHO as the drugs of choice in uncomplicated falciparum malaria, since they are more rapidly effective than any other drug. Because of the risk of encouraging the development of resistance, which has recently been reported in South East Asia, the WHO strongly recommends that artemisinin derivatives should be used together with other antimalarial drugs. Artemether with lumefantrine can be given orally; alternative combinations include with amodiaquine, mefloquine, or sulphonamide–pyrimethamine, although resistance to these agents can occur.

**Table 35.1** Spectrum of activity of drugs used in the treatment of intestinal helminth infections.*

| Drug | *Ancylostoma duodenale* | *Necator americanus* | *Ascaris lumbricoides* | *Strongyloides stercoralis* | *Trichuris trichiura* | *Enterobius vermicularis* |
|---|---|---|---|---|---|---|
| Piperazine | − | − | +++ | − | − | +++ |
| Levamisole | ++ | ++ | +++ | − | − | − |
| Pyrantel pamoate | ++ | ++ | +++ | + | ++ | +++ |
| Albendazole | +++ | ++ | +++ | ++ | ++ | +++ |
| Mebendazole | ++ | ++ | +++ | + | ++ | +++ |
| Tiabendazole | ++ | ++ | ++ | ++ | − | ++ |

* +++, Highly effective; +, poorly effective; −, no useful activity.

Mefloquine, a quinolinemethanol derivative, is usually active against chloroquine-resistant strains and has been successfully used for treatment. However, resistance to mefloquine emerged readily and has limited its use. Moreover, mefloquine use has been associated with neuropsychiatric side effects that may persist for some time owing to the very long plasma half-life of the drug. Halofantrine has a shorter half-life (1–4 days, compared with 2–4 weeks) and fewer adverse reactions but can cause cardiotoxicity with dysrhythmias. The related lumefantrine is safer but is available only in a combination product with artemether.

## 'Benign' malaria

*Pla. vivax*, *Pla. ovale*, and *Pla. malariae* have generally retained susceptibility to chloroquine, which remains the drug of choice in the treatment of these infections. However, to affect a radical cure in *Pla. vivax* and *Pla. ovale* infections, which have a latent exo-erythrocytic phase, it is necessary to also use the 8-aminoquinoline, primaquine. Importantly, patients must be screened for glucose-6-phosphate dehydrogenase deficiency prior to primaquine administration. Low levels of this red blood cell enzyme occur in many populations in endemic areas, and administration of primaquine to such individuals may lead to an acute haemolytic crisis. Primaquine should not be used during pregnancy.

## Antimalarial prophylaxis

Advice on prophylaxis against malaria presents a problem because of the difficulty in predicting drug resistance. Chloroquine has been widely used, but the spread of resistance in *Pla. falciparum* means it is no longer useful. Moreover, it has a bitter taste and more serious side effects such as skin photosensitization and retinal damage may become apparent after prolonged use.

In the United Kingdom, the most commonly recommended agents for antimalarial prophylaxis are mefloquine, doxycycline, or atovaquone–proguanil ('Malarone'). Mefloquine is less used now because of the rise of resistance to the drug and the neuropsychiatric side effects. Doxycycline is generally well tolerated, although can cause gastritis and photosensitivity and is unsuitable for pregnant women and young children. Atovaquone–proguanil is effective and well tolerated but is expensive.

Advice on the choice of prophylactic regimen is under constant review depending on information on drug resistance in individual travel destinations and the availability of new agents. It is therefore wise for anyone counselling a traveller to a malarious area to seek advice from a specialist or make use of the excellent databases held nationally by travel clinics and the expert tropical medicine institutes. The choice of agent—or the decision to take any antimalarial—is a risk assessment that depends on the duration and likelihood of exposure against toxicity.

The most important aspects of prophylaxis are regular medication and continuance of therapy after the last possible exposure in order to eradicate any residual parasites. Prophylaxis needs to continue after leaving the malarious area for 1 week for atovaquone-proguanil and for 4 weeks for other regimens. The reason for the shorter duration with atovaquone–proguanil is that it has the ability to act on the liver and blood stage of the malaria infection, whereas all other regimens only act on the blood stage. It is important for travellers to understand that prophylaxis does not prevent infection entirely and that, if they develop fever, they should always seek medical advice. It is not essential to premedicate patients but it is advisable to start the drugs a week before travelling in order to ensure tolerability. Atovaquone–proguanil only needs to be started 1 to 2 days before travelling. Of great importance, but often neglected, is practical advice to keep exposed parts of the body covered, especially in the evening when mosquitoes are active, and to use insect repellents such as diethyltoluamide (DEET). Screening windows and sleeping under mosquito nets impregnated with insecticide (permethrin) also prevent malaria.

## Amoebiasis

*Entamoeba histolytica* may live harmlessly in the lumen of the gut, usually in the cyst form, or may invade the gut mucosa to cause amoebic dysentery. Secondary spread from the primary intestinal focus sometimes occurs to give rise to distant abscess formation, usually in the liver. The factors that govern the transformation from harmless commensal to invasive pathogen are poorly understood. Over the years, the clinical picture and disease pathogenesis has been further confused by *Enta. dispar*, a non-pathogenic commensal amoeba with morphologically indistinguishable cysts to *Enta. histolytica*.

Acute intestinal amoebiasis is characterized by bloody diarrhoea and abdominal pain. It can be diagnosed by fresh stool microscopy and the demonstration of motile trophozoites with phagocytosed red cells. Serological tests are especially helpful in invasive disease, for example, when trying to distinguish pyogenic bacterial from amoebic liver abscess.

The treatment of symptomless cyst passers, especially those living in endemic areas, is not worthwhile unless there is evidence of recurrent attacks of dysentery. Metronidazole or tinadazole are the first-line therapies and should be continued for 3–5 days. Both give a high cure rate. It is common practice in the developed world to follow metronidazole with a cyst-killing agent, diloxanide furoate, for 10 days. This reduces the risk of ongoing transmission and disease relapse.

Invasion of trophozoites into tissues, especially into the liver, may occur without dysentery, and the first indication of amoebiasis may be a hepatic abscess. Metronidazole or tinidazole therapy needs to be of longer duration than with uncomplicated gastrointestinal disease; although most cases respond within 72 hours, treatment for 5–10 days is recommended. Where there is a very large abscess, surgical aspiration may speed recovery but antibiotics alone are usually sufficient. There is no evidence of drug resistance in amoebae.

## Giardiasis

The flagellate protozoon *Giardia lamblia* is a parasite of the proximal small bowel. There is no invasion of the surface, the trophozoite being attached to the mucosa. Cysts are passed in the stools, and infection is transmitted by contamination of food and water. *Giardia* is a frequent cause of chronic diarrhoea. However, many infections are asymptomatic and, even with a heavy infection in adults, the symptoms may be mild: nausea, flatulence, and steatorrhoea. In young children the condition may give rise to malabsorption. Although worldwide in distribution, this intestinal infection, like most, is more common in less hygienic communities. Giardiasis is fairly common in the United Kingdom as well as being the most frequently imported parasitic disease.

Metronidazole or tinadazole are the treatments of choice, administered in a similar regimen to that used to treat amoebic dysentery. Cases that do not respond to metronidazole/tinadazole may respond to mepacrine (quinacrine) or paromomycin.

## Cryptosporidiosis

*Cryptosporidium parvum* is a common cause of acute diarrhoea in people who have had direct contact with animals or have drunk contaminated water. The disease is generally mild and self-limiting in otherwise healthy individuals, and fluid replacement is all that is usually required. Nitazoxanide appears to be effective if treatment is thought to be necessary. Various drugs, including the macrolide azithromycin and the aminoglycoside paromomycin, have been used (alone or in combination) with modest results against the more severe disease seen in patients with AIDS. Whether nitazoxamide therapy is effective in these patients is presently unclear. Fortunately, the incidence of the disease has declined in this group since effective antiretroviral therapy has become available.

## African trypanosomiasis

African trypanosomiasis (sleeping sickness) is caused by two subspecies of the parasite *Trypanosoma brucei*: *rhodesiensea* and *gambiense*. Both are transmitted by tsetse flies. *Tryp. brucei rhodesiense* is a sporadic disease in east and central Africa, although occasional outbreaks occur. The clinical course of the disease found in this area is more acute than that caused by *Tryp. brucei gambiense*, which is a major health hazard in rural West Africa. Both parasites eventually infect the brain to give the clinical manifestations of 'sleeping sickness'. Before this stage a clinical diagnosis is difficult because of the non-specific nature of the symptoms. However, an early diagnosis is important as treatment is more effective and less toxic at this stage. Laboratory confirmation may be difficult to obtain except in specialized centres because the trypanosomes are often scanty in peripheral blood. Before central nervous system involvement, suramin or pentamidine may be used in therapy but, when a lumbar puncture indicates meningoencephalitis, it is necessary to use an organic arsenical. Melarsoprol has replaced the more toxic tryparsamide for this purpose, although it can cause a haemorrhagic encephalopathy. All the antitrypanosomal drugs are toxic; treatment should be given in hospital and expert advice sought.

An important advance in the treatment of sleeping sickness caused by *Tryp. brucei gambiense* has been achieved with the introduction of eflornithine. This drug is effective even in the late meningoencephalitic stages of the disease but is expensive. *Tryp. brucei rhodesiense* is less sensitive to treatment with eflornithine. Nifurtimox may have a role in the second-line treatment of melarsoprol-refractory disease and in combination chemotherapy.

## Chagas disease

This form of trypanosomiasis is widespread in South America. The causative organism, *Tryp. cruzi*, invades heart muscle, causing myocardial damage which may eventually be fatal. Nifurtimox is a nitrofuran and interferes with the carbohydrate metabolism of the parasite. Adverse effects include gastrointestinal disturbances and neurological complications. These are dose related and rapidly reversible after discontinuation of the drug.

Benznidazole is a nitroimidazole derivate. It is more effective than nifurtimox and is now the drug of choice. It is tolerated better by children than adults. Adverse effects comprise allergic skin reactions (exfoliative dermatitis), gastrointestinal disturbances (weight loss, anorexia), neurological complications (peripheral neuritis), and haematological alterations (bone marrow suppression).

## Leishmaniasis

The parasite *Leishmania* causes cutaneous, mucocutaneous, and visceral (kala-azar) leishmaniasis. About 10 million cases of cutaneous leishmaniasis and 400,000 cases of visceral leishmaniasis occur worldwide each year. Phlebotomine sand-flies transmit leishmaniasis from infected animals to humans or from person to person.

### Kala-azar

Visceral leishmaniasis, kala-azar, is caused by *Lei. donovani*, *Lei. infantum*, and *Lei. chagasi*, all of which are widespread, including the Mediterranean, but 90 per cent of cases occur in north-east

India/Bangladesh, Sudan/Ethiopia/Kenya, or Brazil. Visceral leishmaniasis is a chronic, often fatal, condition characterized by fever, anaemia, and gross splenomegaly. Microscopy and culture of bone marrow or splenic aspirate confirm the diagnosis.

Most patients with visceral leishmaniasis are treated with pentavalent antimonials, amphotericin B, or lipid-associated amphotericin B. Pentavalent antimonials have been traditionally used, although relapse due to drug resistance or inadequate dosage and duration of treatment is not uncommon, especially in India. Sodium stibogluconate or meglumine antimonate is given by the parenteral route in high dosage for at least 30 days but toxic effects such as pancreatitis and cardiac irregularities are common.

Amphotericin B is the first-line drug treatment of kala-azar in India, where resistance to pentavalent antimonials is common. The best amphotericin B regimen is 20 doses of 1 mg/kg on alternate days. Amphotericin B is effective in advanced mucocutaneous leishmaniasis, for which there is a high failure rate with pentavalent antimonials. Liposomal amphotericin is very effective and less toxic but is much more expensive.

Treatment of leishmaniasis continues to evolve. Miltefosine, an oral agent originally developed as an anticancer agent, is now in successful use in India. Paromomycin is an effective alternative agent.

## Cutaneous and mucocutaneous leishmaniasis

Several *Leishmania* species are responsible for cutaneous leishmaniasis. *Lei. tropica* causes anthroponotic cutaneous leishmaniasis in urban areas, *Lei. major* causes zoonotic disease in rural areas, and *Lei. aethiopica* causes cutaneous leishmaniasis in Ethiopia and parts of Kenya. Cutaneous leishmaniasis in the Americas is caused by the *Lei. mexicana* complex and the *Lei. braziliensis* complex. Mediterranean and European cases are usually caused by *Lei. infantum*. Cutaneous leishmaniasis is usually localized and often resolves spontaneously. Topical paromomycin or injections of sodium stibogluconate into the margins of the lesion aid resolution. Mucocutaneous leishmaniasis complicates around 5–10 per cent of cutaneous cases cause by the *Lei. braziliensis* complex and is most common in Peru and Bolivia. It requires systemic treatment with antimonials and may also need surgical intervention. Amphotericin B and miltefosine are alternative agents. Ketoconazole and itraconazole are effective in cutaneous leishmaniasis caused by *Lei. major* or *Lei. mexicana*, but less so against *Lei. tropica*, *Lei. aethiopica*, and *Lei. braziliensis*. Short courses of intramuscular pentamidine are effective in American cutaneous leishmaniasis.

## Co-infection with HIV

Disseminated, visceral leishmaniasis is much more common in those with untreated HIV. Relatively minor cutaneous lesions that would respond to topical treatment or self-heal in the immune competent person can present as disseminated disease that is difficult to cure. Most patients respond well to standard therapy (e.g. amphotericin B) but the incidence of relapse is high unless the HIV is treated and immune suppression lifted.

# Toxoplasmosis

*Toxoplasma gondii* is a ubiquitous organism that normally passes harmlessly from rodents to cats but can cause human infection by ingestion with contaminated food or close contact with infected cats. Toxoplasma infections may cause death or abnormalities in the foetus by transplacental spread during pregnancy. However, many infections pass unrecognized and the parasite may encyst in muscle or brain. Latent organisms then re-emerge in immunocompromised individuals to cause cerebral toxoplasmosis, which may present like a brain abscess in AIDS patients.

The antifolate combination pyrimethamine–sulfadiazine is the usual treatment except during pregnancy, when spiramycin is used. Clindamycin and clarithromycin are alternatives.

## Other protozoan infections

Treatment of infection with intestinal protozoa such as *Isospora belli*, *Cyclospora cayetanensis*, and various microsporidia is poorly defined, although co-trimoxazole (isosporiasis and cyclosporiasis) and albendazole (microsporidiosis) have been successfully used. In patients with AIDS, these opportunist infections usually remit when the CD4 lymphocyte count improves on antiretroviral therapy.

Babesiosis is a rare infection, usually caused by *Babesia divergens* and more common in splenectomized patients. It can be life threatening. There is evidence that the combination of clindamycin and quinine is useful but exchange transfusion may also be needed. Infection with *Bab. microti* in previously healthy persons is usually self-limiting but clindamycin and quinine can be used if therapy is warranted. The combination of azithromycin and atovaquone has also been used with success.

Treatment of infection with the flagellate protozoon *Tri. vaginalis* is considered in Chapter 24.

# Helminth infections

## Nematode infections

### Filariasis

Well over 200 million people harbour filarial worms and, in some areas of the tropics, nearly the whole population is infected. Diagnosis is made by microscopical demonstration of the larval forms (microfilariae) in blood or, in the special case of *Onchocerca volvulus*, in superficial shavings of skin. Some of the blood microfilariae exhibit a curious periodicity in that they are found in peripheral blood during only the day (*Loa loa*) or the night (*Wuchereria bancrofti*). *Brugia malayi* (which is restricted to South East Asia) usually exhibits a less complete nocturnal periodicity. *W. bancrofti* and *Bru. malayi* cause a clinically identical condition (lymphatic filariasis) sometimes resulting in elephantiasis owing to blockage of the lymphatics of the lower trunk. The clinical syndrome is due to a variety of factors depending on degree of exposure and host reaction to the worms and, in any area, a small proportion will have gross elephantiasis. Often by this stage, the disease may be 'burnt out', and an anthelminthic may do little to improve the patient's condition, for which surgical and supportive measures are all that is left. *O. volvulus*, the causative parasite of river blindness, affects large numbers of people in West Africa and Central America. As with the other filariases, many infected persons exhibit only minor symptoms such as skin swelling and itching.

The introduction of ivermectin and albendazole has revolutionized the therapy of filarial infections. These relatively non-toxic drugs are now preferred for the treatment of onchocerciasis and lymphatic filariasis, respectively. One of the benefits of their use is that reactions to treatment are a good deal milder than with the traditional drug, diethylcarbamazine, although ivermectin sometimes gives rise to an encephalopathy in individuals co-infected with *Loa loa*. Ivermectin is administered as a single oral dose, which is repeated annually in endemic areas. Mass treatment with ivermectin, together with vector control, has virtually eradicated onchocerciasis in some districts, and there are hopes that lymphatic filariasis will be similarly controlled with a combination of ivermectin and albendazole. The manufacturers of these drugs are providing them free for control programmes in countries where the diseases are endemic.

## Toxocariasis

Infection with the dog roundworm *Toxocara canis* may cause a condition known as visceral larva migrans, which may result in serious eye infection usually presenting as a visual loss in childhood. Although not a common disease, it is found worldwide and is probably under-recognized. The larvae of the worm migrate to the retina, setting up an inflammatory response. Treatment with diethylcarbamazine has been recommended but hypersensitivity reactions may require steroids to be given as well. Albendazole (or mebendazole) appears to offer an effective and less toxic alternative.

## Intestinal nematode infections

Single doses of the common agents such as piperazine, levamisole, and pyrantel pamoate give acceptable cure rates. Table 35.1 shows the differential activity of these and the oral benzimidazole derivatives, which have a broader spectrum and have largely superseded them but are more expensive. Among benzimidazoles, albendazole exhibits the best broad-spectrum anthelminthic activity. Tiabendazole (thiabendazole) is often poorly tolerated and is best avoided if possible. Ivermectin is the best treatment of *Strongyloides stercoralis* infections, which can cause serious, 'hyperinfection' syndrome with widespread dissemination of the parasite and associated Gram-negative bacteraemia and meningitis.

In warm countries with poor water supplies and inadequate methods of sewage disposal, re-infection with intestinal worms is almost inevitable, although simple health education advice on preventive measures may be valuable.

# Trematode (fluke) infections

## Schistosomiasis (bilharzia)

There are five recognized species of schistosome that affect humans. *Schistosoma haematobium* is the most widely distributed and is found in Africa, Asia, South America, the Caribbean, and the Middle East. *Sch. mansoni* is found in Africa, Asia, and the Middle East. *Sch. japonicum* is restricted to Asia. *Sch. mekongi* and *Sch. intercalatum* are restricted to South East Asia and Africa, respectively.

Schistosome adult worms adopt a more or less benign relationship with the host. In contrast, the eggs cause fibrosis, tissue damage, and the clinical manifestations of schistosomiasis. Acute schistosomiasis—Katayama fever—is most commonly seen with *Sch. japonicum*. Symptoms include fever, malaise, cough, wheeze, and urticaria. The clinical manifestations of chronic infection are dependent on the species. *Sch. haematobium* and, to a lesser extent, *Sch. intercalatum* primarily cause symptoms and signs in the urogenital tract, with haematuria, fibrosis, strictures, and an increased risk of malignancy. Infection with the non-haematobium species (particularly *Sch. mansoni*) leads to egg deposition in the intestinal mucosa and liver. Egg deposition in the liver may lead to hepatic enlargement and, over time, granuloma formation and fibrosis, which can lead to portal hypertension. Splenomegaly, oesophageal varices, and ascites can all occur.

One drug, praziquantel, is effective against all the major types of schistosomiasis and offers the possibility of single-dose therapy for mass treatment campaigns. The drug is extremely well tolerated; the main side effects are abdominal pain, and sometimes nausea and vomiting. In patients with CNS involvement, corticosteroids are often used in conjunction with praziquantel to minimize the inflammation around granulomata. Less useful alternatives include oxamniquine, which is active only against *Sch. mansoni*, and metrifonate (trichlorfon), which is effective against the urinary form, *Sch. haematobium*.

## Other trematode infections

Praziquantel has also transformed the treatment of most other trematode infections, including those caused by the Chinese liver fluke *Clonorchis sinensis* and the lung fluke *Paragonimus westermani*. However, the liver fluke *Fasciola hepatica* does not usually respond to praziquantel. The treatment of fascioliasis is problematic but the veterinary anthelminthic triclabendazole may be effective.

# Cestode infections

## Tapeworms

In addition to its use in trematode infections, praziquantel has emerged as an important agent in the treatment of tapeworm infections, including those caused by *Taenia saginata*, *Tae. solium*, *Diphyllobothrium latum*, and *Hymenolepis nana*. A single oral dose is usually effective, although more prolonged therapy is needed in cerebral cysticercosis caused by *Tae. solium*. In intestinal tapeworm infection, niclosamide is a suitable alternative.

## Hydatid disease

Surgery to remove hydatid cysts after injection of a scolicide such as hypotonic saline, formalin, or cetrimide into the cyst remains the treatment of choice in hydatid disease but is not without risk. Therapy with benzimidazole derivatives, particularly albendazole, has been successful in some cases and may be the only option in inoperable conditions, including disease caused by *Echinococcus multilocularis*.

# Ectoparasites

A variety of arthropods feed on human blood. Some, such as ticks, lice, and mosquitoes, may act as vectors of disease; others, including most mites and fleas, are more of a nuisance. These parasites of the ectoderm are often visible and may produce skin lesions and itching after biting. It is estimated that over half the children in UK schools have head lice at some time, and scabies is common in the elderly in institutions.

## Scabies

The mite *Sarcoptes scabiei* causes scabies in man and is spread by close contact. The commonest sites of infection are the hands, wrists, forearm, and axillae, or the genitalia after sexual contact. The mite burrows into the skin to form tunnels, which are diagnostic of the condition. There is often a more generalized hypersensitivity rash away from the area of penetration. All areas are itchy, and scratching can lead to secondary bacterial infections, including impetigo.

Benzyl benzoate is effective but is unpleasant to use, frequently causes irritation, and is not recommended for children. This has led to the use of the pyrethroid permethrin and the organophosphorus compound malathion. Malathion should not be used repeatedly over a short period. Lindane (hexachlorocyclohexane; now discontinued in the United Kingdom) is strongly suspected to be carcinogenic and should not be used.

The key to treatment of scabies is careful, complete application of the lotion and reapplication if hands have been washed during the period the insecticide is in contact with the skin. The whole body should be covered, with particular attention to hands, fingers, and nails, and left to act overnight, or preferably for 24 hours.

Immunocompromised patients, such as those with HIV, may develop a very heavy infestation that may crust over—so-called Norwegian scabies. Oral treatment with ivermectin can be effective.

## Lice

The most common infestation in the developed world is due to head lice (*Pediculus capitis*). The adult lice pass from person to person during close contact and attach their eggs (nits) to hair. The infestation may spread in schools and the community, and total eradication is probably impossible, though most people develop resistance to re-infection.

There is no ideal insecticide for the treatment of head lice. Lice resistant to permethrin, phenothrin, and malathion, which are the agents in current use, occur; carbaryl is usually effective but there are fears about possible toxicity. 'Wet combing', by passing a fine-tooth comb through hair that has just been washed with conditioner, is useful but should be repeated two to three times a week for several weeks to remove all the lice. Various herbal shampoos such as those containing tea tree oil have advocates but there is little evidence that they are effective. Shaving the head is a drastic measure, which is not recommended.

Pubic lice (*Phthirus pubis*; 'crab' lice) hold tenaciously to pubic hair but can also be found on the head and eyelashes. Aqueous preparations of insecticides such as malathion should be applied overnight to all parts of the body. Pubic lice are generally easier to treat than head lice but it is important to find and treat sexual contacts and to remember that other sexually transmitted infections may be present.

## Key points

- Parasites (protozoa, helminths, and arthropods) tend to cause chronic disease, and many individuals, once infected, remain so for long periods.

- Parasitic infections are particularly common in tropical countries. However, some parasites such as *Tri. vaginalis*, threadworm, and head lice are at least as common in developed countries. Moreover, international travel ensures that infections acquired in the tropics may present to medical practitioners everywhere.

- Falciparum malaria is the most important of all parasitic diseases, killing more people than any other parasite.

- Artesunate is now recommended as the treatment of choice for falaciparum malaria and is more effective than quinine for severe malaria. Artesunate should be combined with another antimalarial to prevent resistance.

## Further reading

Checkley, A. M., Chiodini, P. L., Dockrell, D. H., et al. (2010) Eosinophilia in returning travellers and migrants from the tropics: UK recommendations for investigation and initial management. *The Journal of Infection*, 60(1): 1–20.

Johnston, V., Stockley, J. M., Dockrell, D., et al. (2009) Fever in returned travellers presenting in the United Kingdom: recommendations for investigation and initial management. *The Journal of Infection*, 59(1): 1–18.

Lalloo, D. G., Shingadia, D., Pasvol, G., Chiodini, P. L., Whitty, C. J., Beeching, N. J., Hill, D. R., Warrell, D. A., and Bannister, B. A. (2007) UK malaria treatment guidelines. *The Journal of Infection*, 54(2): 111–21.

# Chapter 36

# The development and marketing of antimicrobial drugs

## Introduction to the development and marketing of antimicrobial drugs

Until the 1990s, most effort towards the discovery and development of new antimicrobial agents was expended on compounds active against bacteria but the demands of the marketplace have caused the emphasis to shift. Of 67 new antimicrobial agents released to the UK market between 1990 and 2004 (Table 36.1), only 26 (39%) were antibacterial agents; in the subsequent 9 years, only 4 of 18 (22%) new antimicrobial agents were antibacterials. Antiviral agents now represent the largest single group of newly marketed compounds. Moreover, nearly all new antibacterial agents are chemically modified variants of existing compounds, although entirely new classes of antiviral and antifungal agents have emerged. Fourteen classes of antibiotics were introduced for human use between 1935 and 1968; since then, only six have been developed (Fig. 36.1). There is a particular lack of new agents with novel targets or mechanisms of action against multidrug-resistant Gram-negative bacteria.

The cost of development of a new antimicrobial, risk of failure to gain regulatory approval (especially considering the number of current agents), and perceived profit margin (unlike drugs prescribed for chronic diseases, antibiotics are typically given for only a few days to each patient) has led to many pharmaceutical companies ceasing development of antibiotics. Only five major pharmaceutical companies (GlaxoSmithKline, Novartis, AstraZeneca, Merck, and Pfizer) still had active antibacterial discovery programmes in 2008. In the same year an investigation of the development pipeline of both small and large pharmaceutical companies found that only 15 of 167 antimicrobial agents had a new mechanism of action with the potential to meet the challenge of multidrug resistance. Most of those were in the early phases of development and thus the chance of these successfully navigating the clinical investigation pathway required for new drugs is slim (Fig. 36.2).

When a new antimicrobial drug is discovered or invented, the first indications of its activity and spectrum are usually gleaned from fairly simple in vitro inhibition tests against a few common representative organisms. Organisms with special growth requirements, such as chlamydiae, mycobacteria, and mycoplasmas, are usually excluded from such primary screening. In vitro screening tests will not detect potentially useful activity if in vivo metabolism of the compound is a prerequisite for the antimicrobial effect (e.g. Prontosil; see 'The foundations of modern chemotherapy' in Chapter 1); nor will such tests reveal agents that might modify microbial cells sufficiently to render them non-virulent or susceptible to host defences, without actually preventing their growth. Furthermore, conventional laboratory culture media occasionally contain substances that interfere with the activity of certain antimicrobial compounds, which may consequently go undetected.

**Table 36.1** Newly marketed antimicrobial agents in 3-year periods 1990–2013 (UK).

| Period | Antibacterial agents | Antiviral agents | Antifungal agents | Antiparasitic agents |
|---|---|---|---|---|
| 1990–1992 | 10 | 1 | 2 | 2 |
| 1993–1995 | 7 | 4 | 1 | 1 |
| 1996–1998 | 3 | 9 | 1 | 1 |
| 1999–2001 | 3 | 8 | 0 | 1 |
| 2002–2004 | 3 | 8 | 2 | 0 |
| 2005–2007 | 3 | 7 | 1 | 0 |
| 2008–2010 | 1 | 4 | 2 | 0 |
| 2011–2013 | 3 | 3 | 0 | 1 |

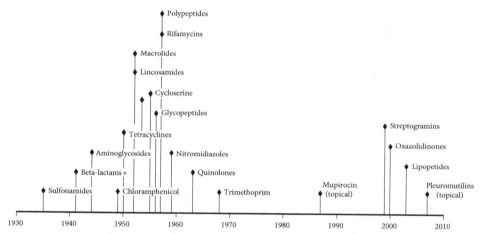

**Fig. 36.1** Antibacterial classes introduced between 1930 and 2010.

Despite these difficulties, in vitro screening offers an extremely simple and generally effective way of detecting antimicrobial activity and has yielded a rich harvest of therapeutically useful compounds over the years. In contrast, the rational design of antimicrobial agents that can disable vulnerable stages of microbial development has not been very fruitful so far, although the use of newer approaches such as genomics, molecular modelling, and combinatorial chemistry offer the prospect that this might change in the future. Indeed, some of the new antiviral agents have been developed by targeting specific viral processes.

## Development of new compounds

Compounds that pass the initial screening tests must be made available in sufficient quantities and in sufficiently pure form to enable preliminary tests of toxicity and efficacy to be carried out in laboratory animals, and more extensive and precise in vitro tests to be performed. Pilot-stage production usually presents little problem, although considerable difficulties may be experienced

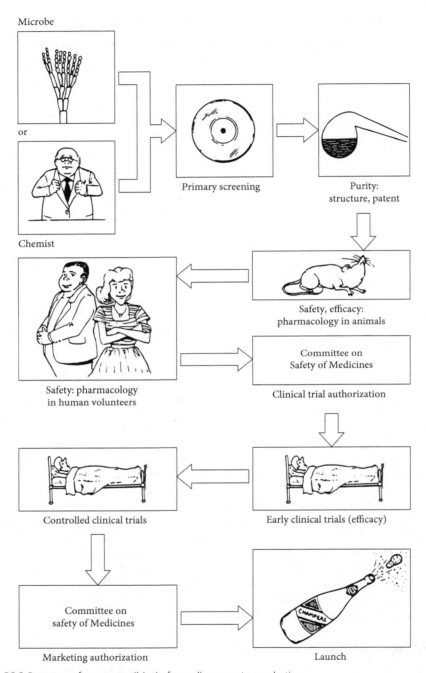

**Fig. 36.2** Progress of a new antibiotic from discovery to marketing.

in scaling up production at a later date, when relatively large quantities of highly purified drug are needed for clinical trials and subsequent marketing.

Animal tests of toxicity, pharmacology, and efficacy are an indispensable part of the development of any new drug but they also have certain limitations. Idiosyncratic reactions may suggest toxicity in a compound that would be safe for human use or, more importantly, adverse reactions peculiar to the human subject may go undetected. The pharmacological handling of the drug may be vastly different from that encountered in the human subject. As regards efficacy testing, animals have important limitations in that experimental infections seldom correspond to the supposedly analogous human condition, either anatomically or in the relationship of treatment to the natural history of the disease process.

If preliminary tests of toxicity and efficacy indicate that the compound is worth advancing further, full-scale acute and chronic toxicity tests are carried out in animals. These include long-term tests of mutagenic or carcinogenic potential, effects on fertility, and teratogenicity. Mutagenicity tests may also be performed in microbial systems (Ames test).

Provided the animal toxicity studies reveal no serious toxicity problems, the first tentative (Phase 1) trials are undertaken in healthy human volunteers to investigate the pharmacokinetic properties and safety of the new drug in man. Although animal data provide only a crude estimate of how the drug may be handled in human beings, if properly interpreted, they allow an estimate to be made for the first human dose-ranging studies. Once these tests have been successfully completed, application may be made to the drug-licensing authority for permission to undertake (Phase 2 and 3) clinical trials.

## Clinical trials

The proof of the pudding is in the eating, and no amount of in vitro or animal testing can replace the ultimate test of safety and efficacy: therapeutic use in human infection. Nevertheless, the clinical trial stage remains, in many ways, the least satisfactory aspect of the testing of any new antimicrobial drug. The reasons for this are not difficult to find: 'infection' is not a static condition in which therapeutic intervention produces an all-or-none effect. Many factors, such as mobilization of the patient's own immune response, drainage of pus, or treatment of an underlying surgical or medical condition, may crucially affect the response to therapy. The patient may improve subjectively, even though the antimicrobial therapy has demonstrably failed to eradicate the supposed pathogen; conversely, the patient's condition may deteriorate despite bacteriological 'success'. Furthermore, ironically, patients recruited into phase 2 and 3 clinical trials of antimicrobial agents may not be truly representative of those for whom the need is greatest. Informed consent is rightly needed to enrol patients into clinical trials but this is frequently very difficult to obtain for sicker patients with serious infections.

## Design of trials

Clinical trials of new drugs are not undertaken lightly. They are difficult to design, tedious and expensive to perform, and fraught with ethical and regulatory pitfalls. Licensing authorities require studies to conform to strict standards of good clinical practice and good laboratory practice. Before undertaking a trial, a detailed protocol is required that defines the conditions for which the new treatment is intended, reasons to include/exclude patients in/from the trial (inclusion and exclusion criteria), the dosage regimens to be used, and the treatment with which it is to be compared.

Phase 2 clinical trials examine different dosages of the investigational drug, and the 'optimum' dosage is then restudied in larger phase 3 studies. In both settings a comparator (established) drug is typically used for some of the recruited patients and there is a key emphasis on collecting detailed information to assure that the new drug is not associated with unacceptable adverse events. Careful consideration should be given as to whether the trial should be open, single blind (treatment known to the prescriber only), or double blind (treatment randomly allocated in a fashion unknown to prescriber or recipient). In general, uncontrolled, open trials are unsatisfactory, except as preliminary indicators of safety and efficacy. They may also be used to gain information on the most appropriate dose of an agent. Controlled, double-blind trials are the most desirable scientifically but are subject to ethical difficulties in that the prescribing doctor does not have full control over the patient's treatment. Placebo-controlled or non-comparative studies are normally acceptable only if adequate treatment is unavailable or controversial.

## Ethical requirements

Ethical considerations need to be taken fully into account. The basic principles that should govern all research involving human subjects are embodied in the Declaration of Helsinki, which was adopted by the eighteenth World Medical Assembly in 1964, with subsequent revisions. In many countries, health authorities have ethical committees that monitor clinical trial protocols. The committee will need assurance that the safety of the new compound has been satisfactorily established and will wish to ensure that written informed patient consent is obtained from trial participants. It will also require adequate safeguards for the detection of unexpected adverse reactions and may have views as to whether a double-blind format or a placebo control is acceptable.

## Statistical considerations

Ambitious trials can fail because insufficient numbers of patients are found to fulfil the criteria required for the study. Alternatively, the condition may be one (acute cystitis is a good example) in which the natural cure rate is so high, and the efficacy of standard treatment so good, that huge numbers would have to be examined to establish the superiority of a new agent, although it may be possible to determine efficacy. It is essential to be reasonably sure, before the trial starts, that sufficient patients can be recruited to satisfy statistical requirements. During the conduct of the trial, regular checks of relevant microbiological, haematological, chemical, and radiological parameters should be made. All findings should be fully documented as soon as the information is available, rather than attempting to glean information from the patients' notes retrospectively, after the trial is completed.

Concerns about the proliferation of similar antibiotics for the same types of infections has recently led the Food and Drug Administration (FDA) to review its guidance on how new drugs are assessed (see 'Drug licensing'). Two issues have been highlighted in particular. First, there is a need to demonstrate that a new drug achieves early demonstrable clinical benefit; for example, fever resolution and lack of progression of skin lesions by the third day of therapy in patients with acute bacterial skin and skin structure infection. Second, controversial discussions are still ongoing over whether companies will be required to demonstrate that a new drug is superior to established treatment rather than simply similar or equivalent (i.e. statistically non-inferior to comparator). This may seem desirable but, in reality, could set the bar so high that it is a further disincentive to drug development.

# Drug licensing

Most countries have enacted some sort of legislation aimed at controlling the marketing of pharmaceutical products. In the United States, federal regulations are administered by the FDA. Within the European Union, a Committee on Proprietary Medicinal Products issues guidelines for harmonizing regulatory requirements among member nations. The European Medicines Agency (EMA), based in London, coordinates drug licensing and safety throughout the European Union, although companies can still seek registration of their products by national regulatory authorities.

In the United Kingdom, executive powers are invested in government health and agriculture ministers, who constitute the Licensing Authority. Ministers are advised directly through the Medicines and Healthcare Products Regulatory Agency (MHRA) of the Department of Health. The MHRA, through its specialist advisory committees, reviews all pharmaceutical products intended for medical or veterinary use. The licensing, manufacture, promotion, and distribution of all medicines intended for human use are supervised by the Commission on Human Medicines, which combines the functions of the Committee on Safety of Medicines (CSM) and the Medicines Commission. The Commission acts as an independent agency in relation to particular issues and concerns, including any challenge to the decisions of the Licensing Authority.

Before clinical trials can be performed on a new drug in the United Kingdom, full toxicological data and a detailed protocol must be submitted to the MHRA. Such applications are scrutinized by the CSM, who must satisfy themselves that all reasonable criteria are met before recommending that a clinical trial authorization should be issued. If the authorization is approved, investigators must undertake to notify any adverse reaction arising during the trial, or any other matter that might reasonably cause the Licensing Authority to doubt the safety or quality of the product.

When clinical trial data have been accumulated, an application for a marketing authorization (formerly called a product licence) may be made. All valid applications are again passed to the CSM for scrutiny. In the United Kingdom new applications are judged solely on the grounds of safety, efficacy, and quality. If marketing authorization is refused, the application may be withdrawn or the applicant may elect to answer the objections raised, either in writing or in person before the committee. Should the application still be refused, the applicant has the right of appeal to the Medicines Commission. Marketing authorizations, once issued, are valid for 5 years in the first instance.

Over the years, the requirements of licensing authorities worldwide (particularly for toxicological testing) have become progressively more stringent. Consequently, the cost of developing a new drug has escalated enormously. The period between the discovery and marketing of a new product is seldom less than 6 years and may be substantially longer, although fast-track procedures have enabled some drugs, notably those used in the treatment of HIV infection, to be licensed much more quickly. Shortening the period is important to the company marketing the new drug, since it maximizes the time during which it can recoup the cost of research and development (which may exceed £500 million) and profit from the discovery while enjoying patent protection. Attempts are being made to harmonize the drug registration requirements of Europe, the United States, and Japan but progress so far has been modest.

# Drug marketing

## Data sheets

All companies marketing products provided for the use of medical practitioners in the European Union are required to produce a Summary of Product Characteristics ('data sheet') giving relevant information about the drug, including the conditions for which its use is licensed, contraindications, and known side effects. Pharmaceutical firms in the United Kingdom collaborate in producing a Data Sheet Compendium, which is freely available to registered medical practitioners (online version: electronic Medicines Compendium is available at <http://emc.medicines.org.uk/>).

## Post-marketing surveillance

Issue of a marketing authorization is no guarantee that a compound is 100 per cent safe, nor even that all adverse reactions have been detected before marketing. Rare, serious adverse events may not be detected among the few thousand patients exposed to the new drug in the phase 2 and 3 studies. Marketing authorization for a new drug may only be granted on the condition that the company initiates a surveillance scheme to check on aspects of drug usage, including safety and/or the detection of resistance emergence. Also, the CSM in the United Kingdom issues postage-paid 'yellow cards' for the notification of adverse reactions. Although the scheme is voluntary, it is important that prescribers and pharmacists collaborate fully with it. Such notifications are particularly important in the first few years in which a new compound is marketed. Copies of the notification form are routinely included with each issue of the *British National Formulary*, and compounds under particular scrutiny are flagged with a black triangle.

## Relationship with the medical profession

In the United Kingdom, the conduct of pharmaceutical companies in marketing their products is regulated by the MHRA. There is also a voluntary Code of Practice drawn up by the Prescription Medicines Code of Practice Authority established by the Association of the British Pharmaceutical Industry in 1993 and re-issued in revised form in 2011 (available at <http://www.abpi.org.uk/Pages/default.aspx>). It covers, among many other things, the content and distribution of advertisements and other promotional literature; hospitality, gifts, and inducements to the medical and allied professions; marketing research; and relationships with the general public and lay communications media.

## Advertisements

The subject of advertising is a perennial bone of contention between health-care professionals and the pharmaceutical industry. The former complain that adverts may cloud their professional judgement; the latter claim their commercial right to exploit their products to their best advantage in the market place and point to the factual data sheets and other information services that they place at the disposal of the medical professions. The truth, as usual, inhabits the middle ground. Advertisements are subject to the usual advertising regulations and may not tell overt lies. Nonetheless, they are intended to sway the prescriber in favour of a particular product. They are clearly cost-effective and there is ample evidence of their influence on prescribing habits.

Doctors and other health-care workers should not delude themselves by claiming that they are uninfluenced by advertisements or other promotional activities. They should make a conscious effort to separate fact from fantasy in advertisements and cultivate a critical attitude, especially towards claims for new products. In particular, prescribers should learn to distinguish between genuine advances and new products, which, though effective, are no better than older, well-tried, and cheaper remedies. They should also be wary of impressive claims ostensibly based on published independent assessments which turn out, in the small print, to refer to unverifiable 'data on file' or papers published by, or on behalf of, the company involved.

## Sources of independent advice

Within the United Kingdom the National Institute for Health and Clinical Excellence and the Scottish Medicines Consortium offer expert independent guidance on the status of medical products. These two bodies have become increasingly influential on if and how newly licensed drugs are used in the NHS, particularly as their reviews can include cost-effectiveness assessments and comparisons with existent agents.

In addition, the *British National Formulary* and children's version (BNF and BNFC, both updated at 12 monthly intervals since Sept 2013), eBNF, and the *Drug and Therapeutics Bulletin* (published by the Consumers' Association), offer reliable sources of objective information to the prescriber. In the United States, the *National Formulary* and the *Medical Letter* provide a similar service. Many health authorities now produce therapeutic guides for use by medical staff in hospital or the community (see Chapter 20). Pharmacies often offer a drug information service to which medical practitioners have access, and most medical microbiology laboratories are able to offer accurate, up-to-date advice on antimicrobial therapy.

Although the marketing of drugs is fairly well regulated throughout the industrially developed world, the same is not true of less favoured countries; in many nations of the world the standards of advertising and marketing often appear to overstep the bounds of what would be considered ethical in more developed countries.

## Drug names

When a new antibiotic is first described in the scientific literature, it usually appears under a number representing the manufacturer's laboratory code for the compound. The reason for using a code is that names proposed by the manufacturer are not always subsequently accepted by the bodies controlling drug nomenclature. These are the British Pharmacopoeia Commission, who recommend a British Approved Name (BAN) to the Medicines Commission in the United Kingdom, the United States Adopted Name (USAN) Council in the United States, and equivalent bodies elsewhere. International agreement is coordinated by the World Health Organization, which specifies or recommends an International Non-Proprietary Name (INN; rINN). Within the European Union, the rINN is now in general use and has replaced the BAN for nearly all drugs used in the United Kingdom. In the case of antimicrobial drugs, conflated names such as co-trimoxazole and co-amoxiclav are still in use in the United Kingdom for combination products, whereas the full names of both components (e.g. trimethoprim–sulphamethoxazole) are preferred elsewhere.

Once the approved name is introduced into the national pharmacopoeia of a country, it becomes the official name. In addition to the approved or official name, the drug may have various proprietary names under which it is marketed and these trade names often differ widely throughout the world, especially if generic versions are available. Approved names try to avoid close nomenclatural similarities but the profusion of 'sulpha-s' 'cefa-s', '-cillins', and '-oxacins' still produces confusion; when the same compound is marketed under different proprietary names, bewilderment is often complete.

## Generic prescribing

There has been a good deal of debate as to whether doctors should use proprietary names in writing prescriptions. On the one hand, it is pointed out that formulations differ so that the pharmacological properties of a drug may vary from product to product. Moreover, adverse reactions caused by a particular formulation may be more easily detected if the product is specified. On the other hand, non-proprietary names are less likely to cause confusion; they remove the necessity of pharmacies keeping a large and varied stock of similar products, and enable the pharmacist to dispense the cheapest version of a particular drug. The BNF sensibly recommends prescribers to use non-proprietary names in all but those few instances where bioavailability problems are paramount. Policies of 'generic substitution', whereby pharmacists can dispense a generic version of a medicine even if a branded product is specified on the prescription, differ widely throughout the world.

## Whither antibiotics?

The number of antimicrobial drugs available to the prescriber is now enormous and, at least as far as antibacterial compounds are concerned, the undoubted value of having a wide and varied choice has been overtaken by the confusion that is caused by the conflicting claims of so many agents with similar or overlapping indications. There are justifiable fears about antimicrobial drug resistance but the fact remains that untreatable infection (due to antimicrobial resistance alone) is thankfully a rare phenomenon at this point. The availability of multiple antibacterial drugs to treat most common infections can present a dilemma over which is the most efficacious or cost-effective agent, remembering that an inexpensive antibiotic can translate into a very costly course of treatment if initial therapy fails.

Most general practitioners rely on a few favourite antibiotics to cover the treatment of most bacterial infections. The WHO includes only a handful of antibacterial agents in its list of essential medicines (Table 36.2). The availability of antimicrobial drugs varies extensively in different countries for reasons that must be commercial rather than therapeutic: for example, over 70 β-lactam antibiotics (including 40 cephalosporins) are on the market in Japan compared with 26 in the United Kingdom; the WHO's essential drugs list has only 12, 8 of which are penicillins.

Chemotherapeutic options for the treatment of non-bacterial infection remain very unsatisfactory. Although great strides have been made in the prevention of viral infection by immunization (Chapter 18), and there have been important developments in antiviral agents, notably for the treatment of HIV and hepatitis C infections, chemotherapy for viral disease is still extremely constrained (see Chapters 5–7). Some sort of effective chemotherapy is available for most fungal, protozoal, and helminth infections but the choice is very limited and, in many ways, unsatisfactory (see Chapters 8 and 9). On a global scale these conditions are responsible for much of the morbidity and mortality from infectious disease that afflicts mankind. A key challenge for the future is to provide for these diseases the same sort of safe, effective chemotherapy that is now available for most bacterial infections, and to make effective therapy for all infections readily available for those who need it most.

## How to encourage new antibiotic development

Antibiotics carry a unique threat in terms of drug development and deployment, in that their use undermines their future value from both the manufacturer's and patient's perspective, as bacteria evolve to become resistant. New antibiotics are urgently needed to address the threat posed by multiply drug-resistant bacteria, especially Gram-negative pathogens (see Chapter 10). However, the commercial viability for such new drugs is doubtful given the current way in which antibiotics are funded. The harsh truth is that the declining financial rewards available in this area have led pharmaceutical companies to divert many of their resources to the more lucrative field of antiviral and, to a lesser extent, antifungal compounds. Quite simply, new antibiotics that are used only very occasionally will need to be priced extremely highly compared with our experience to date, that is, likely thousands of pounds for a course of treatment, instead of tens or hundreds of pounds as we have been used to. Alternatively, the way in which antibiotics are funded has to change.

**Table 36.2** Antimicrobial agents (excluding topical agents) on the WHO model list of essential medicines (2013). Drugs shown in brackets are on the complementary list.

| Antibacterial agents[a] | Antimycobacterial agents | Antifungal agents | Antiviral agents | Antiprotozoal agents | Anthelminthic agents |
|---|---|---|---|---|---|
| Amoxicillin | Clofazimine | Amphotericin | *Antiherpes* | *Amoebiasis and giardiasis* | *Intestinal worms* |
| Amoxicillin + clavulanic acid | Dapsone | Clotrimazole | Aciclovir | Diloxanide[d] | Albendazole |
| Ampicillin | Ethambutol | Fluconazole[d] | *Antiretroviral[g]* | Metronidazole[d] | Levamisole |
| Azithromycin[b] | Isoniazid | Flucytosine | Abacavir | *Leishmaniasis* | Mebendazole[d] |
| Benzathine penicillin | | Griseofulvin | Atazanavir | Amphotericin | |
| Benzylpenicillin | Pyrazinamide | Nystatin | Didanosine | Meglumine antimonate[d] | Niclosamide |
| Cefalexin | | | | Paromomycin | |
| Cefazolin[e] | Rifabutin | | | Sodium stibogluconate or meglumine antimoniate | |
| Cefixime[c] | Rifampicin | | Efavirenz | | Praziquantel |
| Ceftriaxone[f] | | | Emtricitabine | | |
| Chloramphenicol | Streptomycin | (Potassium iodide) | | | |
| Ciprofloxacin[d] | (Amikacin) | | Indinavir | *Malaria[a]* | Pyrantel |
| Clarithromycin[g] | (p-Aminosalicylic acid) | | Lamivudine | Amodiaquine | *Filariasis* |
| Cloxacillin[d] | (Capreomycin) | | Lopinavir + ritonavir | Artemether | Albendazole |
| Co-amoxiclav | (Cycloserine) | | Nevirapine | Artesunate | Diethylcarbamazine |
| Co-trimoxazole | (Ethionamide) | | Saquinavir | | Ivermectin |
| Doxycycline | | | Stavudine | Artemether + lumefantrine | *Trematodes* |
| | | | Tenofovir | Chloroquine | |

*(continued)*

**Table 36.2** (continued).

| Antibacterial agents | Antimycobacterial agents[a] | Antifungal agents | Antiviral agents | Antiprotozoal agents | Anthelminthic agents |
| --- | --- | --- | --- | --- | --- |
| Erythromycin[d] | (Kanamycin) | | Zidovudine | Doxycycline | Praziquantel |
| Gentamicin[d] | (Levofloxacin) | | | Mefloquine | Triclabendazole |
| Metronidazole[d] | | | *Influenza* | Primaquine | (Oxamniquine) |
| Nitrofurantoin | | | Oseltamivir | Proguanil | |
| Phenoxymethylpenicillin | | | | Quinine | |
| Procaine penicillin | | | *Viral Haemorragic Fevers* | | |
| Spectinomycin | | | Ribivarin | (Sulfadoxine + pyrimethamine) | |
| Sulfamethoxazole + Trimethoprim | | | | *Trypanosomiasis* | |
| (Ceftazidime) | | | | Benznidazole | |
| (Clindamycin) | | | | Melarsoprol | |
| (Cefotaxime)[h] | | | | Nifurtimox | |
| (Imipenem + cilastatin) | | | | Suramin | |
| | | | | (Eflornithine) | |
| (Vancomycin) | | | | (Pentamidine) | |

Source: data from World Health Organization (WHO) Model List of Essential Medicines, March 2010 update, Copyright © WHO 2010, available form http://www.who.int/medicines/publications/essentialmedicines/Updated_sixteenth_adult_list_en.pdf.

a. Most of the antimycobacterial, antiretroviral and antimalarial drugs are used in combination and many are available in fixed-dose combination preparations.

b. For genital and ocular chlamydial infections only.

c. For single-dose treatment of uncomplicated ano-genital gonorrhoea only.

d. Examples of a therapeutic group for which acceptable alternatives exist.

e. For surgical prophylaxis.

f. Do not administer with calcium and avoid in infants with hyperbilirubinemia.

g. For use in combination regimens for eradication of *Helicobacter pylori* in adults.

h. 3rd generation cephalosporin of choice for use in hospitalized neonates.

Several possibilities are being actively considered or practised at present given the seriousness of the existent resistance threat. These include the following:

1 Increased public sector funding either to pay for new antibiotics and or to subsidize their development costs; the US Biomedical Advanced Research and Development Authority (BARDA) and the EU Innovative Medicines Initiative (IMI) are two such examples.

2 A reduction of the costs associated with achieving a successful approval to market new a new antibiotic, potentially by simplifying the process and/or lowering the 'barriers' of proof of efficacy that currently exist; for example, the US Generating Antibiotic Incentives Now (GAIN, passed in 2012) act offers the opportunity for an antibiotic drug to be designated as a qualified infectious disease product (QIDP), which means that it is eligible for fast-track review by the regulatory authority (FDA), likely lowering the research and development costs.

3 Extending the patents or other intellectual property rights for new drugs; for example, as set out in the GAIN act.

4 Financial incentives to encourage new drug development, particularly novel agents; several such schemes have been proposed and this remains an area of intensive political debate.

The 2011 European strategic action plan on antimicrobial resistance includes the following key priorities: ensuring that antimicrobials are used appropriately in both humans and animals; preventing microbial infections and their spread; developing new effective antimicrobials or alternatives for treatment; international cooperation to address the risks of antimicrobial resistance; improving monitoring and surveillance of resistance in humans and animals; promoting research and innovation; and, last but not least, improving communication, education, and training. This is a formidable but achievable list of 'must dos', if we are not to undermine the considerable successes in the fight against infection that have been achieved since the discovery of antibiotics (and later vaccines) approximately 80 years ago.

## Key points

- There has been a marked reduction in the number of new antibiotics and especially drugs exploiting novel targets or modes of action.
- Clinical trials of new antimicrobial agents comprise phase 1 (healthy volunteer), phase 2 (dosage investigation), and phase 3 studies.
- Post-marketing surveillance is key to check for rare and potentially serious adverse events.
- Several initiatives aimed at increasing the financial viability of drug discovery have been launched to encourage the development of new antibiotics.

## Further reading

Department of Health. (2013) *Annual Report of the Chief Medical Officer: Volume 2.* <https://www.gov.uk/government/publications/chief-medical-officer-annual-report-volume-2>, accessed 4 December 2014.

ECDC/EMEA Joint Technical Report. (2009) *The Bacterial Challenge: Time to React.* <http://www.ecdc.europa.eu/en/publications/Publications/0909_TER_The_Bacterial_Challenge_Time_to_React.pdf>, accessed 4 December 2014.

Infectious Diseases Society of America (IDSA). (2004) Bad bugs, no drugs. As antibiotic discovery stagnates . . . a public health crisis brews. <http://www.idsociety.org/uploadedFiles/IDSA/Policy_ and_Advocacy/Current_Topics_and_Issues/Advancing_Product_Research_and_Development/ Bad_Bugs_No_Drugs/Statements/As%20Antibiotic%20Discovery%20Stagnates%20A%20Public%20 Health%20Crisis%20Brews.pdf>

Talbot, G. H., Bradley, J., Edwards, J. E. Jr, Gilbert, D., Scheld, M., and Bartlett, J. G. (2006) Bad bugs need drugs: an update on the development pipeline from the Antimicrobial Availability Task Force of the Infectious Diseases Society of America. *Clinical Infectious Diseases*, **42**(5): 657–68.

World Health Organization. (2011) *European Strategic Action Plan on Antimicrobial Resistance.* <http:// www.euro.who.int/__data/assets/pdf_file/0008/147734/wd14E_AntibioticResistance_111380.pdf>, accessed 4 December 2014.

# Appendix: Recommendations for Further Reading

## General texts

Since the availability and use of antimicrobial agents vary widely in different countries, no one book has universal applicability. Among the most authoritative general texts in the English language are the following:

Bryskier, A. (2005), *Antimicrobial Agents—Antibacterial and Antifungals*. Washington, DC: ASM Press.

Finch, R. G., Greenwood, D., Norrby, S. R., and Whitley, R. J. (2010), *Antibiotic and Chemotherapy: Anti-Infective Agents and Their Use in Therapy* (9th edn). London: Saunders, Elsevier.

Greenwood, D. (2008), *Antimicrobial Drugs*. Oxford: Oxford University Press.

Kucers, A, Grayson, M. L., Crowe, S. M., McCarthy, J. S., Mills, J., Mouton, J. W., Norrby, S. R., Paterson, D. L., and Pfaller, M.A. (2010) *The Use of Antibiotics: A Clinical Review of Antibacterial, Antifungal, Antiparasitic and Antiviral drugs* (6th edn). London: Hodder Arnold.

An indispensable guide to the use of all therapeutic drugs for practitioners in the UK is provided by the *British National Formulary*, which is revised twice yearly:

Joint Formulary Committee. (2014) *British National Formulary* (68th edn). London: Pharmaceutical Press.

Comprehensive monographs on antimicrobial agents are to be found in large reference texts on drugs, including the following:

Dollery, C., ed. (1999), *Therapeutic Drugs* (2nd edn). Edinburgh: Churchill Livingstone.

Sebastian, A. (2010), *Antibacterial Chemotherapy: Theory, Problems, and Practice*, Oxford: Oxford University Press.

Sweetman, S. C., ed. (2011), *Martindale: The Complete Drug Reference* (37th edn). London: Pharmaceutical Press. (Also available online.)

## Other useful texts on specific topics

### Antiviral agents and the chemotherapy of viral infections

Butera, S. T., ed. (2005) *HIV Chemotherapy: A Critical Review*. Norwich: Horizon Bioscience.

Driscoll, J. S. (2005) *Antiviral Drugs*. Chichester: John Wiley & Sons.

Richman, D. D., Whitley, R. J., and Hayden, F. G., eds. (2009) *Clinical Virology* (3rd edn). Washington, DC: ASM Press.

Zuckerman, A. J., Banatvala, J. E., Schoub, B. D., Griffiths, P. D., and Mortmier. P., eds. (2009), *Principles and Practice of Clinical Virology* (6th edn). Oxford: Wiley-Blackwell.

### Diseases caused by protozoa and helminths (see also World Health Organization publications below)

Aden Abdi, Y., Gustafsson, L. L., Ericsson, O., and Hellgren, U., eds. (1996) *Handbook of Drugs for Tropical Parasitic Infection* (2nd edn). London: Taylor and Francis, London.

Rosenthal, P. J. (2010) *Antimalarial Chemotherapy: Mechanisms of Action, Resistance, and New Directions in Drug Discovery*. Totowa, NJ: Humana Press.

## Mode of action of antimicrobial agents and mechanisms of resistance

European Commission. (2014) *Key Documents on Antimicrobial Resistance.* <http://ec.europa.eu/health/antimicrobial_resistance/key_documents/index_en.htm>, accessed 4 December 2014.

Franklin, T. J., and Snow, G. A. (2005) *Biochemistry and Molecular Biology of Antimicrobial Drug Action* (6th edn). New York: Springer-Verlag.

Richman, D. D., ed. (1996) *Antiviral Drug Resistance.* Chichester: Wiley.

Salyers, A. A. and Whitt, D. D. (2005), *Revenge of the Microbes: How Bacterial Resistance is Undermining the Antibiotic Miracle.* Washington, DC: ASM Press.

Scholar, E. M. and Pratt, W. B. (2000), *The Antimicrobial Drugs* (2nd edn). New York: Oxford University Press.

Standing Medical Advisory Committee Report. (1998) *The Path of Least Resistance.* London: Department of Health/Public Health Laboratory Service.

Walsh, C. (2003), *Antibiotics: Actions, Origins, Resistance.* Washington, DC: ASM Press.

White, D. G., Alekshun, M. N., and McDermott, P. F. (2005), *Frontiers in Antimicrobial Resistance. A Tribute to Stuart B. Levy.* Washington, DC: ASM Press.

## Laboratory methods

Jerome, K. R., ed. (2010), *Lennette's Laboratory Diagnosis of Viral Infections* (4th edn). London: Informa Healthcare.

Lorian, V., ed. (2005) *Antibiotics in Laboratory Medicine* (5th edn). Baltimore, MD: Lippincott, Williams & Wilkins.

Versalovic, J., Carroll, K. C., Kunke, G., Jorgensen, J. H., Landry, M. L., and Warnock, D. W., eds. (2011), *Manual of Clinical Microbiology* (10th edn). Washington, DC: American Society for Microbiology.

## Antibiotic resistance monitoring

Centers for Disease Control and Prevention, Atlanta, GA. Antibiotic/antimicrobial resistance. <http://www.cdc.gov/drugresistance/>.

European Centre for Disease Prevention and Control (ECDC). (2014) *European Antimicrobial Resistance Surveillance Network (EARS-Net)* <http://www.ecdc.europa.eu/en/activities/surveillance/EARS-Net/Pages/index.aspx>, accessed 4 December 2014. This website has links to various national and international networks.

The British Society for Antimicrobial Chemotherapy (BSAC). (2014) *Resistance Surveillance Project.* <http://www.bsacsurv.org>, accessed 4 December 2014.

## Surveillance of antibiotic prescribing

*European Surveillance of Antimicrobial Consumption (ESAC).* <http://www.ecdc.europa.eu/en/activities/surveillance/ESAC-Net/publications/Pages/documents.aspx>. The website has publications from the project, which has collected and published data about community and hospital use of antibiotics across Europe from 1997 and is now hosted by the European Centre for Disease Control. The Documents page has yearbooks from 2006 with an archive of older reports. There are links to various national and international networks.

## Antibiotic policies and guidelines

European Society for Clinical Microbiology and Infectious Diseases (ESCMID). (2014) *Medical Guidelines.* <http://www.escmid.org/escmid_library/medical_guidelines/>, accessed 4 December 2014. This site has links to guidelines in the fields of clinical microbiology and infectious diseases endorsed by ESCMID and to guidelines from other organisations and societies.

**Health Protection Agency.** Management of infection guidance for primary care for consultation & local adaptation <https://www.gov.uk/government/publications/managing-common-infections-guidance-for-primary-care> (20th January 2015, date last accessed).

**Health Protection Agency & Department of Health.** *Clostridium difficile* infection: How to deal with the problem. <https://www.gov.uk/government/publications/clostridium-difficile-infection-how-to-deal-with-the-problem>

**National Institute for Health and Clinical Excellence (NICE).** (2014) *Find Guidance.* <http://guidance.nice.org.uk/>, accessed 4 December 2014. This site has guidelines on treatment of specific infections and information about implementation:

**Scottish Antimicrobial Prescribing Group:** The Quality Improvement pages include Hospital Prescribing Guidance, Infection Management, Primary Care and Gentamicin and Vancomycin at < https://www.scottishmedicines.org.uk/SAPG/Quality_Improvement/Quality_Improvement> (20th January 2015 date last accessed).

**Scottish Intercollegiate Guidelines Network (SIGN).** (2014) *SIGN 141: British Guideline on the Management of Asthma.* <http://www.sign.ac.uk>, accessed 4 December 2014. This site has guidelines on antibiotic prophylaxis in surgery and treatment of specific infections.

**The British Society for Antimicrobial Chemotherapy (BSAC).** (2014) *Developing Standards for Practice.* <http://www.bsac.org.uk/Standards>, accessed 4 December 2014. This site has guidelines and recommended standards from BSAC Working Parties and links to other educational resources.

## Learning resources about antimicrobial chemotherapy

**PAUSE.** (2014) *Welcome to the Pause Website.* <http://www.pause-online.org.uk/>, accessed 4 December 2014. This website has learning resources (clinical problems and prescribing exercises) created by medical schools in the UK with the aim of teaching prudent use of antibiotics in all clinical contexts. A list of PAUSE resources linked to chapters in *Antimicrobial Chemotherapy* is provided at the end of this chapter.

**Pagani, L., Gyssens, I. C., Huttner, B., Nathwani, D., and Harbarth, S.** (2009) Navigating the Web in search of resources on antimicrobial stewardship in health care institutions. *Clinical Infectious Diseases* **48**(5): 626–32.

**The British Society for Antimicrobial Chemotherapy (BSAC).** (2014) *OPAT: Outpatient Parenteral Antibiotic Therapy.* <http://www.e-opat.com/>, accessed 4 December 2014.

## World Health Organization publications

The World Health Organization issues a wide variety of publications, many of which are available online through the website <http://www.who.int/>. Of particular relevance to antimicrobial chemotherapy are:

**Crompton, D. W. T., Montresor, A., Nesheim, M. C., and Savioli, L.** (2004) *Controlling Disease Due to Helminth Infections.* Geneva: World Health Organization.

**Frieden, T.** (2004) *Toman's Tuberculosis. Case Detection, Treatment and Monitoring* (2nd edn). <http://whqlibdoc.who.int/publications/2004/9241546034.pdf>, accessed 4 December 2014.

**WHO Model Formulary 2014**. Geneva: World Health Organization. The Formulary can be accessed via the Essential Medicines page <http://www.who.int/selection_medicines/list/en/>.

**World Health Organization.** (2004), TB/HIV: *A Clinical Manual* (2nd edn). <http://www.who.int/tb/publications/who_htm_tb_2004_329/en/index.html>, accessed 4 December 2014.

**World Health Organization.** (2005) *WHO Model Prescribing Information: Drugs Used in Parasitic Diseases* (2nd edn). Geneva: World Health Organization.

World Health Organization. (2010) *Guidelines for the Treatment of Malaria* (2nd edn). <http://www.who.int/malaria/docs/TreatmentGuidelines2006.pdf>, accessed 4 December 2014.

World Health Organization. (2014) *Essential Medicines Monitor.* <http://www.who.int/medicines/publications/monitor/en>, accessed 4 December 2014.

World Health Organization. (2014) *Malaria.* <http://malaria.who.int>, accessed 4 December 2014.

## WHO Global strategy for containment of antimicrobial resistance. <http://www.who.int/drugresistance/WHO_Global_Strategy.htm/en/> Journals

Papers dealing with aspects of the use of antimicrobial drugs appear in numerous journals. English language journals specifically devoted to antibiotics and antimicrobial therapy include the following:

*Antibiotics and Chemotherapy*

*Antimicrobial Agents and Chemotherapy*

*Antiviral Chemistry and Chemotherapy*

*Antiviral Research*

*Chemotherapy*

*Clinical Microbiology and Infection*

*International Journal of Antimicrobial Agents*

*Journal of Antibiotics*

*Journal of Antimicrobial Chemotherapy*

*Journal of Chemotherapy*

## Other online resources

Prudent Antibiotic User (PAUSE) learning resources linked to *Antimicrobial Chemotherapy* Chapters (see Table A.1)

**Table A.1** Prudent Antibiotic User (PAUSE) learning resources.

| Antimicrobial Chemotherapy chapter | PAUSE Vignette or Learning Resource |
|---|---|
| 10 The problem of resistance | 012—Sarah Moss |
| | 018—Catheter-related MRSA in a hospital setting |
| | 019—UTI in the community setting |
| 11 The genetics and mechanisms of acquired resistance | 018—Catheter-related MRSA in a hospital setting |
| | 019—UTI in the community setting |
| 16 OPAT: outpatient parenteral antimicrobial therapy | 021—Outpatient Parenteral Antibiotic Therapy |
| 19 Guidelines, formularies, and antimicrobial policies | Prescribing exercises |
| | IVOST (IV to oral switch) protocol and exercises |
| 21 Respiratory tract infections | 001—Pneumonia, 015—Sore Throat |
| 23 Urinary tract infections | 005—UTI Pyelonephritis, 006—UTI in Pregnancy, 007—UTI in the Elderly, 008—Pyelonephritis, 009—Catheter Associated Infection, 019—UTI in the community setting |

**Table A.1** (continued).

| Antimicrobial Chemotherapy chapter | PAUSE Vignette or Learning Resource |
|---|---|
| 25 Gastrointestinal infections | 020—Clostridium difficile associated disease |
| 26 Serious blood stream infections | 002—Septic Shock, 004—Infective Endocarditis, 011—Pancreatitis |
| 27 Bone and joint infections | 013—Foot Infection in Diabetic Ulcer, 014—Septic Arthritis |
| 28 Infections of the central nervous system | 002—Septic Shock |
| 29 Skin and soft-tissue infections | 003—Cellulitis, 013—Foot Infection in Diabetic Ulcer |
| 30 Tuberculosis and other mycobacterial diseases | 010—Tuberculosis, 016—Tuberculosis |
| 33 Management of HIV infection | 017—Needlestick Injuries |
| 34 Treatment of chronic viral hepatitis | 017—Needlestick Injuries |

Source: data from Prudent Antibiotic User (PAUSE), available from http://www.pause-online.org.uk/

# Index

Page numbers in *italics* refer to illustrations; those in **bold** refer to tables

rifamycins 40, 330, 335
rifapentine 40, 330
Rifater 332
Rifinah 332
rilpivirine 62
rimantadine 54–5, 355
ritonavir 62, 370
rotavirus 269, **270**
roundworms **86**
roxithromycin 33

## S

salicylic acid 79, 265
*Salmonella enterica* **270**, 272
   enteric fever 273
   resistance 272
*Salmonella typhi* 7, 272–3
salmonellosis 272–3
   carriage 273
Salvarsan (arsphenamine) 263
*Sarcoptes scabiei* 382
scabies 382
Schatz, Albert 7
*Schistosoma* spp. (schistosomiasis) 87, 381
Scottish Medicines Consortium 391
sepsis 279–80
   assessment 136, 279–80, *280*
   epidemiology 282
   management 286–9, *286*
   meningococcal 307
   neutropenic 342–3, **343**
   *see also* bacteraemia
sepsis syndrome 307
septicaemia *see* bacteraemia; sepsis
septic arthritis 207–300
   antimicrobial therapy 298–9, **298, 299**
septic encephalopathy 314
septic shock 280
Septrin *see* co-trimoxazole
severe acute respiratory syndrome coronaviruses
   (SARS-CoV) 354
sexually transmitted infections 257–66, **258**
   chemoprophylaxis 187
   diagnosis 257–9, *258*
   see also *specific infections*
*Shigella* spp. **270**, 273
shigellosis 273
shingles 351
shunt-associated meningitis 310
sialic acid 55, *56*
side effects *see* adverse reactions
silver nitrate 262
silver sulfadiazine 245
simeprevir 73, 369
sinusitis 230–1
skin
   bacterial infections **242**, 244–5, 317,
     **318, 319**
   burns 244–5
   fungal infections 245–6
   ulcers 245
   *see also specific infections*; topical therapy
sleeping sickness 84, 378

smallpox 9
sodium stibogluconate 84, 379
sofosbuvir 73, 369–70
soft tissue infections 317, **318, 319**
   *see also specific infections*
soil microorganisms, antibiotics from 7–8
sore throat 227–30
specimens
   collection 122–3
   processing 124–5, *124*
   transport 123
spectinomycin 25, 28, 260
spheroplasts 20
spiramycin 85, 380
sporozoa **82**
staphylococci
   endocarditis 291–2
   nasal carriage 244
   resistance 97–8
   *see also specific species*
*Staphylococcus aureus*
   bacteraemia 282, **284**, *287, 288*
   cystic fibrosis 148, 235
   endocarditis 289, 290, 292–3
   gastrointestinal infections **270**, 274
   joint infection 297
   meningitis 310
   osteomyelitis 300
   resistance 93, 112
   respiratory infections 234, 237
   skin and soft tissue infections 244, 317, 319,
     321, 323
   *see also* methicillin-resistant *Staphylococcus aureus*
     (MRSA)
*Staphylococcus epidermidis*
   bacteraemia 282
   endocarditis 292–3
   meningitis 310
stavudine 61
*Stenotrophomonas maltophilia* 235
Stevens–Johnson syndrome 62, 150
Stewart, William 9
streptococci
   endocarditis 291–2
   Group B 185–6, 310
   joint infections 297
   neonatal infection 148, 185–6
*Streptococcus agalactiae* 297
   meningitis 303
*Streptococcus pneumoniae*
   acute otitis media 230
   bacteraemia 282
   endocarditis 289
   immunocompromised patients 340, 346
   meningitis 303, 304, 306, 308
   resistance 98, 112
*Streptococcus pyogenes*
   bacteraemia 282
   joint infections 297
   skin and soft tissue infections 244, 317, 319,
     321, 323
   sore throat 229
streptogramins 34